NURSING HISTORY REVIEW

OFFICIAL JOURNAL OF THE
AMERICAN ASSOCIATION FOR THE HISTORY OF NURSING

ISBN 1062-8061
ISBN 978-0-8261-1772-4

2010 – Volume 18

CONTENTS

10 EDITOR'S NOTE

   PATRICIA D'ANTONIO

   HANNAH LECTURE

12 Nurses Across Borders: Foregrounding International Migration in Nursing History
   CATHERINE CENIZA CHOY

   ARTICLES

29 The Introduction of Deaconess Nurses at the German Hospital of the City of Philadelphia in the 1880s
   CHRISTOPH SCHWEIKARDT

51 "The Relation of the Nurse to the Working World": Professionalization, Citizenship, and Class in Germany, Great Britain, and the United States before World War I
   AELEAH SOINE

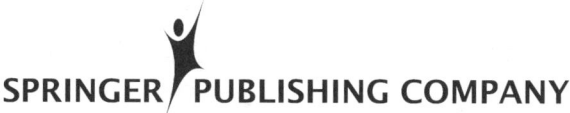

NEW YORK

Reframing Activism: Nursing and Social Action in the United States

81 Guest Editor's Note
MERYN STUART

84 "I am a Trained Nurse": The Nursing Identity of Anarchist and Radical Emma Goldman
CYNTHIA ANNE CONNOLLY

100 Conflict and Compromise: Catholic and Public Hospital Partnerships
BARBRA MANN WALL

118 "Go to Ruth's House": The Social Activism of Ruth Lubic and the Family Health and Birth Center
JULIE FAIRMAN

The Place of Religion as an Interpretive Tool in Nursing History

130 Guest Editor's Note
BARBRA MANN WALL

134 Nursing Body and Soul in the Parish: Lutheran Deaconess Motherhouses in Germany and the United States
SUSANNE KREUTZER

151 Finance and Faith at the Catholic Maternity Institute, Santa Fe, New Mexico, 1944–1969
ANNE Z. COCKERHAM AND ARLENE W. KEELING

Methodology

167 Looking Closely: Material and Visual Approaches to the Nurse's Uniform
CHRISTINA BATES

Notes and Documents

189 Nurse Irene Shea Studies the "Kenny Method" of Treatment of Infantile Paralysis, 1942–1943
Naomi Rogers and Janet Golden

Media Reviews

204 *History of Nursing: Early Years* and *History of Nursing: The Development of a Profession*
Reviewer: Barbara Brodie

207 *Contagion: Historical Views of Diseases and Epidemics*
Reviewer: Jeannine Uribe

209 *Making Visible Embryos*
Reviewers: Winifred C. Connerton and Claire M. Fagin Hall

211 *MCH Timeline: History, Legacy and Resources for Education and Practice*
Reviewer: Elizabeth A. Reedy

213 *Army Nurses of World War One: Service Beyond Expectations*
Reviewer: Jennifer Casavant Telford

Book Reviews

217 *Intensely Human: The Health of the Black Soldier in the American Civil War*
by Margaret Humphreys
Reviewer: Teresa M. O'Neill

218 *This Republic of Suffering: Death and the American Civil War*
by Drew Gilpin Faust
Reviewer: Linda E. Sabin

220 *Florence Nightingale: The Making of an Icon*
by Mark Bostridge
Reviewer: Carol Helmstadter

223   *Die Entwicklung der Krankenpflege zur staatlich anerkannten Tätigkeit im 19. und frühen 20. Jahrhundert: Das Zusammenwirken von Modernisierungsbestrebungen, ärztlicher Dominanz, konfessioneller Selbstbehauptung und Vorgaben preußischer Regierungspolitik [The Development of Nursing into a State-Approved Occupation in the Nineteenth and Early Twentieth Century: The Entwined Influences of Modernization, Medical Domination, Assertion of Confessional (Religious) Independence, and Prussian State Politics]*
by Christoph Schweikardt
REVIEWER: GEERTJE BOSCHMA

225   *Community Nursing and Primary Healthcare in Twentieth-Century Britain*
by Helen M. Sweet with Rona Dougall
REVIEWER: GERARD M. FEALY

228   *Three Generations, No Imbeciles: Eugenics, the Supreme Court, and* Buck v. Bell
by Paul A. Lombardo
REVIEWER: EDWARD SLAVISHAK

229   *Mary Breckinridge: The Frontier Nursing Service and Rural Health in Appalachia*
by Melanie Beals Goan
REVIEWER: KAROL K. WEAVER

231   *An Officer and a Lady: Canadian Military Nursing and the Second World War*
by Cynthia Toman
REVIEWER: STEPHANIE BUCKINGHAM

233   *Armies of Peace: Canada and the UNRRA Years*
by Susan Armstrong Reid and David Murray
REVIEWER: JAYNE ELLIOTT

235 *The W. K. Kellogg Foundation and the Nursing Profession: Shared Values, Shared Legacy*
by Joan E. Lynaugh, Helen K. Grace, Gloria R. Smith, Roseni R. Sena, Maria Mercedes Duran de Villalobos, and Mary Malehloka Hlalele
REVIEWER: BARBARA BRODIE

237 *Unnatural History: Breast Cancer and American Society*
by Robert A. Aronowitz
REVIEWER: LINDA E. SABIN

238 *Cancer in the Twentieth Century*
Edited by David Cantor
REVIEWER: TERESA M. O'NEILL

239 *Mania: A Short History of Bipolar Disorder*
by David Healy
REVIEWER: TOM OLSON

243 NEW DISSERTATIONS

Cover Photo: Sr. Patricia Patton, MMS, a midwifery student at the Catholic Maternity Institute in Santa Fe, New Mexico, holding a newborn. Sr. Patricia studied there between September 1953 and September 1954. This photograph was most likely taken in 1954 after she had several months of didactic instruction and had been an observer during deliveries. By then she would have been ready to attend a birth or care for a newborn, which was what her apron and rolled-up sleeves indicates she was doing. Reprinted courtesy of the Medical Mission Sisters Archives, Fox Chase, Pennsylvania.

Nursing History Review is published annually for the American Association for the History of Nursing, Inc., by Springer Publishing Company, LLC, New York.

Business Office: All business correspondence, including subscriptions, renewals, advertising, and address changes, should be sent to Springer Publishing Company, LLC, 11 West 42nd Street, New York, NY 10036.

Editorial Office: Submissions and editorial correspondence should be directed to Patricia D'Antonio, Editor, *Nursing History Review,* University of Pennsylvania, 420 Guardian Drive, Room 307, Philadelphia, PA 19104–6096. See guidelines for contributors on page 7 for further details.

Members of the American Association for the History of Nursing, Inc. (AAHN) receive *Nursing History Review* on payment of annual membership dues. Applications and other correspondence relating to AAHN membership should be directed to: David L. Stumph, IOM, CAE, Executive Director, American Association for the History of Nursing, Inc., 10200 W. 44th Avenue #304, Wheat Ridge, CO 80033. Phone: (303) 422-2685. E-mail: aahn@resourcecenter.com

Subscription Rates (per Year): Volume 18, 2010. For institutions: $150. For individuals: $85. Outside the United States—for institutions: $150. For individuals: $105. Payment must be made in advance by check (in U.S. dollars drawn on a U.S. bank) or international money order, payable to Springer Publishing Company, LLC, or by MasterCard, Visa, or American Express.

Indexes/abstracts of articles appear in: CINAHL® print index & database, Current Contents/Social & Behavioral Science, Social Sciences Citation Index, Research Alert, RNdex, Index Medicus/MEDLINE, History Abstracts, America; History and Life.

Permission: All rights are reserved. No part of this volume may be reproduced or utilized in any form or by any means, electronic or mechanical, including photocopying (with the exception listed below), recording, or by any information storage and retrieval system, without permission in writing from the publisher. Permission is granted by the copyright owner for libraries and others registered with the Copyright Clearance Center (CCC) to photocopy any article herein for $5.00 per copy of the article. Payments should be sent directly to Copyright Clearance Center, 27 Congress Street, Salem, MA 01970, USA. This permission holds for copying done for personal or internal reference use only: it does not extend to other kinds of copying, such as copying for general distribution, advertising or promotional purposes, creating new collective works, or for resale. Requests for these permissions or further information should be addressed to Springer Publishing Company, LLC.

Postmaster: Send address change to Springer Publishing Company, LLC, 11 West 42nd Street, New York, NY 10036.

Copyright © 2010 by Springer Publishing Company, LLC, New York, for the American Association for the History of Nursing, Inc.

ISSN 1062-8061

ISBN 978-0-8261-1772-4

GUIDELINES FOR CONTRIBUTORS

Nursing History Review, the official publication of the American Association for the History of Nursing, is an annually published and peer-reviewed journal. Original research manuscripts are welcomed in broad areas related to the history of nursing, health care, health policy, and society. The *Review* prefers that manuscripts of approximately 40 pages, inclusive of endnotes.

Submitted manuscripts must be prepared using the guidelines specified in the *Chicago Manual of Style*, 15th edition. Manuscripts must have a title page that contains the full title of the manuscript, the author(s) name(s) as they are meant to appear in print, institutional affiliations and preferred mailing addresses *for all authors*, and relevant contact information for the corresponding author. The title page must be followed with an abstract of approximately 150–200 words.

Manuscripts must be double-spaced and of letter-quality print. They must also use a type size of at least 12 characters per inch or 12 points. Please leave generous margins of at least 1 inch. All pages, including text, notes, and reference pages, must be numbered consecutively. All notes must be double-spaced and placed at the end of the manuscript as endnotes rather than footnotes.

Authors are responsible for securing permissions for all materials and photographs submitted. If more than 500 words of text are quoted from a book, or more than 250 words from an article, or if a table or figure has been previously published, the manuscript must be accompanied by written permission from the copyright owner.

Initial submissions of manuscripts may be sent by e-mail to *nhr@nursing.upenn.edu*. All submissions will be acknowledged when received. *Final versions of manuscripts accepted for publication* should be prepared in MS Word. The final packet must be submitted via e-mail to *nhr@nursing.upenn.edu*. Photographs or other figures accompanying the final manuscript must be attached as TIF files with resolutions of at least 600 dpi. All appropriate permissions and copyright releases must accompany the final submission.

All correspondence regarding manuscripts should be sent to: Patricia D'Antonio, Ph.D., RN, FAAN, Editor, *Nursing History Review*, University of Pennsylvania School of Nursing, 2017 Claire M. Fagin Hall, Philadelphia, PA 19104–4217. Phone: 215/746.8322. Fax: 215/573–2168. E-mail: *dantonio@nursing.upenn.edu* or *nhr@nursing.upenn.edu*

AMERICAN ASSOCIATION FOR THE HISTORY OF NURSING, INC.

Sylvia Rinker
President

Carla Schissel
First Vice President and
Chair, Strategic Planning Committee

Joy Buck
Second Vice President and
Chair, Program Committee

Jean Whelan
Secretary

Kathleen Hanson
Treasurer

Brigid Lusk
Director and
Chair, Publications Committee

Rima Apple
Director and
Chair, Awards Committee

Carol Daisy
Director and
Chair, By-Laws Committee

Barbra Mann Wall
Director and
Member, Finance Committee

Teresa O'Neil
Director, and
Member, Strategic Planning

Arlene Keeling
Past President

Wanda C. Hiestand
Archivist

Marilyn Flood
Chair, Nominating Committee

NURSING HISTORY REVIEW

Patricia D'Antonio, Editor
Barbra Mann Wall, Book Review Editor
Jean Whelan, Media Editor
Elizabeth Weiss, Assistant Editor

Editorial Review Board

Ellen D. Baer Florida	*Carol Helmstadter* Ontario, Canada
Nettie Birnbach Florida	*Wanda C. Hiestand* New York
Eleanor Crowder Bjoring Texas	*Arlene Keeling* Virginia
Barbara Brodie Virginia	*Joan Lynaugh* Pennsylvania
Olga Maranjian Church Connecticut	*Lois Monteiro* Rhode Island
Julie Fairman Pennsylvania	*Sioban Nelson* Toronto, Canada
Marilyn Flood California	*Anne-Marie Rafferty* London, England
Karen Flynn Illinois	*Susan Reverby* Massachusetts
Janet Golden New Jersey	*Naomi Rogers* Connecticut
Christine Hallett Manchester, England	*Meryn Stuart* Ottawa, Canada
Diane Hamilton Michigan	*Nancy Tomes* New York

EDITOR'S NOTE

History and the Humanities

The headline of a recent *New York Times* article spelled out a clear warning. "In Tough Times," it proclaimed, "the Humanities Must Justify their Worth."[1] Reporter Patricia Cohen wrote of colleges and universities canceling or postponing faculty searches in English, literature, philosophy, and religion. She cited statistics that showed how the percentage of humanities degrees conferred stubbornly remains half of what it had been when the fields had a renaissance during the 1960s. And she quoted Andrew Delbanco, the director of American studies at Columbia University. "Although people in the humanities have always lamented the state of the field," he noted, "they have never felt quite as much of a panic that their field is becoming irrelevant." The concern was not that the humanities would disappear. Rather, it was that decisions about what to study in colleges and universities would reflect the prerogatives of class—that only the wealthy could afford the luxury of stepping away from training for particular professions and exploring notions of individual citizenship and social responsibility.

The irony (and perhaps this may be too strong a word), of course, is that this article could not have been constructed without a deep sense of history. Understanding the patterns of inclusion and exclusion in higher education made meaning from numbers. And we see this role of history in what I think of as "meaning-making" all around us. We see it in the resonance of particular historical references deliberately called into play by the first African American president of the United States. We hear it every day as media reporters and commentators struggle to make sense of the global economic crisis by comparing and contrasting our experiences with the experiences of those living through the Great Depression of the 1930s.

This process of meaning-making depends on two interrelated ideas. First, it asks that we see the historical experiences of nurses not as nurses *per se* but rather as emblematic of some broader issue. Second, it asks that we step beyond descriptive experience and attach significance to the broader themes explicated in the narrative. We see these in play in the articles in this issue of the *Nursing History Review*. Both Catherine Cenzia Choy and Aeleah Soine use nurses to deconstruct the nation-state orientation of history, and their work makes meaning of the trope of "international." Similarly, the work of Meryn Stuart, Cynthia Ann Connolly, Barbra Mann Wall, and Julie Fairman uses nurses to consider how individuals understood the social and political implication of their work; and their studies create new meanings about the trope of "activism." Finally, Christoph Schweikardt, Barbra Mann Wall, Susanne Kreutzer, Ann Cockerham, and Arlene Keeling use nurses to explore the intersections of faith and professional service in ways that unpack the trope of religion and spirituality in health care.

This may be a somewhat simplistic way to describe our authors' rich and nuanced historical research. But I am trying to tease out concerns driven by political exigencies dependent on particular moments in time. I am more concerned by those driven by the deeply emotional and human needs served by the universal processes of meaning-making that history does so well. We address essential questions. What does it mean to be a citizen, a professional, and a member of a global community? The need to explore answers to these questions will never disappear.

PATRICIA D'ANTONIO, EDITOR
University of Pennsylvania
2017 Claire M. Fagin Hall
418 Curie Boulevard
Philadelphia, PA 19104

Note

1. Particia Cohen, "In Tough Times, the Humanities Must Justify Their Worth," *New York Times,* February 25, 2009. Available at http://www.nytimes.com/2009/02/25/books/25human.html?scp=2&sq=humanities&st=cse (accessed March 31, 2009).

HANNAH LECTURE

Nurses Across Borders: Foregrounding International Migration in Nursing History

CATHERINE CENIZA CHOY
University of California, Berkeley

Abstract. Although the international migration of nurses has played a formative role in increasing the racial and ethnic diversity of the health care labor force, nursing historians have paid very little attention to the theme of international migration and the experiences of foreign-trained nurses. A focus on international migration complements two new approaches in nursing history: the agenda to internationalize its frameworks, and the call to move away from "great women, great events" and toward the experiences of "ordinary" nurses. This article undertakes a close reading of the life and work of Filipino American nurse Ines Cayaban to reconceptualize nursing biography in an international framework that is attentive to issues of migration, race, gender, and colonialism. It was a Hannah keynote lecture delivered by the author on June 5, 2008, as part of the CAHN/ACHN (Canadian Association for the History of Nursing/Association Canadienne pour l'Histoire du Nursing) International Nursing History Conference.

Without a doubt, health care workers are on the move. In the new millennium, they are moving across national borders in significant numbers, and policy analysts and academics are taking note of the phenomenon. The 2007 conference organized by the health policy journal *Health Affairs,* "Stories Told and Untold: Health Workers on the Move," featured panels on "demographics and living in the diaspora." Physicians comprised the majority of the conference speakers, but nurses play a major role in this global phenomenon. *Nurses on the Move* is the title of Mireille Kingma's 2006 book that highlights the policy and human dimensions of migration and the global health care economy. Kingma observes that "while nursing has been advertised as a 'portable profession' and nurses have always moved from town to town, city to city, and country to country, never has nurse migration been the mass phenomenon we see today. Foreign-educated health professionals represent more than a quarter of the medical and nursing workforces of Australia, Canada, the United Kingdom, and the United States."[1]

For half a century, the Philippines has dominated this trend as the world's leading exporter of nurses.[2] Since 1994, more than 100,000 nurses have left the Philippines to work abroad. Because well-publicized nursing shortages in the United States and the United Kingdom have fueled recruitment of foreign nurse graduates, Filipino physicians have started to enroll in accelerated nursing courses in the Philippines designed for physicians who wish to become nurses to work abroad. According to a 2003 *San Francisco Chronicle* article, as many as 3,000 Filipino medical doctors have left the Philippines as nurses.[3]

Furthermore, the international migration of foreign medical graduates to work as physicians in mid- and lower-level posts in U.K. hospitals and in rural areas and inner cities of Canada and the United States also continues in recent times. A 2005 article by Fitzhugh Mullan on the "metrics of physician brain drain" concludes that international medical graduates "constitute between 23 and 28 percent of physicians in the United States, the United Kingdom, Canada, and Australia. . . . India, the Philippines, and Pakistan are the leading sources of international medical graduates. The United Kingdom, Canada, and Australia draw a substantial number of physicians from South Africa, and the United States draws very heavily from the Philippines."[4]

The loss of professional health providers from poorer countries to richer ones, popularly referred to as "brain drain," is not new. In the late 1970s, reports by Alfonso Mejía, Helena Pizorkí, and Erica Royston culminated in a landmark 1979 study of the global dimensions of physician and nurse migrant flows that illustrated the imbalances regarding their geographical distribution. In the 1970s, approximately 15,000 nurses migrating each year went to eight countries, primarily the United States, United Kingdom, and Canada.[5]

Aside from the sizable percentages of foreign-educated physicians and nurses in specific countries, in the late twentieth century and in the new millennium three new patterns have emerged. First, new source countries for physicians include the Caribbean, Egypt, sub-Saharan African states, Cuba, and the former Soviet Union. China, Thailand, and sub-Saharan African states are exporting more nurses. Second, a new destination for recruited medical professionals is the Gulf states. Third, other health professionals, notably pharmacists and physical therapists, have become more mobile.[6]

The Significance of International Migration for Nursing History

A major contribution of the sociological and policy studies that have dominated research about the international migration of health professionals is that they have brought renewed critical attention to the fact that these movements across national borders matter to the big picture of global health. International migration exacerbates (not solely reflects) the related global inequalities of income distribution and health care delivery.

With some notable exceptions such as Barbara Brush, Margaret Shkimba, and Karen Flynn,[7] nursing historians have paid very little attention to the theme of international migration and the experiences of foreign-trained nurses. Recent nursing historiography articles have pointed to the centrality of the theme of professionalization at the expense of other themes, but another, related explanation for these historical blind spots might be the centrality of the framework of the "nation" in nursing history. Like other historical fields of study, the presumption that the nation defines what counts as history may have had the effect of trivializing foreign-trained nurses.[8] In addition, previous conceptions of international nursing recruitment as a short-term staffing strategy, as well as the xenophobia among some domestic nurses, may have reinforced the idea that foreign-trained nurses were outside the boundaries of nursing history.

The result of these gaps is the erroneous assumption that the international migration of foreign-trained nurses is a recent phenomenon devoid of a substantive past. One of the major arguments I made in *Empire of Care* had to do with the reconceptualization of the temporal origins and historical geography of Filipino nurse migration to the United States. The seemingly late twentieth-century phenomenon of the international migration of Filipino nurses is intimately tied to the early twentieth-century history of U.S. colonialism in the archipelago. The temporal origins of Filipino nurse migration are in U.S. colonial policies in the Philippines, when the colonial government and philanthropic organizations such as the Daughters of the American Revolution (DAR) sponsored a small number of Filipino nursing students to further their nursing education in the United States. Furthermore, although U.S. colonial projects of racial uplift and civilizing missions informed the establishment of nursing schools in the Philippines, they inadvertently prepared Filipino nurses to work abroad, especially in the United States, because they followed patterns of U.S. professional nursing education and included English language fluency in the curriculum.

Nursing history is at an opportune moment to confront these gaps and take them on as legitimate scholarly inquiry. Through international frameworks attentive to the lived experiences of migrant nurses, nursing historians can bring nuance, historical context, and human interest to current discourses of the international migration of health professionals. With few exceptions, these predominantly policy discussions have relegated migrant health professionals to faceless workers and statistics in health care management. Furthermore, these discussions reach a standstill when framed in the ethical debates of human rights—to access quality health care services and to free movement—rights that conflict as when health professionals migrate from poorer countries to richer ones.

Although scholars have noted that the direct consequences of medical migration on the health care delivery systems of the sending countries are difficult to ascertain, the anecdotal evidence powerfully suggests that there are direct links between the two. In July 2004, a *New York Times* article reported that, at the epicenter of the AIDS epidemic, Malawi's largest, 1,000-bed hospital had only thirty nurses remaining and that twenty of these expressed the intention to migrate.[9] In the Philippines, a country popularly perceived as having a nursing surplus for export, at least three hospitals in Mindanao (in the southern part of the archipelago) and two in Isabela province have no nurses.[10]

These cases speak to the growing controversy over the international migration of medical professionals. Sabina Alkire and Lincoln Chen outline the opposing sides of this debate:

> At one extreme are those who define the basic human right of professionals to move, irrespective of occupation. . . . They argue that restriction on labor movements accentuates global economic inequities . . . and argue for more and freer movement. At the other extreme are those who charge Northern countries with exploitive predatory behavior towards Southern countries. They argue that poaching the best and brightest of human resources exacerbates global health inequities.[11]

By bringing attention to the lived experiences of foreign-trained nurse migrants and immigrants, the theme of international migration complements two new approaches to nursing history: the agenda to internationalize its frameworks and the call to move away from "great women, great events" and toward the experiences of seemingly "ordinary" nurses. As Sonya Grypma writes: "Historians of nursing are promoting a 'new historiography' . . . The new historiography rejects nursing's 'cosy professional-centered celebration of its past,' emphasizing issues and themes."[12] Barbara Mortimer's introduction to her edited collection with Susan McGann on *New Directions in the History of Nursing* importantly calls for a new international agenda in nursing history at a moment when "race and ethnicity are pressing issues for the recent history of nursing."[13]

In addition to highlighting the themes of race and colonialism, I believe that the historical documentation of the international migration of nurses would contribute critical insights into the methodology of the new nursing history. Grypma observes that as nursing historiography is undergoing change: "The relevance of the biographic method is being challenged. . . . If the biographic method is to remain relevant in the new non-subject-centered milieu, biography must be approached and written in new ways."[14] By revisioning nursing biography to foreground nurses who have been ignored, misunderstood, or forgotten, Grypma continues, "a wider range of possibilities for biographic study is uncovered."[15]

Ines Cayaban: "A Life Worth Telling"

I would like to present some preliminary research I have been conducting on the life and work of Filipino American nurse Ines Cayaban as one possibility in that "wider range of possibilities" of revisioning nursing biography in an international framework that is attentive to issues of migration, race, ethnicity, and colonialism.

There are still many life histories worth telling, and one example would be that of Cayaban. Born in 1904 in the town of Claveria in the Philippine province of Ilocos Norte, Ines studied nursing at St. Luke's School of Nursing in Quezon City, Metro Manila, and graduated as valedictorian of the class of 1928. In 1931, Ines left the Philippines to further her studies at Columbia University; however, a stopover in Hawaii with a Filipino family Ines knew from the Philippines led to her working and living in Hawaii for the remainder of her life. She married a Filipino American she met in Hawaii, and they had a son, Dante. Ines worked first as a public health nurse at Palama Settlement for low-income and immigrant communities, then as a health educator and home nursing program director for the Hawaii Cancer Control Society, and as a supervisor of several community outreach programs such as the Tuberculin Skin Testing Service.

What makes the study of Ines Cayaban's life possible is the 1981 publication of her autobiography, *A Goodly Heritage*.[16] Conventional archival material on Filipino nurses is scarce. Nursing archives at Boston University and the University of California, San Francisco, do not have specific collections or boxes or even folders on this particular group. When Filipino and other foreign-educated nurse migrants appear in these collections, they rarely do so as multidimensional beings with agency. Furthermore, Filipino American nurses themselves hold archival material about their life histories and ethnic organizations in personal, not public collections, contributing to the challenge of conducting traditional archival research on their history. Thus, much of the history of migrant health workers must be researched ethnographically, through oral interviews, for example.

In this context, the significance of the publication of Ines's autobiography is magnified. The book provides a personal lens through which to view Filipino nurses' experiences during the first two decades of U.S. colonial rule in the Philippines (roughly the 1900s through the 1920s); Filipino American life in Hawaii in the 1930s; public health and plantation nursing in Hawaii; and perhaps most important and accurately how a Filipino American nurse recollected particular events and experiences related to these movements and time periods.

I wish to emphasize three key points about Ines's life history: First, in nursing historiography, although a nursing diploma could mean different things to women, a path to professional leadership for some and a skilled craft for others, for Filipino nurses beginning in the early twentieth century it signified a route to the United States. I have argued in my book that Filipino migration to the United States, often undertaken during this period to pursue further nursing education, followed a pattern of women geographically moving to become more socially and economically mobile, in this case, to assume nursing supervisory and educational positions upon their return to the Philippines.

One theme that distinguished Filipino migration from other nurses' mobility was the colonial context, a U.S. presence in the form of Americanized education at the elementary school level and beyond; American manufacturing; the U.S. military; and American popular culture. This multilevel presence in the Philippines appears throughout Ines's recollections of her youth, shaping an intimate understanding of and relationship to the United States. Ines writes that she started to learn English as soon as she entered public school, emphasizing that "the Philippine educational system is patterned after the American system."[17] In another recollection, U.S. colonial public education and American business production are linked: "While attending the intermediate grades," Ines recalls, "I was one of the handicrafts students selected by the school to crochet narrow laces for an American business firm. The order was placed through the Board of Education and the pupils were chosen for the quality of their work and the speed with which they met the deadline."[18]

The presence of the U.S. military in her small hometown of Claveria during World War I informs her curiosity about racial diversity in the United States: "Many of the soldiers were young, fair-looking Americans; others were dark-skinned men who they called Negroes."[19] And despite the historically violent role played by the U.S. military in the establishment of colonial rule in the archipelago,[20] Ines's autobiography notes instead her nostalgic childhood impression of the military presence: "The best friends of the children were the Army cooks wearing long white aprons and towering white caps. They used to hand out delicious crunchy cookies and biscuits to passers-by."[21] The introduction of sports such as baseball also created happy memories of her childhood. In high school Ines played third base on a team and in her writing called attention to her enjoyment of such "physical pursuits."[22]

Nursing was also part of this multilevel U.S. colonial presence in the Philippines, a presence highlighted not only by American nurses in the archipelago, but also by returning Filipino nurses who had studied in the United States. In her recollections of how and why she became a student nurse, Ines writes about the influence of returned Filipino nurses from abroad:

> One day in December [1924] . . . news spread all over town that a well-educated nurse had arrived from Manila to spend the holidays with her family and friends. She was the principal of the School of Nursing at St. Luke's Hospital . . . Her name was [Escolastica] Aguinaldo. . . . [She] took her post-graduate studies in nursing at Columbia University in New York City under a Rockefeller Foundation grant. It was her going to America more than her position as a nursing educator that intrigued me.[23]

As the final sentence above illuminates, the allure of going to the United States profoundly shaped her decision to enter the nursing profession. For Ines, the traditional calling of the nurse, youthful ambition, and the emerging Filipino trend to go to the United States complemented one another. In the chapter of her autobiography devoted to how she became a nurse, Ines writes:

> I had an intense desire to serve people of all ages, particularly the needy and the sick. . . . Also in those days, it was the fad to go to America and return home with a special profession. Shortly after World War I, many Filipino youths developed a great interest in going to the United States, especially those who had contacts with American soldiers during the war. I was among the ambitious women aged twenty who had dreams of seeing America the Beautiful. The question in my mind was how and when.[24]

What Ines refers to as a "fad to go to America and return home with a special profession" needs to be contextualized in the history of U.S. colonial educational programs. The colonial government established the *pensionado* program, beginning in 1903, that sponsored an elite group of several hundred Filipino young men and a few young women to further their education in the United States and return to the Philippines to assume positions in the U.S. colonial government and educational institutions. Ines's reference to the increasing numbers of "Filipino youths who developed a great interest in going to the United States after World War I" refers to the historical migration of several tens of thousands of self-supporting Filipino students who followed in the wake of the *pensionados*.[25]

These student movements provide an important context for understanding Filipino nurses' international mobility during the early twentieth century. Filipino nurse migration to the United States during this period may have been an elite experience of Filipino "women worthies" to the extent that their numbers pale in comparison to the masses of Filipino nurses migrating today, and because many of these women led distinguished careers in nursing upon their return to the Philippines. Yet, however small, it was still a *collective* experience that inspired, encouraged, and facilitated international migration. Ines writes that her plan to the United States materialized in the advice given to her by returned nurse Escolastica Aguinaldo:

> I had the rare opportunity of meeting Mrs. Aguinaldo. . . . My first remark to her was that I had an intense desire to follow in her footsteps—to enter the portals of Columbia University. Her quick answer was, "Be a nurse, a real good nurse with high scholastic grades. The sponsor will give you free transportation, free board and lodging, and a small additional allowance. Come home after two years and pay back your scholarship by working for at least two years." She added, "Being a topnotcher in nursing school would do the trick." . . . I could not afford to miss the boat. My only passport to the USA was a nursing certificate of high standing.[26]

This collective experience of young Filipino women going to the United States in the early twentieth century also emerges in other parts of Ines's autobiography. For example, she intended to leave the Philippines to further her studies at Columbia University in April 1931 but waited for three Filipina friends who were also going to the United States so that they could travel together. One was also a nurse and another was a social worker leaving for postgraduate work at the University of Minnesota.[27] On Ines's stopover in Hawaii, her host family was the Esquerases family; Pilar Esquerases (née Bacungan) had been Ines's head nurse at St. Luke's Hospital in 1925. By the end of 1925, Pilar left for Hawaii as a recruit of the Hawaiian Sugar Planters Association (HSPA), which employed bilingual professional workers and registered nurses from the Philippines to help the Filipino male laborers in the plantations adjust to their new environment, maintain their health and well-being, and ensure their productivity. Assigned to different plantation hospitals, these Filipino nurses were an example of the early twentieth-century institutionalization of Filipino international nurse recruitment and an interesting topic for further study: the role of Filipino nurses in Hawaiian plantation medicine.

The second key point about Ines's life history that I want to emphasize is that it gives us a window to view the ways that salient issues of race and racism—intersecting with issues of gender, class, empire, and migration—informed her life experiences. Although most of her autobiography does not explicitly refer to race and racism, three moments in the text are best understood with attention to these issues. The first moment concerns Ines's initial plan to go to the United States in 1928; the second relates to the legal status of Filipinos in the United States before World War II as "U.S. nationals" who were ineligible for U.S. citizenship; and the third refers to her cross-country travel experiences in 1960.

Following Escolastica Aguinaldo's advice of becoming a "topnotcher" at a prestigious nursing school in order to go to the United States with a scholarship, Ines graduated from St. Luke's as valedictorian of the class of 1928 and planned to leave the Philippines in July to pursue graduate studies at the University of Chicago under a scholarship from the DAR. However, the terms of her scholarship contract were changed after the wife of an Episcopalian minister in Mindanao died in childbirth. Ines explains that "instead of the original grant providing for free travel expenses and accommodation at a university student's residence, I was told to accompany the widower and take care of the newborn baby on the ship. During the year or years of study, I was to stay with a family and do housework and other chores to earn my board and lodging."[28] In other words, the terms of the "scholarship" were changed to a form of paid domestic labor. The situation calls to mind Paul Kramer's concept of "inclusionary racial formation."[29] U.S. colonial institutions and other sponsors may have believed that Filipinos could eventually become civilized beings and racial equals (hence their inclusion in education abroad programs) but only under American tutelage and supervision. In the meantime, that tutelage legitimized the inferior treatment and in this case subservient labor of Ines to care for the more pressing needs of the White widower and infant. The contradiction of nursing as a gendered female and subservient class of skilled labor embedded in the notion of being "ordered to care" is racialized in this historical example.

In her memory of this event, Ines displays defiance and critique of this racialized and gendered treatment, although she does not label it as such. She emphasizes instead that the missionaries did not treat her with respect and suggests that her family and nursing supervisors informed and supported her decision to reject this "opportunity" of going abroad:

> It was not so much the terms of the new contract that annoyed me as the way the missionaries peremptorily acted. They expected me to follow everything they wanted me to do without giving me sufficient time to deliberate and make a proper decision. Authoritatively, the superintendent told me of the change and wanted me to say "Yes" right away. Her negative approach incensed my pride and after conferring with other nursing executives in Manila and with my family, I refused the award on July fourth, three days before the scheduled sailing date.[30]

July fourth ironically, symbolically, and coincidentally refers to the date of U.S. independence from Britain and later, in 1946, the date given by the U.S. government to mark Philippine independence from the United States.

If the DAR could not control Ines's mobility, it could also not control the other Filipino nurses who would go under their auspices: The nurse sent in Ines's place "and two other scholars of DAR subsequently failed to return to the Philippines to fulfill their obligation of working in nursing institutions for two full years after their graduate work was completed because they got married."[31] Ines would go on to work at Dagupan Hospital in the province of Pangasinan. She describes herself as "an ambitious woman in a hurry to go to America,"[32] but clearly not at the cost of her dignity and self-respect.

The absence and presence of race and racism in Ines's autobiography is both frustrating and fascinating. Asian American historiography beginning in the late 1960s has greatly enriched our knowledge about anti-Asian racism in the United States and late nineteenth- and early twentieth-century Asian immigration restriction and exclusion, which affected Filipino Americans through programs such as the 1934 Repatriation Program. Yet, Ines omits discussion about anti-Filipino sentiment in her chapter on "Hawaii in the 1930s" and describes feelings of ambivalence:

> At the outbreak of the great depression, many Filipinos in Hawaii returned to the Philippines lured by the prospect of free transportation provided by the Territorial government and the Hawaiian Sugar Planters Association. As interpreter and assistant to those who were assigned to persuade Filipinos to go home, I had mixed emotions over the repatriation program, but I did not discourage those who were offered the free trip; neither did I favor their going. I left it up to them to decide and to weigh the pros and cons of their return. My concern was for the criteria used in selecting

those to be sent home. Priority was given to those who had TB and/or were under welfare support.³³

Although this passage does not speak to the racist, anti-Filipino, and anti-Asian sentiment of the Repatriation Program, it does suggest that Ines questioned the socioeconomic motives behind repatriation to remove the sick and those unable to work from the United States and back to the Philippines. Though such motives can be explained historically in the context of the Great Depression, in her writing Ines displays her common sense knowledge that disease travels but realizes that treatment is not transnational:

> I wrote the authorities at the Bureau of Health in Manila to inform them that many of those being repatriated had active tuberculosis, in the hope that they would provide a follow-up program for these TB cases. The reply to my letter stated that there was to be no follow-up program. So the repatriates from Hawaii, whether healthy or ill, went about their own individual ways.³⁴

I was thus surprised to read in one of the later chapters of Ines's autobiography, entitled "My Travels," explicit descriptions of racial prejudice that she, her husband Jesus, and her son Dante encountered during a 1960 cross-country trip from the East to the West Coast of the United States. Though the last section details a 1973 European vacation with a Filipino nurse friend that recounts their exciting visit to popular tourist attractions throughout Europe, most of the chapter details the 1960 trip and presents the reader with the juxtaposition of travel as forms of both downward and upward mobility. Ines describes the racialized incidents this way:

> When we reached Virginia, we stopped overnight at a small motel. The motel did not have a dining room; however we were told that there was a restaurant two miles farther where we could take our breakfast. . . . Twenty, perhaps thirty minutes passed. I was getting hungry and impatient. Finally I stood up and approached a waitress at the counter, only to be told that they were no longer serving breakfast. "At this time? At eight-thirty in the morning?" I demanded in disbelief, and she answered "Yes." My husband stood angrily and remarked that he was sure we were being denied service because the restaurant employees thought we were blacks. He took his overcoat and told me and our son that we were leaving. I refused to leave and insisted that I be allowed to use their telephone so that I could call our congressman in Washington D.C. I told that waitress that we were from Hawaii. . . . At that she sincerely apologized and begged us to sit down and be served. She covered our table with linen and gave us good service. I was proud of our victory over prejudice and felt satisfied that I gave the waitress a piece of my mind on the subject of being non-Christian and cruel to others, especially to the blacks and browns.³⁵

The restaurant incident is not an isolated one. She continues:

> Somewhere in Arkansas we decided to stop for lunch at a seafood restaurant.... As soon as we were seated in the restaurant, Daddy ordered and we settled to wait for what we hoped would be the gourmet treat of the day. The minutes ticked by... twenty... thirty.... Incensed, I stood up to tell the waitress that we had waited long enough and that if they were discriminating against us, I would call our congressman to report about it.... This time it was I who ate my meal angry and upset.[36]

Discriminatory treatment is a recurring motif in this chapter. Ines recollects:

> Dante and J.O. decided that at the next stop we would go to a larger and better motel even if we had to pay more.... It was a motel in Abilene, Texas.... We saw the motel of our choice with a lighted sign above the gate: "Room Available." Imagine our surprise when the manager at the reception desk said there was no room. I was so disgusted and angry that I told the man to his face that I knew he was refusing us because of the color of our skin. I informed him that we were Filipinos, naturalized American citizens and residents of the new state of Hawaii where Aloha is always extended to anyone, regardless of race, color, age or creed. Then I added my strategy of calling Washington, D.C. It worked.... By then I was used to such crises and forgave the manager when he apologized and explained that he was just carrying out the motel's regulation not to accept black people. I said something that may have sounded foolish but which I thought was important: that hotel and motel managers should learn something about the various races and peoples of the world and know what "human relations" means so that situations like this can be avoided. I capped this off by saying that we American people had won World War II with the help of other nations, regardless of racial origin and color, and that it was about time the whole world put a stop to racial prejudice.[37]

Ines's writing in these passages suggests that her own views of racial tolerance were informed by the antiracist agendas of World War II and a Christian worldview, but they were also informed by her cross-racial work as a public health nurse in Hawaii. Yet, though her status as a public health nurse, symbolized by her nurse's uniform, may have translated to upward mobility for her in Hawaii—"I have always considered my nurse's uniform as a mark of authority and a professional symbol which not only protected me but demanded recognition and respect"[38]—without the uniform and in the U.S. south, the color of Ines's skin marked her as racially inferior.

It is also important to note salient absences in this chapter and throughout the book. Ines's reference to "the new state of Hawaii where Aloha is always extended to anyone, regardless of race, color, age or creed" speaks to important differences in racial contexts across various regions of the United

States, but it also problematically erases racialized violence in Hawaii's history, including racism against Filipinos.

The third key series of moments in Ines's autobiography that speak to issues of race and racism refer to Ines's brief discussions of U.S. citizenship, more specifically how both she and her husband Jesus were excluded from particular kinds of employment because of their ineligibility for U.S. citizenship before World War II. For example, Ines writes that, even though Jesus Cayaban had obtained his bachelor's degree in education from the University of Hawaii, he "was not allowed to teach after his graduation because he was not an American citizen at the time."[39] And, after Ines's job as a district nurse at Palama Settlement was terminated because its public health nursing department was taken over by the Territorial Board of Health, she could not qualify for the civil service examination for employment in this official health agency because she was not and could not become a U.S. citizen. She does not refer to their "second-class" racialized and colonial status in the United States as "U.S. nationals," who may be permanent residents who are intimately part of their local communities, but with limited rights. This liminal state of Filipinos in the United States refers to what historian Mae Ngai calls "impossible subjects" in her study of illegal immigration and the making of modern America—subjects who are a social reality but a legal impossibility.[40]

In this context, I think it is noteworthy that at the end of her autobiography is Ines's lengthy resume. After traditional sections on education, employment, and civic activities, the very final line reads: "Naturalized American citizen in 1947." This line bears witness to the fact that foreign-educated nurses have become a permanent part of their local communities. Ines would return to visit the Philippines several times before her death in 1997, and she would maintain pride in her Filipino roots. As she wrote in her autobiography, perhaps directed to an audience of Filipino American youth: "Be proud of your heritage as Filipino, as well as being a good American."[41] She saw no contradiction in dual loyalties and identities.

The final key point I wish to make about Ines's life history is that it offers us some documentation of the ways Filipino American nurses contributed to health care delivery in the diaspora, in this case the United States, with cross-racial and cross-cultural sensitivity. Although my approach to research and writing is scholarly, I also believe in the importance of bringing scholarly work to the general public, and I think that parts of Ines's autobiography speak to a melancholy from contemporary Filipino health workers in the diaspora, and perhaps other foreign-educated health workers as well, that they are "unsung heroes" who hunger for public acknowledgment and understanding of their contributions to health care delivery. Indeed, the 2008 outrage by the

Filipino American community over a joke in the popular TV series *Desperate Housewives* that ridiculed the professional ability of Philippine-educated doctors speaks to this melancholy regarding current one-dimensional perceptions of foreign-educated health workers and the hunger for more nuanced and accurate portrayals.[42]

For example, though the story of foreign-educated health professionals, both doctors and nurses, working in AIDS wards has yet to be told, Ines's autobiography provides a glimpse into foreign-educated health workers' contributions regarding cancer prevention and education in Hawaii. In 1949, Ines joined the Hawaii Cancer Control Society Education Department:

> My function as health educator and supervisor of the home nursing program was both interesting and challenging. At that time the word cancer was spoken in hush-hush tones and although cases (morbidity) were far below that of tuberculosis in Hawaii, the mortality rate was high and there was much fear of having the disease. Among women, there was a great feeling of shame because of the prevalence of breast and uterine cancers. . . . What I wish to point out is that during the early days of our cancer control programs, non-Caucasian women were ashamed to have a pelvic examination, especially in having a smear taken from the cervix for the Pap test. The Filipino women were very shy at being examined "down below," particularly by a male physician. It took quite a long time to convince them that periodic pelvic examination was very essential in discovering cancer in its early stages, and insuring a high rate of cure. . . . Like the Filipino women, the Japanese women were also shy in submitting themselves to breast and pelvic examinations.[43]

According to Ines, health education involved giving talks before groups of people—professionals and nonprofessionals, adults and young adults—regardless of race, color, or creed. It also included radio programs, television talks, and a good many articles in the press. For some years, she gave weekly cancer talks in the Ilocano dialect on three radio stations.

Ines expressed pride in this challenging work: "We appeared before plantation camp people . . . the participants would ask questions not only about the subject of the evening but also about TB, nutritional disorders, gout, diabetes, arthritis, heart trouble, high blood pressure, stroke, diet and others. At the end they would ask, 'When are you coming again?' It made me feel good."[44]

Although contemporary discourses in the Philippines position Filipino nurses in the diaspora against their would-be Filipino patients in the Philippines, the above passage speaks to the fact that foreign-trained nurses can simultaneously contribute to health care delivery systems abroad and to the broader Filipino community.

CATHERINE CENIZA CHOY
Associate Professor, Department of Ethnic Studies
University of California, Berkeley
506 Barrows Hall, MC 2570
Berkeley, CA 94720–2570

Acknowledgments

I thank the Canadian Association for the History of Nursing and the Associated Medical Services History of Medicine Program for their generous support of the Hannah Lectures. I am also grateful to Geertje Boschma, Judith Young, Carol Helmstadter, the conference sponsors, and the organizing and program committees for their work regarding the 2008 CAHN/ACHN International Nursing History Conference.

Notes

1. Mirielle Kingma, *Nurses on the Move: Migration and the Global Health Care Economy* (Ithaca, N.Y.: Cornell University Press, 2006), 2.
2. See Barbara L. Brush, Julie Sochalski, and Anne M. Berger, "Imported Care: Recruiting Foreign Nurses to U.S. Health Care Facilities," *Health Affairs* 23, no. 3 (2004): 78–87, and Catherine Ceniza Choy, *Empire of Care: Nursing and Migration in Filipino American History* (Durham, N.C.: Duke University Press, 2003).
3. M. H. Alipalo, "Doctors Leaving Philippines to Become Nurses—for the Money," *San Francisco Chronicle*, November 5, 2003, cited by Brush, Sochalski, and Berger, "Imported Care."
4. Fitzhugh Mullan, "The Metrics of Physician Brain Drain," *New England Journal of Medicine* 353, no. 17 (2005): 1810–18.
5. Alfonso Mejía, Helena Pizorkí, and Erica Roynston, *Physician and Nurse Migration: Analysis and Policy Implications* (Geneva: World Health Organization, 1979), 43–45.
6. See Tim Martineau, Karola Decker, and Peter Bundred, *Briefing Note on International Migration of Health Professionals: Leveling the Playing Field for Developing Country Health Systems* (Liverpool: Liverpool School of Tropical Medicine, 2002), and Sabina Alkire and Lincoln Chen, "Medical Exceptionalism in International Migration: Should Doctors and Nurses Be Treated Differently," draft paper for Global Migration Regimes workshop sponsored by Institute of Future Studies, Stockholm, in collaboration with Common Security Forum colleagues at the Center for History and Economics, King's College, Cambridge, and the Global Equity Initiative, Harvard University, and in cooperation with the World Health Organization, 2004.

7. See Barbara Brush, "Exchangees or Employees? The Exchange Visitor Program and Foreign Nurse Immigration to the United States, 1945–1990," *Nursing History Review* 1, no. 1 (1993): 171–80, and Margaret Shkimba and Karen Flynn, "'In England We Did Nursing': Caribbean and British Nurses in Great Britain and Canada, 1950–70," in *New Directions in the History of Nursing: International Perspectives*, eds. Barbara Mortimer and Susan McGann (New York: Routledge, 2005), 141–57.

8. See Prasenjit Duara, "Transnationalism and the Challenge to National Histories," in *Re-Thinking American History in a Global Age*, ed. Thomas Bender (Berkeley: University of California Press, 2002), 25–46.

9. Celia W. Dugger, "An Exodus of African Nurses Puts Infants and the Ill in Peril," *The New York Times*, July 12, 2004.

10. See Jaime Z. Galvez Tan, "The Brain Drain Phenomenon and Its Implications on the Health Care System," paper presented at the Dr. Alfredo J. Ganapin Advocacy Forum Series III, "Policy Issues on Skilled Migration: The Case of Filipino Nurses," Quezon City, Philippines, 2005.

11. Sabina Alkire and Lincoln Chen, "Medical Exceptionalism in International Migration," draft paper for Global Migration Regimes workshop.

12. Sonya J. Grypma, "Critical Issues in the Use of Biographic Methods in Nursing History," *Nursing History Review* 13 (2005): 171.

13. Barbara Mortimer, "Introduction: The History of Nursing: Yesterday, Today and Tomorrow," in Mortimer and McGann, *New Directions in the History of Nursing*, 9.

14. Grypma, "Critical Issues in the Use of Biographic Methods," 171.

15. Ibid., 173.

16. Ines V. Cayaban, *A Goodly Heritage* (Wanchai, Hong Kong: Gulliver Books, 1981).

17. Ibid., 24.

18. Ibid., 25.

19. Ibid., 28.

20. See Paul A. Kramer, *The Blood of Government: Race, Empire, the United States, and the Philippines* (Chapel Hill: University of North Carolina Press, 2006), and Stuart Creighton Miller, *"Benevolent Assimilation": The American Conquest of the Philippines, 1899–1903* (New Haven, C.T.: Yale University Press, 1982).

21. Cayaban, *A Goodly Heritage*, 28.

22. Ibid., 30.

23. Ibid., 42.

24. Ibid.

25. See Barbara M. Posadas and Roland L. Guyotte, "Unintentional Immigrants: Chicago's Filipino Foreign Students Become Settlers, 1900–1941," *Journal of American Ethnic History* 9, no. 2 (Spring 1990): 26–48.

26. Cayaban, *A Goodly Heritage*, 42–43.

27. Ibid., 65.

28. Ibid., 56.

29. Kramer, *The Blood of Government*, 192.

30. Cayaban, *A Goodly Heritage*, 56.

31. Ibid.

32. Ibid., 57.

33. Ibid., 117.

34. Ibid.
35. Ibid., 125–26.
36. Ibid., 126–27.
37. Ibid., 127–28.
38. Ibid., 82.
39. Ibid., 75.
40. Mae M. Ngai, *Impossible Subjects: Illegal Aliens and the Making of Modern America* (Princeton, N.J.: Princeton University Press, 2004).
41. Cayaban, *A Goodly Heritage*, 96.
42. See Benito M. Vergara, Jr., *Pinoy Capital: The Filipino Nation in Daly City* (Philadelphia: Temple University Press, 2009), 153–54.
43. Cayaban, *A Goodly Heritage*, 102–3.
44. Ibid., 105.

ARTICLES

The Introduction of Deaconess Nurses at the German Hospital of the City of Philadelphia in the 1880s

CHRISTOPH SCHWEIKARDT
Institute for History, Theory and Ethics in Medicine
RWTH Aachen University
Germany

Abstract. In 1884, seven deaconesses from Iserlohn, Germany, came to the Philadelphia German Hospital to take over nursing care and hospital administration. This article deals with the preparation and implementation of deaconess rule at the German Hospital and conflicts during the tenure of the first two Sisters Superior, Marie Krueger (1826–1887) and Wanda von Oertzen (1845–1897). Recruitment of the deaconesses took place within a network of relations between German and American motherhouses. Before their arrival in Philadelphia, the benefactor of the German Hospital, John D. Lankenau (1817–1901), had committed himself to hospital rule by the Sister Superior. A Deaconess Committee was created to deal with the opposition of the Medical Board. Introducing deaconesses to the Philadelphia German Hospital led to a major change of medical personnel and allowed the hospital to develop a new corporate identity.

Religious women played an important role in health care during the nineteenth century.[1] On the Protestant side, the Kaiserswerth deaconess movement was the "first non-Catholic attempt to harness evangelical energy of women in a public role."[2] German pastor Theodor Fliedner (1800–1864) founded the deaconess movement in the small town of Kaiserswerth in 1836 to revive the biblical female diaconate. Nursing, though by no means the only activity of deaconesses, developed into one of their most important fields of work.

In 1849, William Alfred Passavant (1821–1894),[3] an American Lutheran minister who dedicated his life to the founding and administration of benevolent institutions, introduced deaconesses from Kaiserswerth to Pittsburgh, Pennsylvania. He met with very limited success, however. Between 1849 and 1891, there were only about twelve consecrated deaconesses in Pittsburgh, half of whom still belonged to the Kaiserswerth Motherhouse.[4]

Deaconesses were introduced to Philadelphia in 1884 with the express purpose of serving the nursing needs of the German Hospital of Philadelphia. The Philadelphia Motherhouse, founded two years later, soon became the largest motherhouse in the United States, with a maximum of 127 sisters in 1936.[5] It played a leading role as the center of the American Deaconess Movement.[6] The first deaconesses of the motherhouses in Omaha and Baltimore received their training in Philadelphia.[7] By 1899, seven Lutheran motherhouses had been established in the United States, in Philadelphia, Brooklyn, Omaha, Minneapolis, Milwaukee, Baltimore, and Chicago.[8]

The introduction of deaconesses to Philadelphia merits special attention. In 1906, this move was characterized as "one of the most radical changes that the German Hospital had experienced. Prior to that year the patients were nursed and the entire household taken care of by paid help, who showed woeful lack of interest in their work."[9] Also, the first seven deaconesses from Germany had been members of an "independent" deaconess community.[10] Deaconesses who organized themselves independently outside the traditional motherhouse were a rare exception in Germany. Finally, the arrival of the deaconesses went hand-in-hand with pivotal decisions on hospital organization and the position of the Sister Superior. This article focuses on the circumstances of the deaconesses' arrival in Philadelphia and examines the conflicts that occurred during the tenure of the first two Sisters Superior.

The research was facilitated by a broad range of primary sources from the Barbara Bates Collection at the University of Pennsylvania School of Nursing in Philadelphia, the Lankenau Hospital Archive Center records in Wynnewood, Pennsylvania, the Evangelical Lutheran Church in America Archives in Elk Grove, Illinois, and the Archives of the Fliedner Foundation in Düsseldorf-Kaiserswerth, Germany. They include annual reports, anniversary publications, pastors' memoirs, and sisters' personal files as well as hospital and motherhouse Boards of Trustees minutes.

Patient Care at the German Hospital before the Arrival of the Deaconesses

The German Hospital of Philadelphia was founded in 1860 by philanthropic citizens to serve German immigrants who spoke little or no English.[11] It was located at Twentieth and Norris streets. During the Civil War, the U.S. government took possession of the hospital for the care of sick and wounded soldiers, so the hospital opened for civilian patients in 1866. In 1872, with growing demand, the hospital moved to Corinthian and Girard avenues. The hospital expanded rapidly, so new buildings and additions to existing ones were needed. These improvements were largely the gift of the wealthy immigrant businessman John D. Lankenau (1817–1901), whose name the hospital was later to bear.[12]

In the early 1880s, the Medical Board consisted of nine physicians: four specialists in internal medicine, four surgeons, and one eye and ear specialist.[13] These men served as visiting physicians and supervised the house officers, young physicians seeking clinical experience after graduation from medical school.[14] Assistant physicians worked for the dispensary of the Surgical, Medical, and Gynecology Clinics, and Clinic of Eye and Ear Diseases.[15]

Hospital administration lay in the hands of a warden or matron. From 1878 onward, the hospital employed married couples.[16] Charles S. Turnbull, who served on the Medical Board in 1878,[17] had vivid reminiscences of the nursing and hospital administration during his time at the German Hospital:

> Mrs. Salm, the Warden's wife, served as Matron, and a handsome typical German she was. She not only superintended the house but also the kitchen and the German cooking and genuine "Reid-Hof" cooking it was—because she often put on the apron and did the cooking herself. She looked after the nurses; these she hired from outside, or recruited from the ward as recent importations convalesced. These German immigrants by the way, usually made excellens [sic] nurses and servants, but this was before the days of Special Education, and at a time when asepsis and antisepsis were unknown quantities. Many were the shortcomings on the part of the hireling, necessarily employed, and now we can only suppose it to have been—for the patients—the "survival of the fittest."[18]

In retrospect, Adolph Spaeth (1839–1910), pastor of St. Johannes Church and professor at the Philadelphia Seminary,[19] recalled that the main problem of the hospital was that, generally, not competent and reliable attendants but "schiffbrüchige Existenzen"—persons whose life had been shipwrecked—had been hired as stopgaps at the bedside.[20] It was this condition Lankenau and his allies were determined to alter.

32   CHRISTOPH SCHWEIKARDT

Setting the Stage: The Change of Hospital Board Representation and the Search for Deaconesses in Germany

John Lankenau has been characterized as "perhaps the greatest Lutheran layman in nineteenth-century America."[21] He was born in Bremen in 1817 and came to Philadelphia in 1836. Having become a wealthy businessman, he married Mary J. Drexel, sister of rich, successful Catholic Anthony J. Drexel (1826–1893). Lankenau was elected to the Board of Trustees of the German Hospital in 1866 and served as its president from 1869 until his death in 1901.

Improvement of nursing services at the German Hospital lay at Lankenau's heart and may well have been the main impetus for the 1884 introduction of deaconesses. Lankenau was thoroughly dissatisfied with the inadequate nursing care by ward attendants. Pastor Spaeth also remembered a cold and distant relationship between church and hospital. Arriving at the hospital outside visiting hours for pastoral care of ill or dying patients, he himself had been denied access.[22] According to Spaeth, Lankenau's Catholic brother-in-law had encouraged Lankenau to steer the hospital toward the Protestant Church.[23] Lankenau's sister, who lived in Bremen, specifically recommended that he introduce deaconesses from Germany.[24] In all likelihood, Lankenau came to the conclusion that the internal administration of the hospital had to be taken over by deaconess service. This move had to be prepared by changes to the hospital charter, to give Lutheran pastors a say on the Board of Trustees.[25] So a group of church-minded men, consisting of Lankenau, German consul Charles H. Meyer (d. 1898),[26] other Hospital Board trustees, and pastors moved to guide the hospital into the interests of the Lutheran Church.[27]

In 1880, Meyer asked Spaeth to become a trustee. After some consideration, Spaeth accepted and became a trustee in 1881.[28] The first ground had been broken. Lankenau then proposed more far-reaching changes to the charter of the German Hospital, which came into effect in 1882. Three of the sixteen seats on the board were to be occupied by ministers who were recognized by the Evangelical Lutheran Ministerium of Pennsylvania and Adjacent States. Aside from Spaeth, Dr. William Julius Mann (1819–1892), pastor of Zion Church and also a professor at the Philadelphia Seminary, and Frederick Wischan, pastor of St. Paulus Church in Philadelphia, were elected.[29]

However, in their search for deaconesses from Germany for the German Hospital, Lankenau and Meyer did not succeed in recruiting sisters from any of the established German motherhouses. Finally, Pastor Carl Wilhelm Theodor Ninck (1834–1887)[30] from the Hamburg Deaconess Motherhouse told them of a small independent community of deaconesses in Iserlohn, where they ran the town hospital.

During the summer of 1883, the deaconesses considered Meyer's request to come to Philadelphia. Oberin (Sister Superior) Marie Krueger expressed concerns as to their future position at the German Hospital. The Iserlohn Hospital House Rules of 1872 put the Sister Superior in charge of the internal administration of the hospital.[31] So Lankenau promised her in a letter dated October 29, 1883, that the entire leadership of the Philadelphia German Hospital would be given to her charge—provided that she would be completely able to administer competently this burdensome office in all avenues and with all the associated demands.[32] He also explained that the warden and his wife did honest work to the best of their powers but lacked ability. This lack of real ability was so manifest that the warden had already resigned and stayed only out of consideration for Lankenau and the institution until the sisters took over the administration.[33]

Ultimately, seven sisters, Marie Krueger, Magdalene von Bracht, Wilhelmine Dittmann, Alma Kohlmann, Marianne Kraetzer, Pauline Loeschman, and Friedericke Wurzler, agreed to come to Philadelphia. Meyer, who visited Iserlohn in April 1884, offered them free transportation home in case they could not tolerate the climate. He also promised a vacation trip to their home country after five years.[34]

The Controversy with the Medical Board

The seven pioneering sisters arrived in Philadelphia in June 1884 to take over hospital duties. According to Sister Magdalene von Bracht's reminiscences, there were twenty-seven patients in the hospital when the deaconesses arrived. On the men's wards there were two male attendants, on the women's wards one female attendant. The large wards were bare brickwork, and the walls had not yet been painted. Sister Marie took over administration, Sister Marianne kitchen and household, Sister Wilhelmine and Sister Friedericke operations and male patients, Sister Magdalene and Sister Alma the women's ward. Sister Pauline, trained as a kindergarten teacher, helped everywhere. She felt dissatisfied and left after a few weeks, and Sister Friedericke returned to Germany after a year due to a lung condition.[35]

Difficulties ensued not only with household management, which the deaconesses were meant to replace, but also with the Medical Board. In this regard, the institutional framework built up to support the deaconess cause and the subsequent policy pursued merit special attention. At a hospital Board of Trustees meeting—probably in June or early July 1885—[36]Adolph Spaeth moved to appoint a Deaconess Committee.[37] The committee, inaugurated on July 18, 1885, included eight of the sixteen members of the Board of Trustees: Lankenau and Meyer, the three pastors Spaeth, Mann, and Wischan, and John C. File, J. Henry Tilge, and Gustave A. Schwarz.[38] These men were sympathetic to and understanding of the deaconess cause.

At the first meeting, the Sister Superior was unanimously elected to the Deaconess Committee.[39] Changes were to be pushed through against the resistance of those trustees and physicians who did not approve of Lankenau's plans. Spaeth called the Deaconess Committee "a state within the state." The committee met shortly before the Board of Trustees meetings and prepared the strategy of the church-minded faction.[40] At the third meeting, on August 29, 1885, Lankenau was elected chairman of the Deaconess Committee, where he served as treasurer as well.[41] From the very beginning, the committee pursued the foundation of a deaconess motherhouse according to the Kaiserswerth model.[42] It acted as predecessor of the Board of Trustees of the Mary J. Drexel Home and Philadelphia Motherhouse of Deaconesses.[43] After incorporation, Lankenau served as the president of this Board of Trustees as well.

On October 31, 1885, the Deaconess Committee gave the mandate to Meyer to present a plan for reorganization of the Medical Board: Only physicians who in advance declared full agreement with deaconess rule should be elected to serve in the hospital.[44] Meyer stated this principle in a draft for a letter later sent by the Board of Trustees to the board. To serve on the Medical Board of the German Hospital, physicians had to provide written acknowledgment of their willingness to conform to the following rules:

> The Oberin must be looked upon as the executive head of the Hospital and Household. All admissions and discharges of patients, or permits for temporary absence must pass through her hands, desired changes of patients must be arranged by her, purchases of any kind must be authorized by her; hence it is greatly desired that the Medical Staff should address recommendations for admission of patients, complaints or observations of every nature directly to her. . . . The present Rules and Regulations for the government of the Medical Board are suspended in every instance where they come in conflict with the above rulings.[45]

In short, the visiting physicians faced the choice of complying with the regulations set by the Sister Superior, resigning, or risking not being re-elected by the Board of Trustees in 1886.[46] The Deaconess Committee felt in a stronger position than the physicians. It was convinced that even if the whole Medical Board resigned, some of the best physicians in the city would be ready to replace them.[47]

Step by step, physicians who did not wish to cooperate with the deaconesses left the Medical Board.[48] Others who were unpopular with the Deaconess Committee left, and a few left for unrelated reasons. Surgeon James M. Barton had been reproached with coming during lunch time and opening disgusting wounds, so that not only the patient concerned but all the others lost their appetite.[49] He resigned his position because it was impossible for him to make visits between 9 and 11 in the morning.[50] Frank Woodbury, seen as an obstinate opponent of the deaconesses,[51] left in 1886. Marcus Franklin, visiting surgeon since 1874 and in many ways unpopular with the Deaconess Committee, left in 1886 as well, when his "extensive private practice demanded his entire attention."[52] J. Solis Cohen, who had regarded it beneath him to comply formally with the Board of Trustees demands concerning the deaconesses, left in 1887. James Collins, who had, in the eyes of the Deaconess Committee, exposed surgical patients to unnecessary suffering by reluctant, indecisive, and wrong treatment and who had kept them improperly long in the hospital,[53] also left in 1887.

In 1885, the Board of Trustees decided to create the post of chief resident physician.[54] "His duties were to assume charge of the Resident Physicians and the Assistants in the various Dispensaries."[55] The church-minded faction of the board succeeded in the appointment of Dr. George A. Bodamer, a member of the parish of St. Johannes.[56] Bodamer served as chief resident physician until 1889[57] and thereby as liaison between the sisters and the resident physicians. Bodamer knew John B. Deaver (1855–1931) as an excellent surgeon. Spaeth gave Bodamer credit as the first to call strong attention to Deaver. Deaver applied in 1885 to become visiting surgeon at the German Hospital with the prospect of cooperating with deaconesses in charge of the hospital patients. The Deaconess Committee agreed. In 1886, Deaver was elected to the Medical Board as replacement for Dr. Marcus Franklin.[58] He carried on for decades a fruitful career at the German Hospital that would make him world famous.

The Philadelphia German Hospital also changed its bylaws to formalize deaconess command. The new 1887 bylaws stated:

> The Hospital is to be conducted by Deaconesses according to the rules of the Order of Deaconesses, as practiced in Germany, governed by a Sister Superior, or Oberin. . . . The Oberin must be respected as the executive head of the Hospital and Household. She has to see that the rules and regulations of the Hospital, as well as the prescriptions of the physicians, are carried out, and she is the direct head and superior of the deaconesses and sister probationers serving in the Hospital. . . . The Oberin shall appoint or discharge all servants, nurses, or mechanics employed by the

Hospital. All admissions or discharges of patients, all permits for temporary absence, all changes of patients from one ward or room to another, must be authorized and arranged by her. . . . The Oberin shall attend officially at the monthly meetings of the Board of Trustees, of the Committee on Deaconesses, and at the weekly meetings of the Visiting Committee, as an advisory member; and all resolutions concerning the internal administration of the Hospital shall be communicated to her for further action.[59]

The Death of Oberin Marie Krueger

The turmoil was not over after the controversy with the Medical Board. In 1887, Marie Krueger died suddenly. Her death was attributed to heart failure.[60] According to the Deaconess Committee, she had taken a too hot bath that had led to severe scalding. This, in turn, caused a latent heart condition to become acute.[61] Her judgment had been impaired: She had taken the bath while she was disturbed due to "passionate opium consumption."[62]

Krueger had belonged to the Kaiserswerth Deaconess Motherhouse. Kaiserswerth deaconesses including Krueger had been in charge of poor children in Iserlohn from 1856 until 1867.[63] When the motherhouse called the deaconesses to give up this task, she separated from the motherhouse to run the Iserlohn poorhouse and hospital (Armen- und Krankenhaus) independently.[64]

Meyer informed Kaiserswerth directing pastor Julius Disselhoff (1827–1896)[65] that Krueger had been urged to resign during the year before her death, and that the search for a successor in Germany had already started.[66] In his reply to Meyer, Disselhoff used strong language: He wrote that Krueger had been a very gifted person, but that her gift had been a seduction that had led her away from the humility of a deaconess. In Disselhoff's eyes, she had formerly dissociated herself from the Kaiserswerth Motherhouse on purpose, in blatant disobedience and a selfish display of self-will.[67] His letter also stated that, before leaving for Philadelphia, she had asked forgiveness, which he had granted her, but that he had not been able to enter into an official relationship with her again.[68]

Obviously, Disselhoff still felt hurt by Krueger, because he concluded toward the end of his letter: "Wholeheartedly, I wish, honored Consul, that you will find a Christian virgin or widow as directress of your young deaconess motherhouse who has not only the necessary talent, but above all humility, which is not made-up, and transparent integrity. A deaconess who is to lead a deaconess motherhouse must be above all deaconess from tip to toe. Otherwise she cannot educate deaconesses."[69] It was left to pastor Adolph Spaeth to convince Disselhoff, on a journey to Germany in 1886, that the irregular conduct of one sister should not impair the recognition of the Philadelphia Motherhouse.[70] The Kaiserswerth General Conference did vote to admit Philadelphia to membership conditionally in 1888, the year after Krueger's death.[71]

The Board of Trustees decided that the memory of Marie Krueger was to be held in honor.[72] In 1891, Chief Resident Physician Carl Frese mentioned a "short illness" before her death together with her great merits in developing the hospital, which were "gladly recognized."[73] Later, abundant praise was lavished on her and even an act of providence was invoked. In 1934, the fiftieth anniversary of the deaconesses' arrival was celebrated.[74] The anniversary publication recalled Lankenau's praise forty-seven years earlier: "Deeply moved, Mr. Lankenau paid her the highest tribute at the next Board meeting and said: '. . . She was a woman of greatest energy and endowed with most comprehensive administrative gifts. It was she who completely reorganized the German Hospital and raised it to such a high degree of perfection.'"[75] On the seventy-fifth anniversary in 1959, Theodore Bachmann wrote:

> Under Sister Marie Krueger's able administration, the hospital's reputation was rising rapidly. Top physicians were attracted, and the nursing service set the highest standards. Suddenly, however, on November 30, 1887, Sister Marie died. The blow severely tested the faith of those who had come to depend so much upon her exemplary leadership. To one of the bereaved Sisters, the pastor in Iserlohn, who had known Sister Marie well, wrote words of encouragement. Never, as he put it, had he met "a woman more distinguished, intellectually more alert, or of firmer character." To which he added, "Trust Him who, in His overruling providence, has never made a mistake!"[76]

Marie Krueger's Successor: Wanda von Oertzen (1845–1897)

Though Krueger's resignation as Sister Superior was pursued behind the scenes, obviously none of the deaconesses at the Philadelphia Motherhouse was found suitable to succeed her. So Lankenau and Meyer turned to Germany to find a suitable successor. Again, pastor Ninck in Hamburg turned out to be an important counsel. Ninck directed them to Wanda von Oertzen. By the time of Marie Krueger's death, the search for a successor had already been narrowed down to her.[77] A handwritten "Lebenslauf" (Curriculum Vitae) of Wanda von Oertzen, dating from 1888, is preserved in her personal files, so we know which qualifications she brought to Philadelphia.[78]

Von Oertzen was a daughter of Baron von Oertzen, who died in 1849.[79] She had worked for thirteen years at the Deaconess Seminary Salem (Stift Salem) without being consecrated as a deaconess. She enjoyed the freedom of travel and visiting her family. According to her CV, her elder brother had objected to her consecration, fearing the moral pressure on consecrated deaconesses, and foreseeing that the time would come when she would have to return to care for her mother.[80] But she did train as a nurse in Kiel in the summers of 1885 and 1886 under Friedrich von Esmarch (1823–1908), one of the most famous surgeons of the nineteenth century. She clearly made a favorable impression there, because she became the deputy to the surgical ward head nurse.[81] Called to Philadelphia as Sister Superior, she was educated as a deaconess in the Hamburg Deaconess Motherhouse of directing pastor Ninck for less than three months before leaving for the United States in May 1888.[82]

Spaeth at first objected to the appointment of von Oertzen. In his eyes, she could not prove regular deaconess training in one of the recognized German deaconess motherhouses. Not until February 1888 had she agreed to enter the deaconess motherhouse of pastor Ninck to get training. Spaeth withdrew his objection only after being reassured by a German colleague as to the suitability of her character and her working capability. More than once, he recalled in his memories, she had openly told him: "I just lack deaconess education!" On the other hand, Spaeth admitted that her excellent training as a nurse had enabled her "to take up a position in the hospital which also impressed our physicians."[83]

Another severe conflict occurred between Wanda von Oertzen and Philadelphia Motherhouse Rector Augustus Cordes. Cordes had been assistant to Pastor Ninck in Hamburg before being called to Philadelphia in 1888.[84] Spaeth had become acquainted with Cordes in 1887 in Germany. Cordes had a former deaconess as his wife, and, according to Spaeth, he was in every respect excellently gifted and prepared for the office of rector.[85]

In a letter to Kaiserswerth on May 8, 1891, Cordes reported a veritable crisis, for which he named two main causes. First, the Board of Trustees laymen were, in Cordes's eyes, with only one exception "unkirchlich"—"not churchly." Cordes seems to use this term to describe a lack of respect or understanding of the proper role of the church and his own role as motherhouse rector. They sought to interfere with the inner organization of the motherhouse and to enforce measures against his conscience. It was unfortunate, Cordes wrote, that Lankenau also belonged to this group. Second, Cordes complained that the Oberin was no "deaconess mother," that she was unsuccessful at winning the trust of the sisters, and that a considerable number of sisters intended to leave.[86]

From the Board of Trustees minutes we know that Cordes challenged Oberin von Oertzen in a letter dated June 13, 1892. She had to give up her post, he wrote, or else he would resign. The Board of Trustees accepted Cordes's resignation after a statement from the Sister Superior that she had given the matter thorough consideration and did not see a reason to step down. Meyer moved that the trustees present fully approve the answer of the Sister Superior, which they did unanimously.[87]

Later, Meyer explained in a letter to Disselhoff:

> You know the faults our Sister Superior is reproached with, which, however, are neutralized by her eminent qualities in such a way that we could not let her go in order to keep our otherwise so appreciated pastor Cordes. I am convinced that a mature man, who by nothing but dignity and firmness fills her with respect, could very well work in harmony besides and with her, in particular, when the fields of work are distributed correctly.[88]

Wanda von Oertzen stayed, and Cordes was succeeded by the Rev. Carl Goedel, who was installed in July 1893.[89] After von Oertzen's death, Lankenau "gave a lasting expression of the love and respect for her by placing a memorial tablet in the beautiful vestibule of the Motherhouse."[90]

Why did the Board of Trustees of the Motherhouse back the deaconesses and their Sister Superior against all odds? Although it is difficult to prove, it is likely that the personal bond between Lankenau and "his" deaconesses—a bond forged through common faith as well as mutual confidence and obligation—can hardly be overrated.[91] A level of trust had to be established for the women to leave Germany and come to work in the United States.[92] So the beginnings of personal trust and mutual obligation can be traced back to their decision in Germany. There is a photograph of Lankenau sitting with several deaconesses on the porch of his summer home in New Jersey (see Figure 1).

Clearly Lankenau would not have invited the deaconesses to use his home as a retreat and had them photographed there if he did not genuinely feel affection for them.[93] We also know that Lankenau bequeathed the motherhouse a large part of his fortune.[94] Aside from this, we have to take into account that the Deaconess Committee, which included Lankenau and the Lutheran pastors of the Board of Trustees, had seen itself as the basis for the deaconess project in the United States.[95] This meant strong commitment for their mission in the face of adversaries who did not share their vision.

After von Oertzen's death in 1897, her responsibilities were divided: Sister Emilie Schwarz became Sister Superior, and Sister Magdalene von Bracht, one of the original seven, took over the direction of the hospital.[96] Until 1909

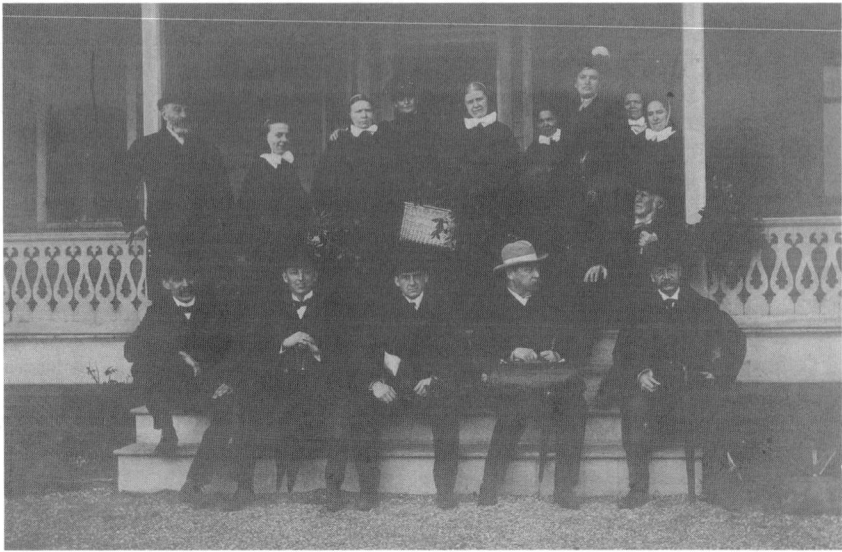

Figure 1. John D. Lankenau with deaconesses and visitors at his summer home in Cape May, New Jersey, in 1901. Lankenau, the only person sitting in the second row, is on the far right. I wish to thank Bonnie Dorwart for this photo. Reprinted courtesy of the Archive of Lankenau Hospital, Annenberg Conference Center for Medical Education, Wynnewood, Pennsylvania.

Sister Magdalene von Bracht served as Directing Sister of the German Hospital, a position that "included the superintendency of the Hospital as well as direction of the Nursing Staff."[97]

Conclusion

In the 1880s, Protestant Germany offered the deaconess motherhouse tradition, an established, highly esteemed, and expanding institution where nursing care was one of the most important fields of work. But the painstaking search for deaconesses from Germany for the Philadelphia German Hospital in the early 1880s shows the scarcity of deaconesses who could be recruited for the New World. So 1884 marked a turning point for the hospital, when Lankenau and his allies transplanted the pioneering deaconesses to Philadelphia, to be followed by the deaconess motherhouse institution.

The German Hospital profited from the nursing skills and experience of the first two Sisters Superior. Marie Krueger brought thorough experience in hospital administration, Wanda von Oertzen skills as a surgical nurse. The deaconesses formed the core of new corporate identity of the hospital, which included a major change of medical personnel. With the 150th anniversary of Lankenau Hospital coming up in 2010, an interesting area of research would be to what extent and how the corporate culture of the hospital, as it was established in the 1880s, was preserved and how it adapted to the changing needs of the medical marketplace.

The introduction of the deaconesses was made possible by exceptional institutional and personal circumstances. Lankenau's wealth, his generosity as a benefactor of the Deaconess Motherhouse and the German Hospital, as well as his unrelenting support of the deaconesses until his death in 1901, proved a decisive factor in the future direction of the German Hospital. Lankenau's commitment together with the fact that he chaired the Board of Trustees of the hospital, its Deaconess Committee, and later the Board of Trustees of the Motherhouse, resulted in the powerful position of the Sister Superior, a position that enabled her to prevail in conflicts with physicians and pastors. This was a position much stronger than could be expected of an Oberin in Germany, especially in the ensuing conflicts. Lankenau's 1883 letter shows that he had pledged a strong commitment to the leadership of the Sister Superior at the German Hospital before their arrival in the United States. He and the German Hospital offered career opportunities to deaconesses who had controversial personalities, at least in the eyes of the pastors concerned.

Sioban Nelson argued that the deaconesses had a subordinate position within their own organizational structure and did not have a public face for those outside the hospital.[98] However, the 1887 bylaws made the Sister Superior an advisory member of the Board of Trustees of the German Hospital, which meant that she could argue her position at the monthly meetings. Also, the Board of Trustees of the German Hospital, which existed before the arrival of the deaconesses, was not the organizational structure for the deaconesses proper. The decision-making body for the deaconesses was the Board of Trustees of the Mary J. Drexel Home and Philadelphia Motherhouse of Deaconesses and its predecessor, the Deaconess Committee of the German Hospital. Formally, deaconess work at the German Hospital meant that the motherhouse sent its sisters into a field of work outside the direct responsibility of its Board of Trustees. This, however, did probably not matter much as long as Lankenau was alive and chaired both committees. The lack of a public face in the annual reports of the hospital may well have served to avoid irritating not like-minded trustees.

In 1917, the German Hospital changed its name to "Lankenau Hospital" when the one hundredth anniversary of Lankenau coincided with the anti-German sentiment that swept the country when the United States entered World War I.[99] Today, Lankenau Hospital, having meanwhile moved to the suburban community of Wynnewood,[100] honors its pioneer women religious: To the left of the main entrance, between the portraits of "leaders of the past" John Lankenau and John Deaver, is a picture of the first seven deaconesses.

PRIVATDOZENT DR. CHRISTOPH SCHWEIKARDT, MA
Institute for History, Theory and Ethics in Medicine
RWTH Aachen University
Wendlingweg 2
D-52074 Aachen
Germany

Acknowledgments

I wish to express my gratitude to Professor Patricia D'Antonio, Dr. Friederike Baer, Archivist Götz Bettge, Archivist Annett Büttner, M.A., Professor Bonnie Dorwart, Professor Julie Fairman, Curator Gail Farr, Dr. Norbert Friedrich, Archivist Catherine Lundeen, Professor Joan Lynaugh, Archivist Tanja Marschall, Archivist Nancy Miller, Dr. Otto Plassmann, Archivist John Peterson, Dr. Susanne Kreutzer, Dr. Robert Lamparter, Professor Heinz Rodegra, Sister Marilyn Stauffer, Professor Jean Whelan, Professor Barbra Mann Wall, doctoral student Lisa Zerull, and the anonymous reviewers of *Nursing History Review* for their contributions, as well as the Barbara Bates Center for the Study of the History of Nursing, University of Pennsylvania, Philadelphia, for the Alice Fisher Society Summer Fellowship 2007, which made this research possible. I also wish to thank Alison Anderson, Ph.D., for editing the English text.

Notes

1. On women religious as nurses see, e.g., Sioban Nelson, *Say Little, Do Much: Nurses, Nuns, and Hospitals in the Nineteenth Century* (Philadelphia: University of Pennsylvania Press, 2001); Barbra Mann Wall, *Unlikely Entrepreneurs: Catholic Sisters and the Hospital Marketplace, 1865–1925* (Columbus: Ohio State University Press, 2005). For the nineteenth century see, e.g., Catherine Prelinger, *Charity, Challenge, and Change: Religious Dimensions of the Mid-Nineteenth-Century Women's Movement in Germany* (New York:

Greenwood Press, 1987); and Silke Köser, *Denn eine Diakonisse darf kein Alltagsmensch sein: Kollektive Identitäten Kaiserswerther Diakonissen 1836–1914* (Leipzig: Evangelische Verlags-Anstalt, 2006). Doctoral student Lisa Zerull, University of Virginia, is currently working on a project on deaconesses at the motherhouse in Baltimore. From a church historian point of view, Jennifer Wiley Legath, Princeton University, is working on a Ph.D. thesis on the American deaconess movement between 1880 and 1930. A shorter version of this paper appears in the proceedings of the 2008 Annual Conference of the Rhenian Circle of Medical Historians (Rheinischer Kreis der Medizinhistoriker): *Medizingeschichte im Rheinland: Beiträge des "Rheinischen Kreises der Medizinhistoriker,"* ed. Dominik Groß and Axel Karenberg (Kassel: Kassel University Press).

2. Nelson, *Say Little, Do Much*, 126.

3. On Passavant's eminence see, e.g., Robert H. Fischer, *A Servant of All People: The Legacy of William Alfred Passavant (1821–1894), Pioneer in the Church's Ministry of Mercy* (Chicago: Lutheran School of Theology at Chicago, 1997).

4. Frederick Weiser, *Love's Response: A Story of Lutheran Deaconesses in America* (Philadelphia: Board of Publication of the United Lutheran Church, 1962), 56.

5. Frederick Weiser, "The Origins of Lutheran Deaconesses in America," *Lutheran Quarterly* 13, no. 4 (1999): 423–34, 431. Weiser lists the names of the motherhouses with the numbers of deaconesses (both consecrated and probationer) for 1899, 1940, and the highest report (number of deaconesses together with the year when the maximum was attained).

6. Nelson, *Say Little, Do Much*, 138.

7. Martin Lehfeldt, *Fifty Years Pioneer Work for the Female Diaconate Within the Lutheran Church in U.S.A.* (B. Div. thesis, Hartwick Theological Seminary, New York, May 1938), 35.

8. On the Lutheran deaconess movement, see Ann Doyle, "Nursing by Religious Orders in the United States. Part IV—Lutheran Deaconesses, 1849–1928," *American Journal of Nursing* 29, no. 10 (Oct. 1929): 1197–207. On deaconess motherhouses of other Protestant congregrations, see Ann Doyle, "Nursing by Religious Orders in the United States. Part V—Deaconesses, 1855–1928," *American Journal of Nursing* 29, no. 11 (Nov. 1929) 1331–43, and Ann Doyle, "Nursing by Religious Orders in the United States. Part VI—Episcopal Sisterhoods, 1845–1928," *American Journal of Nursing* 29, no. 12 (Dec. 1929), 1466–84.

9. Albert G. Miller, "History of the German Hospital," in *History of the German Hospital of Philadelphia and Its Ex-Resident Physicians*, ed. Albert G. Miller (Philadelphia: J.B. Lippincott, 1906), 17–66, 41.

10. Mary J. Drexel Home and Philadelphia Motherhouse of Deaconesses, *The Mary J. Drexel Home and Philadelphia Motherhouse of Deaconesses: Fortieth Anniversary 1884–1924* (Philadelphia: [The Home], 1924), 8.

11. Carl Frese, *Geschichte des Deutschen Hospitals: Zum 25jährigen Jubiläum seiner Eröffnung 1866: Auf Anordnung des Verwaltungsrats zusammengestellt von Carl Frese, M.D., Oberhausarzt* ([Philadelphia], 1891), 3.

12. Roberta West, *History of Nursing in Pennsylvania: Completed and Edited Under the Direction of the Pennsylvania State Nurses' Association* (Harrisburg, Pa.: Evangelical Press, 1939), 441–42.

13. *Vierundzwanzigster Jahresbericht des Deutschen Hospitals der Stadt Philadelphia 1883* (Philadelphia: Druck vom Globe Printing House, 1884), 5; *Fünfundzwanzigster*

Jahresbericht des Deutschen Hospitals der Stadt Philadelphia 1884 (Philadelphia: Druck vom Globe Printing House, 1885), 3, 9.

14. The twenty-fourth Annual Report gives the name of two house physicians, Charles L. Weed and Augustus Stabler. *Vierundzwanzigster Jahresbericht 1883*, 5. The twenty-fifth Annual Report gives three names, E. G. Rehfuß, Charles Collmar, and H. L. Whitney. *Fünfundzwanzigster Jahresbericht 1884*, 3.

15. In 1883, four so-called "Primärassistenten" worked in the four clinics. *Vierundzwanzigster Jahresbericht 1883*, 25.

16. Frese, *Geschichte des Deutschen Hospitals*, 36.

17. Frese, *Geschichte des Deutschen Hospitals*, 35.

18. Charles S. Turnbull, "Reminiscences," in *History of the German Hospital of Philadelphia and Its Ex-Resident Physicians*, ed. Albert G. Miller (Philadelphia: J. B. Lippincott, 1906), 162–66, 164.

19. Frederick Weiser, "Serving Love: Chapters in the Early History of the Diaconate in American Lutheranism" (D.Theol. dissertation, Department of Church History, Lutheran Theological Seminary, Gettysburg, Pa., 1960), 50.

20. [Adolph Spaeth], Zur Geschichte des Diakonissen-Mutterhauses in Philadelphia aus den Erinnerungen eines Philadelphia Pastors (To the History of the Deaconess Motherhouse in Philadelphia from Remembrances of a Philadelphia Pastor), original document 1908, English translation 1982 (hereafter Spaeth, Erinnerungen), 7. Archives of the Evangelical Lutheran Church in America, Elk Grove, Illinois (hereafter ELCA Archives), ULCA 60/1/1, Record Group 60, Mary J. Drexel Home and Philadelphia Motherhouses of Deaconesses, History, Historical Files 1860–1982, Box 1 of 1, Folder 3.

21. Evangelical Lutheran Church in America, Deaconess Community of the ELCA, John Diederich Lankenau, http://www.elca.org/Growing-in-Faith/Vocation/Rostered-Leadership/Deaconess-Community/Our-History/Past-Deaconesses/Lankenau.aspx (accessed May 23, 2008).

22. Spaeth, Erinnerungen, 5–6.

23. Spaeth, Erinnerungen, 8: "Und nun hatte dieser Präsident den Mut auf dem betretenen Wege einen Schritt weiter zu gehen und die Kirche mit dem Hospital in Verbindung zu bringen, obwohl er sich keinen Augenblick darüber täuschte, daß er bei der Mehrzahl seiner Verwaltungsräte auf keine sonderlichen Sympathieen in dieser Richtung rechnen durfte. Er hat mir selbst in späterer Zeit erzählt, wie er zu diesem Schritt ganz besonders von seinem römisch-katholischen Schwager Drexel animirt wurde! Wahrlich, eine seltsame Fügung Gottes, daß von solcher Seite der erste Wink kam, der schließlich zur Gründung unseres Diakonissen-Mutterhauses führen sollte!" Another recollection points in the same direction: "One day, so we were told by his co-worker, the late Mr. Gustave A. Schwarz, when he returned from the hospital almost in despair, one of his brothers-in-law said to him: 'John, nothing will come of your hospital until you get your Church to work with you. Why don't you ask the Lutheran Church to help you?'" *Mary J. Drexel Home Fortieth Anniversary*, 8.

24. Miller, "History of the German Hospital," 41: "For several years President Lankenau, in consequence of a suggestion made to him by his sister, Mrs. H. Lukas, of Bremen, had been considering the introduction of a number of Deaconesses from Germany to take the place of the paid helpers."

25. Miller, "History of the German Hospital," 41, implies this interpretation.

26. Miller, "History of the German Hospital," 63.

27. Weiser, *Serving Love*, 50.
28. Spaeth, Erinnerungen, 5–6.
29. Weiser, *Serving Love*, 50–51.
30. Karl Heinz Voigt, "Carl Wilhelm Theodor Ninck," in *Biographisch-bibliographisches Kirchenlexikon*, ed. Traugott Bautz (BBKL Nordhausen, 2005), 24: col. 1121–32, http://www.bautz.de/bbkl/n/ninck_c_w_t.shtml (last update January 24, 2005, accessed May 23, 2008).
31. Hausordnung und Dienstanweisung für die Diakonissen und Probeschwestern im städtischen Armen- und Krankenhause zu Iserlohn, 3. ELCA Archives, ELCA 127/6/1, Deaconess Community of the ELCA, Personnel, Deceased Personnel Files (hereafter DPF), 1884–2003, Van-Wagner, L. Box 29, Folder: Von Bracht, Magdalene, 1850–1941 (hereafter Personal File von Bracht).
32. John D. Lankenau, letter to Marie Krueger, October 29, 1883, 1. ELCA Archives, PA 213/1 Personal Papers John Diederich Lankenau (1817–1901), Box 1 of 16; folder 24: JDL Business Correspondence, John D. Lankenau to Oberin Marie Krueger—Offering Deaconess work.
33. Lankenau letter to Krueger, October 29, 1883, 2.
34. Some Reminiscences of Sister Magdalene von Bracht, "From Iserlohn to Philadelphia" (title of the English version; there is no title to the handwritten German version), 1–2. ELCA Archives, DPF, Personal File von Bracht.
35. Some Reminiscences of Sister Magdalene von Bracht, 5–7. Spaeth, Erinnerungen, 10–11, remembered that one Sister left after one week.
36. Miller, "History of the German Hospital," 44. Miller gives February 1885 as the date the members of the Deaconess Committee were named. However, it is unlikely that they would have waited months before starting their work.
37. Spaeth, Erinnerungen, 12.
38. Diaconissen Comité (hereafter Deaconess Committee) meeting, July 18, 1885, 1. ELCA Archives, ULCA 60/3/2, Minutes 1885–1922, Protocoll des Philadelphia Diaconissen Mutterhauses, Board of Directors Minutes. M. J. Drexel Home + Phila. Motherhouse of Deaconesses (hereafter PPDM); Spaeth, Erinnerungen, 12.
39. Deaconess Committee meeting, July 18, 1885, ELCA Archives, PPDM, 1.
40. Spaeth, Erinnerungen, 12–13: "Um einen festen zielbewußten Plan und eine innere Geschlossenheit in die ganze Diakonissenbewegung zu bringen, machte ich im Hospital-Verwaltungsrat den Vorschlag, ein stehendes Diakonissen-Kommittee zu ernennen, das die genze Sache leiten und regelmäßig in den Monatsversammlungen des Verwaltungsrats über seine Maasnahmen berichten solte. Am Abend des 18. Juli 1885 trat dieses Kommittee zum ersten Mal zusammen und hielt nun bis zum Januar 1888 im Ganzen 32 Sitzungen, die für die Organisation des Diakonissenwerks in Verbindung mit dem Hospital von grundlegender Bedeutung waren. Folgende Männer gehörten dazu: J. D. Lankenau, Chas. H. Meyer, W. J. Mann, A. Spaeth, F. Wischan, J. C. File, J. H. Tilge, G. A. Schwarz. In den ersten drei Versammlungen führte ich den Vorsitz, da dann auf meinen Antrag Herr Lankenau diese Stelle einnahm, der zugleich auch als freigebiger und zuverlässiger Schatzmeister fungirte. Es war dieses Kommittee, ehrlich gestanden, ein Staat im Staate des Hospital-Verwaltungsrats. Die Hälfte aller Trustees gehörte ihm an, und es waren gerade die Männer, bei denen man am ehesten ein Verständniß und eine Sympathie mit der Diakonissen-Sache erwarten durfte. Alle wichtigen Maasregeln des Hospitals, die sich auf die Diakonissen-Sache bezogen, wurden in diesem Kommittee sorgfältig vorbereitet, das seine Sitzungen immer kurz vor der monatlichen Versammlung

des Hospital-Versammlungsrats hielt, und dann immer in einheitlicher geschlossener Front vor den Board trat und dort seine Wünsche und Pläne vertrat und durchsetzte. Es waren Kampfeszeiten. Aber es war eine gute heilige Sache, für die wir stritten und wir haben immer mit ehrlichem, offenen Visier gekämpft. Wer heutzutage die geachtete und geschätzte Stellung unsrer Diakonissen im Hospital ansieht, kann es kaum begreifen wie wir dazumal uns wehren mußten auf Schritt und Tritt, und allerlei Widerspruchsgeistern den Segen des Diakonissendienstes gleichsam aufzudrängen genötigt waren."

41. Deaconess Committee meeting, August 29, September 26, 1885, ELCA Archives, PPDM, 4, 6.

42. Deaconess Committee meeting, July 18, 1885, ELCA Archives, PPDM, 1.

43. On November 21, 1885, the Deaconess Committee authorized Lankenau to appoint the "Incorporatoren" of the future Mary J. Drexel Home and Philadelphia Motherhouse of Deaconesses. Deaconess Committee meeting, November 21, 1885, ELCA Archives, PPDM, 10, 12.

44. Deaconess Committee meeting, October 31, 1885, ELCA Archives, PPDM, 9.

45. Board of Trustees of the German Hospital of Philadelphia, letter to the Members of the Medical Board. ELCA Archives, PPDM, 17. No date is given, but according to the Deaconess Committee meeting of February 20, 1886, ELCA Archives, PPDM, 24, the letter was dated December 14, 1885.

46. Spaeth, Erinnerungen, 13–14: "Die älteren Herren sahen die ganze Arbeit unsres Diakonissen-Kommittee's mehr oder weniger als einen Eingriff in ihre eigene Domäne an und ließen sich nichts sagen. So blieb schließlich nichts übrig, als den Aerzten das Ultimatum zu stellen und ihre Wiederwahl in das medizinische Kollegium davon abhängig zu machen, ob sie die neue Ordnung der Dinge annehmen oder ablehnen wollten."

47. Spaeth, Erinnerungen, 14: "Wir konnten es in dieser Sache wohl auf eine Krisis ankommen lassen, denn wir waren dessen versichert, daß, wenn auch unser ganzes medizinisches Kollegium uns gekündigt hätte, wir sofort einige der ersten Aerzte der Stadt bereit gefunden hätten, an ihre Stelle zu treten und in gutem Einvernehmen mit unsern Schwestern zusammen zu arbeiten." See also Deaconess Committee meeting, December 19, 1885, ELCA Archives, PPDM, 14–15.

48. Spaeth, Erinnerungen, 14: "So wurde denn allmählig unser medizinisches Kollegium von allen den Elementen gesäubert, die sich feindlich und unverbesserlich unsern Diakonissen entgegenstellten."

49. Deaconess Committee meeting, January 23, 1886, ELCA Archives, PPDM, 19.

50. Deaconess Committee meeting, February 20, 1886, ELCA Archives, PPDM, 22.

51. Deaconess Committee meeting, February 20, 1886, 23.

52. Albert G. Miller, "1870–1873 Marcus Franklin," in *History of the German Hospital of Philadelphia*, ed. Miller, 94–95; Frese, *Geschichte des Deutschen Hospitals*, 35. Miller gives the year as 1885.

53. Deaconess Committee meeting, December 19, 1885, ELCA Archives, PPDM, 14.

54. Albert G. Miller, "1885–1889 George A. Bodamer," in *History of the German Hospital of Philadelphia*, ed. Miller, 112–13, 112 summarily speaks of the "authorities of the German Hospital," which must have been the Board of Trustees as the decision-making body.

55. Miller, "History of the German Hospital," 47.

56. Spaeth, Erinnerungen, 14: "Ein wichtiger Schritt in unsrer medizinischen Reformbewegung war auch die Anstellung eines bezahlten Oberarztes im Hospital, dem die

freiwilligen Hausärzte, die frisch von der Universität kamen, unterstellt sein sollten. Nach heißen Kämpfen gelang es uns, Dr. Geo. Bodamer, ein Kind der St. Johannis-Gemeinde, an diese Stelle zu bringen, und damit eine gesunde und zuverlässige Vermittlung zwischen den jungen, unerfahrenen Hausärzten und den Schwestern zu schaffen. Und es war Dr. Bodamer, der uns zuerst mit allem Nachdruck auf Dr. Deaver aufmerksam machte, der dann später die chirurgischen Leistungen des Hospitals auf eine zuvor unerhörte Höhe bringen sollte."

57. Miller, "1885–1889 George A. Bodamer," 113.

58. Deaconess Committee meeting, February 20, 1886, ELCA Archives, PPDM, 22–23.

59. *By-Laws of the German Hospital of the City of Philadelphia: Incorporated April 2, A.D. 1860* (Philadelphia: Globe Printing House, 1887), 41, Art. XIX.

60. Charles Meyer uses the term "Herzlähmung." Charles H. Meyer, letter to Julius Disselhoff, December 8, 1887, 1. Archives of the Fliedner Foundation Düsseldorf-Kaiserswerth (hereafter FlA), AKD 329, Philadelphia, Diakonissen-Mutterhaus 1880–1894 (hereafter AKD 329 PDM).

61. Deaconess Committee, extraordinary meeting, December 3, 1887, ELCA Archives, PPDM, 74.

62. Two lines and parts of two others are erased on page 74 of the minutes of the extraordinary Deaconess Committee meeting on December 3, 1887. The text of pastor Disselhoff's letter to Charles H. Meyer, dated Kaiserswerth December 20, 1887, which was copied to the minutes, was not erased. Disselhoff stated that the truth had propelled his correspondent to hint that opium had been the cause of her burns: "Die Nachricht von dem plötzlichen Tode der früheren Diakonissin Marie Krüger, welche Sie, verehrter Herr Consul, mir in Ihrem Schreiben vom 8 ds mittheilen, hat mich um so tiefer ergriffen, als die Wahrheit Ihnen gebot die Verwirrung der Verstorbenen in Betreff des leidenschaftlichen Opium Genußes anzudeuten." ELCA Archives, PPDM, 77. A draft copy of this letter is also preserved in the personal files of Marie Krueger at the Fliedner Archives in Kaiserswerth.

63. Heinz Rodegra, "Zur Geschichte des Deutschen Hospitals in Philadelphia (USA)," *Historia Hospitalium* 14 (1981–1982): 179–90, 187.

64. The first Iserlohn address book, published in 1866, mentions Marie Krueger as "Diakonissin (Oberin) im Armen- und Krankenhaus." Tanja Marschall, Iserlohn Town Archives, email to the author, October 9, 2007. The date July 1867 is mentioned in FlA, Pflegerinnenbuch 1836–76, fortlaufende Nr. 185, Diakonissen-Verzeichnis 1836–76, fortlaufende Nr. 62. Disselhoff's letter to Meyer of December 20, 1887, gives the year 1867. ELCA Archives, PPDM, 78.

65. On Disselhoff, see Friedrich Wilhelm Bautz, "Julius Disselhoff," in *Biographisch-bibliographisches Kirchenlexikon*, ed. Traugott Bautz (BBKL Hamm 1990), 1: cols. 1331–32, http://www.bautz.de/bbkl/d/disselhoff_j.shtml (last update February 17, 2005, accessed May 23, 2008).

66. Charles H. Meyer, letter to Julius Disselhoff, December 8, 1887. FlA, AKD 329 PDM.

67. Disselhoff, letter to Meyer, December 20, 1887: "Wir wissen aus früherer Zeit, daß die Verstorbene eine reich begabte Natur war. Diese Begabung war ihre Verführung. Sie hat wie Sie vielleicht durch Herrn Professor Dr Spaeth wissen, offenbarem Ungehorsam und in selbstsüchtiger Eigenwilligkeit seiner Zeit von unserm Diakonissen-Mutterhause mit Absicht und Bewußtsein sich losgesagt." ELCA Archives, PPDM, 77.

68. Disselhoff, letter to Meyer, December 20, 1887, 77–78: "Ehe sie nach Philadelphia abreiste hat sie ihren Irrthum brieflich bekannt und um Verzeihung gebeten. Ich habe sie nicht bloß schwarz auf weiß, sondern von Herzens-Grund meiner Verzeihung versichert, und in diesem Sinne seitdem an sie gedacht, und gedenke auch jetzt ihrer in diesem Geiste, wenn auch eine amtliche Verbindung mit ihr sachlich nicht möglich war."

69. Disselhoff, letter to Meyer, December 20, 1887, 79: "Von ganzem Herzen wünsche ich Ihnen, verehrter Herr Consul, daß Sie zur Vorsteherin Ihres jungen Diakonissenhauses eine christliche Jungfrau oder Witwe finden, welche nicht nur die nötige Begabung, sondern vor allen Dingen ungeschminkte Demut und durchsichtige Lauterkeit besitzt. Eine Diakonissin, welche ein Diakonissen Mutterhaus leiten soll, muß vor allen Dingen von der Sohle bis zum Scheitel Diakonissin sein, sonst kann sie keine Diakonissen erziehen."

70. Spaeth, Erinnerungen, 22: "Unsre Oberin war eine frühere Kaiserswerter Schwester gewesen und hatte sich von ihrem Mutterhause getrennt. Die Folge davon war eine ziemlich kühle Haltung gegen die Schwesternschaft, die sich unter ihrer Leitung in Iserlohn gesammelt hatte und dann zu uns nach Philadelphia übergesiedelt war. Freilich ließ mich das der selige Disselhoff, Fliedners Nachfolger in Kaiserswert, nicht persönlich entgelten. Ich war über Pfingsten in seinem Diakonissenhaus. Am Sonntag Abend, nachdem wir zusammen gemütlich zu Tisch gewesen, gingen wir hinaus in den Garten, auf den Wall, und wandelten dort wohl zwei Stunden im ernsten Gespräch, wobei ich für Philadelphia plädirte und die weitgreifende Bedeutung des in Philadephia begonnenen Werkes für ganz Amerika darzutun suchte. Es gelang mir auch am Ende, von Disselhoff das Versprechen zu bekommen, daß die vorgekommene Unregelmäßigkeit einer einzelnen Schwester kein Hinderniß werden dürfe, wenn es sich um förmliche Anerkennung und um freundliches Zusammenarbeiten zwischen Kaiserswert und Philadelphia handeln sollte. Es hat auch nicht lange gedauert, so hat unser Mutterhaus Aufnahme in die General-Konferenz der Diakonissenhäuser gefunden, die sich alle drei Jahre in der Wiege des deutschen Diakonissenwerkes, in Kaiserswert versammelt."

71. Weiser, *Serving Love*, 55.

72. Minutes, Deaconess Committee, extraordinary meeting, December 3, 1887. ELCA Archives, PPDM, 74.

73. Frese, *Geschichte des Deutschen Hospitals*, 10.

74. The arrival of the deaconesses in 1884, not the foundation of the motherhouse two years later, was taken as the date for calculating the anniversaries. Mary J. Drexel Home and Philadelphia Motherhouse of Deaconesses, *Mary J. Drexel Home and Philadelphia Motherhouse of Deaconesses: Fiftieth Anniversary 1884–1934* (Philadelphia: [The Home], [1934]).

75. *Mary J. Drexel Home Fiftieth Anniversary*, 26.

76. Theodore E. Bachmann, *The Story of the Philadelphia Deaconess Motherhouse, 1884–1959* (Gladwyne, Pa., 1960), 11.

77. Charles H. Meyer, letter to Julius Disselhoff, December 8, 1887. FlA, AKD 329 PMD.

78. Lebenslauf von Wanda von Oertzen aus dem Hause Roggow, March 19, 1888. ELCA Archives, DPF, PMD, Van-Wagner, L., Box 29, Folder: Wanda von Oertzen. Biographical information, death notices, funeral sermon, program. Correspondence re: Sister von Oertzen, n.d., 1888, 1897, 1954.

79. Lebenslauf von Wanda von Oertzen, I.

80. Lebenslauf von Wanda von Oertzen, II.
81. Lebenslauf von Wanda von Oertzen, III.
82. See Spaeth, Erinnerungen, 29.
83. Spaeth, Erinnerungen, 29: "Da wir nun kein Zeugniß darüber hatten, daß Wanda von Oertzen eine wirkliche regelmäßige Ausbildung in einem anerkannten Diakonissen-Hause Deutschlands erhalten hatte, und da sie erst im Februar sich bereit erklärte, in die Diakonissenanstalt von Pastor Ninck in Hamburg einzutreten, um sich als Diakonissin ausbilden zu lassen, so hatte ich meine großen Bedenken über ihre Berufung. Erst als ich ein Schreiben von Konsistorialrat Krummacher in Stettin erhielt, der sich sehr günstig über ihren Charakter und ihre Leistungsfähigkeit aussprach, zog ich meine Einsprache gegen ihre Berufung zurück. Ich darf das jetzt hier ganz offen mitteilen, denn ich habe Wanda von Oertzen gegenüber nie ein Hehl davon gemacht, daß ich solche Bedenken gehabt hätte. Und in der ihr eigenen Offenheit hat sie auch mehr als einmal später zu mir gesagt: Mir fehlt eben die Diakonissenschulung! Was sie hatte, und was sie in der Geschichte unsres Hauses zu einer für jene Zeit höchst bedeutenden, vielleicht unentbehrlichen Kraft machte, das war ihre vortreffliche Schulung als Krankenpflegerin, die sie unter Esmarch genossen, und die sie befähigte, im Hospital eine Stellung einzunehmen, die auch unsern Aerzten imponirte."
84. *Mary J. Drexel Home: Fortieth Anniversary*, 13.
85. Spaeth, Erinnerungen, 30.
86. A. Cordes, letter probably to Julius Disselhoff, May 8, 1891. FlA, AKD 329 PMD.
87. Versammlung des Verwaltungsraths des Mary J. Drexel Home etc., June 23, 1892. ELCA Archives, PPDM, 179–80.
88. Charles H. Meyer, letter to Julius Disselhoff, 18 September 1892: "sie sind mit den Fehlern bekannt welche unsrer Oberin vorgeworfen werden die aber durch ihre eminenten Eigenschaften derart aufgehoben werden daß wir sie nicht konnten gehen lassen um unsern sonst so geschätzten Pastor Cordes zu behalten. Ich bin überzeugt daß ein gereifter Mann der ihr durch nichts als Würde und Festigkeit Respect einzuflössen versteht, sehr gut neben und mit ihr in Harmonie arbeiten kann namentlich bei correcter Vertheilung der Arbeitsfelder." FlA, AKD 329 PMD.
89. Lehfeldt, *Fifty Years Pioneer Work*, 33.
90. *Mary J. Drexel Home: Fortieth Anniversary*, 16.
91. On this point, I am grateful for the views given by Bonnie Dorwart, Marilyn Stauffer, and Lisa Zerull during email correspondence, April 2008.
92. Lisa Zerull, email to the author, April 7, 2008.
93. Bonnie Dorwart, email to the author, April 8, 2008.
94. Last Will and Testament of John D. Lankenau of the City of Philadelphia, 6–9.
95. Minutes, Deaconess Committee meeting, July 18, 1885, ELCA Archives, PPDM, 2: "Es wird hervor gehoben, daß unser Diaconissen Comité die Basis für die Entwickelung des Diaconissenwerkes in Amerika bilden muß."
96. Weiser, *Serving Love*, 62.
97. Weiser, *Serving Love*, 73, gives the date 1908, but the funeral sermon gives 1909. See Funeral Sermon "He Leadeth Me!" 3 ELCA Archives, DPF, Personal File Magdalene von Bracht. West, *History of Nursing in Pennsylvania*, 446. The early twentieth century brought marked changes. Student nurses in increasing numbers from the new

training school at the German Hospital took over a large part of the care for the patients. This process merits its own study. See Barbara Bates Center for the Study of the History of Nursing, School of Nursing, University of Pennsylvania Lankenau Hospital School of Nursing Records, MC 88, Lankenau Hospital Training School.

98. Nelson, *Say Little, Do Much*, 139.

99. In the 1917 minutes of the Board of Trustees of the German Hospital, a draft resolution gives as one motive to change the name from German Hospital to Lankenau Hospital that—in spite of the loyalty of all the staff—the name could be a hindrance to the hospital in fulfilling its duties. Minutes of the Board of Trustees 1916–1917, Meeting June 18, 1917, Lankenau Hospital Archive Center, German/Lankenau Hospital, Minutes of the Board of Trustees.

100. Lankenau Institute for Medical Research, History: A Tradition of Research, http://www.limr.org/PDF/NEWSQUICKLINKS/LIMRHistory.pdf (accessed May 23, 2008). See also Lankenau Hospital homepage, http://www.mainlinehealth.org/lh/ (accessed May 23, 2008).

"The Relation of the Nurse to the Working World": Professionalization, Citizenship, and Class in Germany, Great Britain, and the United States before World War I

Aeleah Soine
University of Minnesota

Abstract. Campaigns for state nursing registration in the United States and Great Britain have a prominent place in the historical scholarship on nursing professionalization; the closely related German campaign has received less scholarly attention. Applying a transnational perspective to these three national movements highlights the collaborative and interrelated nature of nursing reform prior to World War I and recognizes the important contribution of German nurses to this dialogue and agenda. Focusing particularly on the years 1909–12, this article depicts a generation of German, American, and British nurses who organized national and international nursing associations to realize state registration as a stepping stone to other markers of professional recognition, such as collegiate education, full political citizenship, social welfare, and labor legislation. However, the consequent reliance of these strategies on nation-states as arbiters of citizenship and professional status undermined the shared ideological foundation of international and national nursing leaders. This article contributes to a more multinational understanding of how these international nursing leaders transcended and were confined by the limits of their nation-states in the years leading up to World War I.

On June 26, 1913, Lavinia Dock gave her final address to the American Nurses' Association. Her paper, "The Status of the Nurse in the Working World," challenged the middle-class nature of professional identity that had set nurses of respectable means apart from—and in fact above—the working class.[1] Dock called on nurses to jettison this nineteenth-century legacy and instead to recognize the tripartite demands of the worker—"education, hours of work, wages"—as issues of shared relevance between professional nurses and the world of workers. She supported her radical assessment of protective labor legislation with the claim of manipulation inherent in "the sentiment too often skillfully suggested by hospital directors personally interested, that a 'profession' must not become tainted with 'trade unionism' . . . [which would] destroy professional ethics. All solemn pharisaism! And hospital directors know it is."[2]

The suggestion that nurses were being exploited by hospital administrators makes palatable the formerly inconceivable idea that nurses would embrace working-class alliances over professional solidarity with physicians and administrators. Though remaining devoted to education and female enfranchisement as the primary vehicles toward professionalization, Dock was also integrating tenets of protective labor legislation into the foundations of nursing professionalization. The significance of this message was not its foresight or effectiveness but rather its unique ability to convey the essential combination of professional aspirations and complications of gender, class, and nation-state formation that characterized the transnational nursing professionalization movement in the early twentieth century, as it prepared to embark on a new path.

In the decade before World War I, the International Council of Nurses (ICN) and the transnational professionalization movement it represented reached the height of their collaborative success in pursuit of state registration for nursing. Registration was a logical strategy for nurses to follow based on the precedents of physicians, lawyers, and professors in Europe and the contemporary professionalization efforts of the female-dominated occupations such as social work, elementary education, and midwifery.[3] In the quarter-century prior to World War I, nursing registers were developed in twenty-two of the twenty-six German states,[4] thirty-two of the forty-eight American states, and various other nation-states belonging to the ICN.[5] Great Britain, however, still had no such system of nursing registration at this time.[6] This uneven attainment of nursing registration between 1909 and 1912 challenged the ideological unity among nursing leaders in Great Britain, the United States, and Germany.[7] Because nursing leaders saw professionalization as an ongoing campaign for national associations, training schools, nursing registration, and postsecondary education, the potential for transnational collaboration diminished as their common goals and measures of success became increasingly reliant on the particular laws and customs of individual nation-states.

The national nursing traditions of Germany, Great Britain, and the United States had acknowledged common roots in the Protestant deaconess motherhouses founded in the 1830s. All three also continued to have direct connections with the Nightingale reforms of the 1860s and 1870s, and they were among the charter members of the ICN.[8] Because of the ongoing tradition of interaction among these national nursing organizations and their shared ICN leadership in the early twentieth century, this article conceives of their professionalization efforts as a form of transnational project that cannot be fully captured by a merely comparative model of analysis.[9] Rather, it demonstrates how the agenda of the transnational movement for nursing professionalization was increasingly shaped by changing ideas about national identity, citizenship, and class within women's associations and professions.

By 1912, designing and implementing postsecondary educational programs was at the forefront of the agenda to professionalize nursing. However, state registration had by then changed the relationship between female nurses and the state in unintended ways and fueled growing tension in their collaborations. Because many of the most outspoken nursing leaders recognized that professionalization required state cooperation, and that raising the bar of professional requirements would become continually more difficult unless women gained the right to vote or a compelling influence in legislative bodies, they pursued an elite agenda that sought national unity and political citizenship as modern forms of leverage in the interest of nursing reform.[10]

Meanwhile, nursing reformers were increasingly distracted from the forefront of professionalization by a growing recognition that overwork, illness, and social insecurity were threatening working nurses and any cross-class sense of sisterhood or common professional identity among nurses. The lack of cross-class unity was a particularly dangerous threat as unaffiliated local and national nursing organizations sought protective labor legislation and broader nursing recruitment, which undermined the leadership of the transnational movement.

On both fronts, the implementation of a registered nursing system required too much adaptation to the increasingly divergent political and social considerations within nation-states; they simply could not continue to sustain a common transnational model of nursing based upon a shared sense of professional identity and goals. Instead, they began to proceed on the courses most adapted to their national context at the time.

Nursing and the Emergence of Twentieth-Century Nation-States

At the turn of the twentieth century, both well-established and newly founded nation-states grappled with the changing face of modern citizenship.

Economically, industrialization and urbanization had created labor unrest and growing working-class consciousness, which led eventually to greater government regulation of labor practices and social welfare provisions. Politically, these economic conflicts and solutions created the foundation for a new type of politics that moved away from the nineteenth-century doctrine of liberalism, or unfettered free market capitalism, and toward a belief in the state's power and obligation to protect the safety and welfare of its workers and consumers.

The extent and nature of the intervention varied greatly among Great Britain, Germany, and the United States; historians have noted that there was no automatic or easy connection between economic development and democratization.[11] Industrialization began earliest in Great Britain, yet the British state still resisted universal suffrage for men of lesser means and women entirely in the early twentieth century. Labor organizations, militant suffragettes, and colonial uprisings throughout the vast British Empire weakened the once confident national identity of the British people and their state. The liberalism that had been touted by the British industrial elites throughout the nineteenth century gave way to a series of concessions that introduced successive expansions of enfranchisement, protective labor legislation, and the beginning of a state welfare system.[12] Yet, even in an era of greater state regulation, the registration of nurses remained difficult to procure for a group that lacked the professional consensus, consistent message, and powerful lobby of the opposing hospital administrators and physicians.[13] For example, Dr. Sydney Holland, the "time-worn enemy of registration" according to Lavinia Dock, was the primary oppositional witness in the parliamentary hearings on state registration and carried with him a petition signed by many of the prominent physicians and their nurses in London.[14]

German industrialization came almost a century later, but the German government was much quicker to implement labor legislation, offer social welfare provisions, and extend universal male suffrage, although the motivation and extent of these gestures can be debated. In Germany, national unification occurred formally in 1871 with the end of the Franco-Prussian War, and a major industrial boom followed shortly thereafter. Having defeated Austria, Denmark, and France, Prussia was able to expand its borders, incorporating some swaths of land against the preference of their inhabitants, but in the end securing for itself a large German nation-state and empire ruled from Berlin. Yet the awkward combination of power concentrated in the hands of the emperor and the concession of many important powers to the individual German states (*Länder*) continued to undermine national unity and orderly administration.[15] For nurses, this unpredictable political milieu not only disenfranchised women and excluded them from political associations and universities for most of the imperial era (1871–1918) but also made the practical implementation of state registration after three years of training and collegiate education particularly difficult. Unlike the situation in Great Britain, the passage of a Prussian state registration bill in 1906 was in large part due to the early and independent support of German doctors. However, the same physicians blocked later attempts to increase the required training period from one to three years, which demonstrated the level of political influence held by medical practitioners and administrators versus nurses.[16] As an adaptation, nursing reform fell under the umbrella of issues taken up by the professionally and maternally oriented women's movement, which often chose socially acceptable discourses of maternalism and charity that drew on feminized ideologies of social motherhood and domesticity to disguise conflicts with the state over women's increasing visibility in the public sphere.[17]

As in Great Britain, the United States federal government was hesitant to depart from its liberal devotion to the free market and resisted the development of a welfare state. However, American feminists had begun to offer maternalist arguments for the improvement of nursing and for state involvement in the registration of nurses as a result of their trans-Atlantic correspondence and collaboration.[18] The key differences in American and European women's appeals to their natural maternal capacities was that American women more urgently saw such strategies as making demands that would lead to women's suffrage, full citizenship, and control over a system of state welfare and social reform.[19] Sandra Lewenson has effectively demonstrated how female social reformers of the Progressive Era (1890–1913) in the United States saw suffrage, social reform, and control of their personal and professional lives as intimately connected.[20] Though a small group of German social reformers joined their American counterparts in a movement of social justice feminists, widespread political campaigns were not characteristic of German nursing reformers or continental European social reformers more generally.[21]

However, the reconciliation of welfare and liberalism at this time in Europe created alternative opportunities for German maternalists to shape the roles available to women in the new industrial economy while not necessarily advocating for women's suffrage. For example, the associations under the umbrella of the League of German Women's Associations often tackled issues of women's sexuality, social welfare programs, and professional opportunities for women to an extent not seriously considered or implemented in the United States until the New Deal of the early 1930s, after the attainment of suffrage.[22]

With regard to nursing professionalization, the federalist structure of the United States government presented many of the same obstacles to nursing reform as in Germany. Here, too, state registration was under the purview of individual state rather than federal jurisdiction, meaning that nursing reformers had to pass their registration and regulation bills through not just one legislative process, but 48 separate legislatures. However, the decentralized nature of the American and German states may have been advantageous to nursing reformers, because a few successful examples could provide compelling evidence in the campaigns of other states. The passage of state registration in the largest and most powerful German state of Prussia was followed by all but a few purposely resistant states within two years. Meanwhile, in Great Britain, the all-or-nothing system of centralized state governance and administration placed the burden on the Parliament alone to implement a national register.

Professionalization Through Registration

The ICN was an organizational body representing a transnational movement dedicated to the professionalization of nursing. It grew out of conversations first at the World's Fair Exhibition in Chicago (1893) and then at the International Council of Women's (ICW) designated section on the "Professions" in London (1899), which served to establish a common understanding of female professionalization that was not limited to one discipline. Rather, the process of creating women's professions was based on the shared goals of contributing to the individualization and socialization of women in an industrialized society through artistic and scientific endeavors. In keeping with the middle-class character of professionalization more broadly, middle-class women and members of the ICW counted themselves among the professionals seeking individualization and their working-class counterparts as being the recipients of their professional expertise and socialization efforts.[23] The ICN not only adopted this understanding from the ICW but also added markers of professionalization that were distinct to nursing, such as goals for training programs and registration laws.[24] The ICN's successes over its first decade brought a sense of great accomplishment and pride as nurses began to see the fruits of their faith in a democratic, feminist, and transnational nursing tradition of their own making.

In 1909, the ICN Congress returned to its institutional origins in London in what was planned to be a grand celebration of the triumphant success of nursing professionalization throughout its member countries, but especially in the nation of the ICN's founding and leadership—Great Britain. The meeting was dominated by the recognition of a generation of elite women who led the way for nursing to become a respectable female profession. When Agnes Karll, president of the German Nurses' Association (Berufsorganisation der

Krankenpflegerinnen Deutschlands),[25] assumed the ICN presidency for the next three-year period, she accepted her new position by sending a dedication and greeting to Florence Nightingale in honor of her pioneering nursing work and early connection to German nursing. Later in the day, Isabel Hampton Robb of the United States urged a resolution in favor of state registration and proclaimed the growing sentiment that "the last word on State Registration had been spoken"[26]—a reference to the recent wave of successful nursing registration bills in ICN member nations and in various U.S. and German states.

However, the 1909 London International Congress of Nurses also marked a point of transition for the ICN and the transnational nursing professionalization movement it represented. The ICN shifted its organizational center from Great Britain to Germany in terms of both leadership and location. The contrast between the jubilant backdrop of the 1909 London Congress and the more subdued 1912 Congress in Cologne is in many ways striking. Ethel Fenwick, the organization's founder and first president (1904–7), fell short of realizing her triumphant vision of British state registration and regulated training requirements even after the London Congress. The eventual disappearance of celebrated British and American personalities symbolically brought to a close the era of reform dedicated to improving hospital training schools and implementing state registration and began a new era focused on professional unity, political engagement, and postsecondary education. In fact, several prominent nursing leaders from the British Empire and United States most closely identified in continental Europe with nursing reform had died between the two meetings, most notably Isabel Hampton Robb; Isla Stewart, a founding member of the ICN from Great Britain; Clara Barton, well-known volunteer nurse in the Franco-Prussian War and founder of the American Red Cross; and Florence Nightingale, who continued to be honored by the organization in spite of their disagreements over state registration and women's suffrage.[27]

Furthermore, state registration in all member states no longer seemed imminent, as Great Britain, the center of registered nursing campaigns for over two decades, still had no state-sponsored registration system. The significance of this setback was not lost on Ethel Fenwick. In the first 1912 issue of the *British Journal of Nursing* (*BJN*) her front page editorial outlines the agenda for the new year, including her plea that a state registration bill be passed before the international congress in Cologne so that British nurses could meet their international colleagues "with the right to use a legal title, instead of still being forced to own that, though the registration of trained nurses was first proposed in this country, others have outstripped us in attainment."[28]

Deaths and defeat for British nurses were clearly not what Agnes Karll had hoped for during her presidency, but elevating German nursing to the international prominence of British and American nursing was definitely among her goals. In February 1912, she wrote to American leader Lavinia Dock, "I always meant this Congress *to be the turning point for German* nursing. As I can tell Germany about the College for Nurses on 1st of March in Berlin and afterwards in Cologne the year 1912 may mean a great deal for our profession in Germany."[29] Her other writings reaffirm again and again her hope that the 1912 Congress would facilitate a "turning point" for German nurses seeking to join Great Britain and the United States as recognized partners in the international nursing professionalization movement.

The Cologne Congress was also a turning point for the ICN nurses more broadly. Divisions between members now able to speak on the effects of state registration and those who had no such success to speak of sparked an escalated sense of competition among national members. Nurses wishing to showcase their progress in creating postsecondary programs in nursing clashed with those wishing to stay focused on improving training and examination. As the fruits of the first major victory became apparent, the sense of unity and common purpose started to decay.

By 1912, the expectations of nursing leaders no longer focused predominantly on state registration and three-year training schools. Rather, the Cologne Congress marked the consolidation of a new path in nursing professionalization that built on the goals of the past but placed much greater emphasis on building a shared professional identity, female political participation, and collegiate education. German nurses in particular intended to demonstrate to the international community that they were prepared to strengthen the regulatory policies of the German state, that they were supporters of women's suffrage and collaborators with their national and the international women's movement, and that they had made a realistic commitment to implementing education beyond a three-year nurse training course.

Professionalization Through Education

In early twentieth-century nursing, the pillars of professionalization were organization, state recognition, and education. Though state registration continued to take priority in the association's first decade, the ICN leadership always saw it as a stepping stone toward the higher ideal of collegiate education. In the organizational phase of the ICN, founder and British nursing leader Ethel Fenwick described the vision for their association:

> I claim that the time has come when nurses need their educational centre, their endowed colleges, their chairs of nursing, their university degrees, and State Registration, and the present seems the psychological moment to come to the public, not as strangers, but as professional workers known and trusted through the length and breadth of the land, and to urge that, as nurses pour out on its behalf a skill and devotion for which gold is no real recompense, the public shall now prove its appreciation and interest in the noble work of nursing by giving something of its wealth to place nursing education and the status of trained nurse on a strong financial basis.[30]

With the symbolic attainment of state registration and the growing acceptance of women in colleges and universities, nursing leaders demanded a significant shift in the orientation of the nursing platform to a growing list of educational reforms.

The first foray of nurses into postsecondary education came in 1899 with a course in Hospital Economics offered at Teachers College, Columbia University. The course was not specifically in nursing, but instructed nursing superintendents in how to teach nursing subjects in a training school.[31] Over the next decade, this program was incrementally expanded as Adelaide Nutting gradually paved the path of nursing into the academy with her increased commitment from part-time instructor to the first professor of nursing in 1907 and head of the new Department of Nursing and Health in 1910. Nutting's major priorities included revising the three-year curriculum in nursing, separating nursing schools from hospitals, and gaining the recognition of universities for nursing education.[32]

Meanwhile, Nutting and other American nursing leaders were consulted by a group of physicians in Minnesota seeking to reform medical education along similar lines and who, at the urging of Dr. Richard Olding Beard, added a school of nursing to their plans for a university-based medical school at the University of Minnesota. The first university-based school of nursing opened in 1909 under Superintendent Bertha Erdmann. The Minnesota school was tied closely to the nursing leadership at Teachers College. On her appointment as superintendent, Erdmann was sent immediately to Teachers College for graduate education until the school opened.[33] Her successor Louise Powell also highlighted the connection between the University of Minnesota and Teachers College, as she was chosen for the position based on the recommendation of Nutting, who had been her mentor.[34]

As president of the ICN from 1909 to 1912, Agnes Karll paid close attention to educational trends in the United States. The International Education Committee of the ICN received a prime time slot in the Cologne conference program. Being paired with Karll's own report on the effects of state registration gave the distinct impression that the president was symbolically celebrating the success of one phase in nursing professionalization while she introduced the embarking of the ICN on the next. Her own plan to expand postsecondary nursing education in Germany, despite cultural barriers to the entrance of women and nursing into the universities, was modeled closely on Teachers College and was finally realized in the opening of a postsecondary program in nursing at the Women's College of Leipzig in 1912. For Karll, this program was the "crowning achievement"[35] of German nursing professionalization, as she described it:

> The purpose of training is to give state registered nurses with at least five years of practical experience (of which at least three years were spent in a hospital) the opportunity both to deepen and to expand their specialized and general knowledge, in order that they are able to satisfy the demands that are put before matrons and ward supervisors . . . the theoretical training is provided at the College for Women in Leipzig.[36]

Though German women were banned from universities until 1908, the possibility of creating a collegiate program of nursing was not unrealistic. Because of the stratified system of German education, secondary and postsecondary trade or professional training programs existed alongside universities and carved out a respectable niche for nursing at these alternative educational institutions. Of course, this would later have negative ramifications, as nursing developed its preparatory tradition outside the university system, where it largely remains today.[37] As university degrees became signature symbols of social capital and professional credibility, this exclusion of nurses from the German university prevented some of the upward social and professional mobilization of nurses that took place subsequently in the United States and Great Britain. From the perspective of 1912, however, German nurses saw the founding of a theoretical and practical training program in the context of a postsecondary education program as a major step forward that kept them competitive with their allies, even if they were not at the forefront. The discussions surrounding the College for Women in Leipzig demonstrated that the university programs in the United States had opened the door to a new era in nursing professionalization, in which collegiate education would begin to edge state registration out of the limelight. For German nurses, this was a short-lived tenure at the helm of the transnational nursing reform movements before their progress was eclipsed by World War I.

Political circumstances inhibited nursing programs from developing in universities, yet the space made available in the College for Women served as a platform for integrating preparation and theoretical instruction similar to those in the programs of other countries. Karll describes the nursing curriculum at Leipzig as "mandating comprehensive social and legal, pedagogical, scientific, historical, literary historical and philosophical lectures and practicum."[38] More specifically, this curriculum prepared nurse superintendents with three levels of biology, hygiene, chemistry, and physics, plus various history, psychology, discipline-related sciences, and practical courses in discipline-related social welfare and law. Furthermore, at the time, this program would have been considered an advanced course aimed at nurses already equipped with the experience equivalent to a three-year practical training program. At the end of the four semesters, a diploma would be issued to students successfully completing all coursework, complying with character expectations, and passing the final examination.[39]

In all three national cases, the combined power of state registration and higher education was twofold: it both bestowed a guarantee of social respectability and professional qualification and acted as a gatekeeper for which such recognition would be granted. Though the first aspect was the capstone of an earlier generation's program of reform, the new generation was even more fixated on raising the level of exclusivity, experience, and expertise required to become part of such a recognized group. The transnational professionalization movement in nursing seemed close to attaining such state and educational guarantees of professional status, but the practical considerations of instilling a unity of purpose and a shared identity among nurses of varying backgrounds and experiences proved more difficult. As nurses found out, a strategy that called on the nation-state to be the arbiter of respectability and capability also called on groups of nurses within each nation-state to forge a common vision of nurses as female professionals and citizens.

Professionalization Through Citizenship

The emphasis on state registration that dominated nursing reform from the late 1880s to the 1910s grew out of conversations among both physicians and nursing matrons in Great Britain. Nursing reform was an issue receiving serious contemplation by physicians, politicians, and nurses in the 1880s, but opinions differed over whether regulation of nursing should remain under the purview of hospitals or be taken over by an independent external body such as the state or an autonomous nursing association.[40] In the early years of the British Nurses' Association, Dr. and Mrs. Bedford Fenwick poured a great deal of their efforts into bringing supportive physicians into the association. In a speech in 1887, Ethel Fenwick stated, "A great crisis has come for the Nursing Profession, and no steps can be taken to meet it without the assistance and advice of leading medical men." She ended her speech with a reference to the bylaws of the British Nurses' Association that discussed the potential number of physicians in the governing bodies of the association, so that "the *medical profession may always have a controlling voice in the management* of the Association."[41]

For anyone familiar with Ethel Fenwick's speeches and actions later in her life, this support for physician intervention is truly out of character, but the executive committee consisted of both physicians and matrons, with physicians filling the ranks of vice presidents and being guaranteed various means of influence over the association, including membership for all interested "medical men," physician and surgeon approval over the terms of registration, and essentially veto power by the "medical men" as a group against measures proposed within the association.[42] Typical of nineteenth-century strategies in nursing and professional reform, seeking broad membership and alliances was meant to grant legitimacy and acceptance for new pursuits in the short term, but it often had the effect of pushing reformers to the periphery of their own movements in the long term.

Even in the short term, the strategic incorporation of physicians in the British Nurses' Association could not diminish the overall opposition of the medical community. By the time the principle of state registration was widely accepted enough for a bill to reach Parliament, debates over implementation and standards split the collaborative relationship apart, leading to several new nursing organizations independent of physician interests. Conflicts between nurses and physicians/hospital administrators made clear that it was physicians who had the ear of legislators and parliamentarians, or even were themselves members.

As nurses experienced marginalization from the process of regulating their own work and qualifications, many became more convinced of the need for suffrage as a foundation for professionalization. This gravitation toward endorsement of women's suffrage was a marked ideological shift from the earlier era of Nightingale nursing schools and the International Red Cross, which tried to elevate the role of the nurse above politics. However, the very nature of success of state registration campaigns demonstrated to nurses that elevating their role as nurses could only be attained through politics and that their exclusion from the political process was undermining their original objectives.

German nursing leaders of the late imperial era (1880–1918) intuitively recognized this dilemma between the political citizenship that promised them greater influence over their own professional regulation and the social citizenship that had already secured their legitimate and respected role in imperial German society. Because the nursing professionalization movement based its strategies on the emulation of male professions such as medicine, education, and law, it is not surprising that attaining political citizenship through suffrage and education was a central tenet of the new path following the passing of the previous generation.

As members of the International Council of Women, through which nursing leaders first collaboratively discussed and founded the International Council of Nurses, Ethel Fenwick and Lavinia Dock were characteristically sympathetic to the cause of suffrage. They were also not hesitant to use the ICN as a platform for advocating women's suffrage. Fenwick regularly edited a column in the *BJN* called "Outside the Gates," which focused on the political position of nurses as women and disenfranchised citizens.[43] Dock used her column in the *American Journal of Nursing* (*AJN*) as well to highlight news from the suffrage movement, but her introduction of a resolution supporting suffrage to the ICN created open drama in the 1909 international meeting. The first resolution failed because a few American delegates were unsure of the propriety of endorsing a political position on behalf of colleagues who had not been asked their opinion on the issue.[44] The hesitancy of others to follow the lead of Fenwick and Dock reflected the contentiousness of women's suffrage among nurses at this time. Although suffrage was a popular cause, many nurses believed that open and public agitation for it would undermine their sense of moral authority, social respectability, and, more pragmatically, professional alliances with male reformers.

German leader Agnes Karll was much less vocal or publicly devoted to the cause of suffrage in her own country. In a letter of September 14, 1911, she felt that the suffrage movement had not yet established a significant foothold among German women, and she feared, "If I had not to be so careful in the interest of our nurses, I would talk much more about it, but I needt risqué [sic] to make enemies for them," suggesting that open advocacy of the position would alienate some potential members of the German Nurses' Association. But she also told Dock in the same letter, "I feel more strongly every day, that [in Votes for Women] lies the only help for our ghastly conditions. . . . I shall be at the front, if the real fight for Votes should begin in Germany in my lifetime. I am sure of that."[45]

But for Dock, suffrage was in no way an issue to be left for the future. In her May 1912 column in the *AJN*, she called on American nurses to come together in unanimously supporting the suffrage resolution to be introduced in Cologne (and to avoid another embarrassing debacle of a suffrage resolution being both submitted and defeated by American nurses). She offered that

Great Britain and Ireland had already committed their delegates to the cause and that state registration and suffrage were closely linked, with six nurses currently in prison for "the cause of setting women free."[46] The rest of the column details the imprisonment of militant suffragettes in England and alludes to the growing gulf between "our lordly Law-makers" and decent women, further insinuating to nurses that the ringleaders against these suffragists were rumored to be medical students from Guy's and London Hospital—two institutions also notoriously opposed to the cause of state registration.[47]

By tying the lack of women's suffrage to the exploitation of nurses, Dock was able to rally the support of some nurses to the cause of suffrage and some suffragists to the cause of nursing professionalization. This twin strategy characterized the new generation of nursing leaders, who put their faith in the ICN and the transnational movement it represented and pursued a unique direction in nursing reform that was present neither in the generation before nor in the one after it. Still, the gradual alignment of the nursing reform movement with the suffrage movement was not without growing pains, and in the interim often further marginalized nursing leaders from physicians, administrators, and even many working nurses.

By the time of the 1912 Congress, the position of the German Nurses' Association and ICN under Karll's leadership was still ambiguous on suffrage because of her conscious hesitation about alienating any potential supporters to the cause of professionalization, but both the international records and German Nurses' Association journal provided ample space for suffragists to make their case known. The 1909 Congress in London was marked by the continued influence of older nursing ideologies emphasizing the moral authority, social respectability, and essentially apolitical nature of proper nurses, as demonstrated in the failed prosuffrage resolution. Opponents of the resolution were upset at the organization's willingness to jeopardize its nursing reform agenda by advocating for controversial political issues. Yet, by the 1912 Congress, the same prosuffrage resolution barely caused a ripple before being passed.

The role that suffrage and the women's movement played in creating a common foundation for diverse organizations of middle-class nurses, especially in Germany, was realized much more broadly during those three years. Lavinia Dock reported her "great interest" in "The Woman in Household and Profession," a traveling exhibition designed for the German Women's Congress in March 1912, which demonstrated the synthesis of various secular and religious nursing associations in Germany. For example, German Catholic nuns contributed a visual presentation highlighting the work of sixty-four orders of nursing sisters, who had set up efficient hospital wards for civilians and soldiers. Eight of the orders even had training programs for secular nurses.[48] The German Women's Congress also hosted a session on the role of the state and society in nursing, which featured papers not only from the German Nurses' Association, but also from the Red Cross, the Kaiserswerth Deaconess Motherhouse, and the Catholic orders that provided an overview of the organization of nursing in Germany.[49]

Though the conflicts between the German Nurses' Association and the religious nursing orders in Germany should not be minimized, they also had much in common in 1912. They all made priorities of providing care for nurses in sickness and old age, expanding preparation and training beyond a year, and raising the social respectability of nurses in society. In spite of the rhetoric, German statistics suggest that Protestant deaconesses and Catholic sisters were also seriously plagued by a lack of social insurance and stricter state regulation despite their public claims to private social welfare programs.[50] However, an even greater priority of the Kaiserswerth administration was to protect the privileged social position of the deaconess nurses that was gained by the ideological commitment to charitable rather than remunerative labor. The German Nurses' Association's efforts to raise nurses' salaries (and subsequently their class status) ideologically undermined the image of nursing as an occupation of Christian charity that had provided the original key to the deaconesses' success in Germany, but it also highlighted the growing reality of sickness and poverty among both unaffiliated and religious nurses excluded from legal protections afforded to most male workers.

By characterizing nursing as a particularly female profession, reformers also built upon a sense of nursing autonomy in which they claimed that nursing was not a medical profession and thus presented no threat to the authority of doctors, but that therefore neither should nursing be controlled by doctors. Creating a professional identity for nurses was a project with roots far back into the nineteenth century; the explicitly professional concept of nursing, now emphasizing collegiate education and state recognition at the Cologne Congress, showed an intentional distancing from such nineteenth-century concepts as "social motherhood."[51] It gravitated instead toward an ideological mixture of equal rights feminism, socioeconomic and racial superiority, and commitment to educational advancement.[52] Together, these characteristics depicted a new concept of the female professional, in which an educated woman of middle-class background would gain recognition as a good nurse through her educational experience and scientific training. National and international nursing leaders saw it as their priority to downplay references to respectable women's innate nursing capacities, hoping that such notions would be thoroughly extinguished by legislation requiring minimum standards for nurse training and examination, and by increasing a sense of professional loyalty among nurses rather than to particular doctors or institutions. However, in pursuing such an agenda, nursing leaders often alienated themselves from the nurses they hoped to represent and exacerbated the underlying ideological conflicts within nursing and early twentieth-century health care more broadly.

As organizations began to move away from seeing these professional markers as goals and toward seeing them as standards, nursing leaders exposed the class divisions and socioeconomic tensions between them and the working nurses they claimed to represent. The question of adequate remuneration had to be delicately balanced in a way that both demanded that the traditional privileges of social respectability, recognized expertise, and public service characteristic of the existing male professions be applied to nursing, and also defended nurses against the labels of wage labor and commercialism that were especially distasteful for elite women. In the effort to claim for themselves a professional sense of respectability and social position, nursing leaders no longer were willing to seek compromises for the sake of professional unity. Rather, international nursing leaders were more prepared to leave behind the nurses who would not or could not measure up to the higher expectations of professionalization. The goal for this new generation of nursing reformers was to establish solidarity among nursing "sisters" against hospital administrators, physicians, and nurse supervisors. However, such efforts required cross-class cooperation and laid bare the class-specific nature of nursing reform. As a result, the new generation of nursing leaders was compelled to peer under the bar they had themselves set.

Professionalization through Social Welfare and Labor Legislation

In 1912, C. W. Saleeby, a British doctor and author, observed, "The modern nurse . . . may be of widely variable social antecedents, and the public has not yet learnt whether to regard her as an ally, if not almost an equal, of the doctor—or, on the other hand, as a domestic servant, who gives herself airs."[53] This significant variation in the class background and social status of nurses was an ongoing challenge to professionalization.[54] Superintendents or matrons, who managed staff nurses in hospital or other institutions, were usually of an educated middle-class background, had completed a three-year course of training, and provided the elite stratum of nurses who could afford the time and money to write papers and travel internationally on behalf of their professional cause.[55] The nurses under their management worked physically and mentally strenuous hours as nurses and probationers in hospitals and private duty and may have felt their situation better represented by industrial labor organizers in opposition than in alliance with the higher-class superintendents.

Although national and international nursing associations claimed to represent all nurses within their scope, only graduates of three-year training programs were eligible for membership in the national councils and therefore also the ICN. Given that nursing registration in Germany required only one year's training and few three-year programs existed, Karll thought this requirement exacerbated artificial divisions among nurses committed to reform rather than bringing them together to work for their shared cause. Three-year programs were common enough in Great Britain and the United States that nursing leaders had little sympathy for nurses who did not join one of their affiliated professional associations. The frustrations on both sides of the divide were spilled out on the pages of the British and American nursing journals in 1912, as a series of letters between nurses and the editor of the *BJN* made clear. A nurse identifying herself as A.C.F. first wrote to the British editor:

> Can you tell me how I am to attend the International Congress at Cologne?—I do not belong to a League. If I went "on my own" should I be recognized—and be invited to social functions? I am a great believer in international intercourse between classes of workers—but at the hospital where I trained we were discouraged from joining any nurses' societies, and from reading the professional nursing journals.[56]

The editor's response stated that the treatment of nonmembers had not yet been decided, but that all three-year trained nurses should join the Society for the State Registration of Trained Nurses or its Scottish or Irish counterparts.[57] Two weeks later, another letter was printed in the journal from "One who loves unity," suggesting that the editor's response did not sufficiently recognize the pressures working nurses felt about joining a professional organization:

> I dare not belong to the Society for State Registration because our Matron and Committee do not approve of it.... It does seem unfair that we nurses in England seem to be the only ones who have no freedom of action—in every other country in the world, even China and Japan, they are not such serfs as we are. When the splendid International Congress was held in London in 1909 we were not permitted to take any part in it—and unless one risks one's livelihood one has just to grin and bear it.[58]

This time, the editor's response angrily admonished the writer and other nurses who did not join the association for fear of losing their position: "It is only those who have sufficient courage to risk loss of work, for what is right, who ever are free to do their duty. Personally, we have little sympathy for those who consider their immediate self-interest before everything." A couple of months later, Lavinia Dock referenced the second letter in her "Foreign Department" section of the *AJN*. Softening the tone of the British editor, Dock optimistically posited that "this nurse would surprise herself by the good results of showing a little more spirit, if she would try . . . our advice to the nurse is: 'Dare to revolt!'"[59]

In some ways, this particular example characterizes the stratified structure of British and American nursing organizations in the early twentieth century and the mixed attitudes among nursing leaders toward integrating a wider spectrum of interests into their organizational platforms. The best known and most active nursing associations were heavily dominated by superintendents or matrons. The American Society of Superintendents of Training Schools in the United States and Canada, which became the National League of Nursing Education (NLNE) in 1911, dedicated itself mainly to the expansion of educational and professional possibilities for the elite among North American nurses.[60] In Great Britain, the Society for State Registration began working explicitly and uncompromisingly for state registration after some nurses became frustrated with the hesitation of the Royal British Nurses' Association[61] to support a bill for state registration. The Matrons' Council, also founded and led by Ethel Fenwick, could be considered the counterpart to the NLNE and was even more selective in membership and ambitious in agenda than the Society for State Registration.

By contrast, Lavinia Dock was a known advocate of organizing the support for trained nurses beyond superintendents and worked to broaden the movement's appeal rather than make it more exclusive. Her address to the Sixteenth Annual Convention of American Nurses warned nurses already affiliated with the professional association "that the nurse is a worker no one can deny. However, professionally she may build her career, however distinguished and noble she may make it . . . she is still closely related to the world of workers whom we may call toilers."[62] Though Dock was not proposing lowering professional standards in the name of inclusivity, she was suggesting that the professional association had an obligation to consider the interests of working nurses in the national representative body. The pragmatist in Dock recognized the potential of working nurses to undermine the professionalization movement if they continued to feel more loyalty to their own hospitals than to the national nursing association. Meanwhile, the social reformer in her brought a genuine sympathy for the social ills afflicting the industrial working class, even if such sympathy was laced with an aura of middle-class paternalism.

Interestingly, the conflicts between the national organizations and working nurses were more often the product of clashes among superintendents than between superintendents and working nurses directly. The sense of autonomy and competition among hospital training schools inhibited the development of professional loyalties among nurses at different institutions. Thus, a community of physicians, matrons, and working nurses often developed out of a sense of pride or loyalty to a particular hospital program, in contrast and competition with the programs and personnel of other hospitals. As for the letters quoted above, Dock characterized the "disunity" of British nursing as arising from the strife between the Matrons' Council and more conservative elements in British nursing.[63] The Matrons' Council, like the NLNE, was often accused of being exclusive and personality-driven.[64] Superintendents from less prestigious hospitals or training schools resented its concentration of power and disregard for internal dynamics that varied from institution to institution. Often superintendents were merely enforcing the will of physicians and hospital administrators on the nurses under them, out of the same fear and insecurity that kept their charges from rebelling.

In Germany, nurses were also distributed across the class spectrum, from the legions of nursing aides (male and female) who provided domestic service and some patient care in hospitals and homes to the aristocratic members of Red Cross-affiliated women's associations who offered their services as patrons, managers, and volunteer nurses. In 1912, the German Nurses' Association estimated that active German nurses were divided among Catholic orders (26,000), Protestant motherhouses (12,000), Red Cross motherhouses (4,500), the Evangelical Diaconate (1,800), and those with no institutional affiliation (30,000). It was this last group that the German Nurses' Association hoped to represent, but the requirement that members hold a three-year training certification limited the actual membership to about 3,000 German nurses.[65]

The other significant subgroup in nursing was male nurses, who according to 1909 occupational figures numbered 12,881, about 19 percent of the total number of nurses in Germany, though only about 9 percent of those in religious orders.[66] By these numbers the German Nurses' Association looks insignificant in the grand scheme of German nursing, but its privileged position in relationship to nurses outside Germany and its relatively recent founding gave the impression that it was growing in numbers, prestige, and influence.[67] The effect was that though the German Nurses' Association envisioned drawing other nursing organizations under its umbrella, other organizations and unaffiliated nurses saw their own interests as in opposition to those of the professionalization movement.

Divisions and conflict among nursing factions over race, class, and ideological underpinnings were not unique to Germany. The American Nurses'

Association (ANA) had been the nationally representative body for only a year, and though more broadly representative than the NLNE, it was also considered to be dominated by a handful of prestigious large hospital training schools.[68] Though the ANA could claim to represent 20,000 nurses at the time of its 1912 annual convention, the organization had no individual members but counted nurses through its association with training schools and alumni associations.[69] The number of nursing delegates or members at that convention was only 340, although the difficulty of traversing the vast geographic territory of the United States must have contributed to the relatively low representation.[70] In addition, the NLNE was restricted to superintendents, and its membership delineated clearly the sharp class distinctions between nursing leaders and the working nurses who were excluded from their ranks.

Racial separation also contributed to a lack of unified representation of American nurses. From 1908 to 1951, African American nursing leaders coordinated their own representation through the National Association of Colored Graduate Nurses, but discrimination continued to bar its members from working in a vast majority of American hospitals or playing significant roles in broader nursing associations.[71] Two African American nurses attended the 1912 ICN Congress, which elicited great excitement from among its members, but their presence was perhaps more a curiosity to the White European and American women who tried to point to their professional success than an indicator of potential for their own colonial nursing projects.[72]

The overwork of nurses was a systematic condition throughout European and North American hospitals in the nineteenth century. Not surprisingly, one of the five themes at the 1912 Congress and the topic of the keynote address was "The Overstrain of Nurses," by Dr. Herman Hecker. Hecker based his assessment on Prussian statistics from 1909 to make the case that nurses have fewer legal protections against labor exploitation than factory workers in Germany. As evidence he cited that a nurse works an average of fourteen hours per day, including Sundays, and more than 40 percent of questioned nurses worked fourteen to eighteen hours per day.[73] By the conclusion of the Congress, Lavinia Dock reported that the ICN had passed a resolution "condemning the system of overwork which prematurely ruins the health of nurses in some continental countries."[74] Her attempt to isolate the problem of overwork as a continental problem is interesting, given a similar dilemma in American nursing, in which nurses most often worked alone in private duty, 84–168 hours per week, in a position more often treated like a servant than a professional.[75] Even more ominous was the implicit agreement of German medical personnel, who articulated the answer to Germany's "mortality" problem with the call for, "as in England and the United States, strict selection of healthy probationers free from hereditary taint."[76] Though the problems of nursing mortality and unhealthy working conditions were common in European and North American countries, the elite composition of American and British nursing associations allowed them more easily to overlook the conditions of working nurses—a circumstance German leaders never had the (mis-)fortune of experiencing.

Agnes Karll was well acquainted with the effects of overwork, and exploitation of nurses was a personal issue to which she was especially devoted. Her own career as a nurse reformer began after her short tenure as a private duty nurse left her too physically debilitated at the age of thirty-one to continue active nursing without another means of economic support. Her situation prompted her to begin working with Deutsche Anker, an insurance company, to provide health and disability insurance to German nurses starting in 1899.[77] During a lecture tour in fall and winter 1911, Karll conveyed her shock over nurses' physical and mental health to Dock: "So many nurses and I almost never realized how sorely they need us, than this time . . . and how they die, that is simply heart-rending. So many suicides! And so many dreadfully ill and most die much to[o] young. How I long for your book about 'fatigue and overwork!'"

Suicide might seem a particularly odd example of the physical and social challenges facing nurses, but the individual stories make clear the contribution of broader contemporary social problems. The growing pains of industrialization had only begun to be dealt with in Germany, following late nineteenth-century industrialization of its society. In one particular case, an otherwise well-regarded young nurse in Berlin injected a patient with the wrong drug. After she was infamously skewered by the German press, she committed suicide. Left unreported was that on that particular day the nurse had come off duty at 3 a.m. only to be back on duty by 8 a.m. that same day. This so-called half-night duty was a common strategy for circumventing early labor legislation that mandated a period of rest after a night shift but not after a half-night shift. Nurses routinely were on duty from 8 p.m. until 2 or 3 a.m. and then returned to the wards at 8 a.m. for a full day shift. Such cases were not isolated incidents. According to the German Nurses' Association 1910 statistics, five of twelve deaths among its members were due to suicide, a significant increase from the already troubling nine of thirty-five deaths attributed to suicide since the association was founded in 1903. Thus, the German Nurses' Association recorded approximately 24 percent of its members' deaths between 1903 and 1911 due to suicide, with the other 76 percent attributed to diseases and accidents.[78]

Perhaps less severe, but more prevalent than death was the estimated 30 percent of nurses and 53 percent of probationers whose careers ended in invalidism according to a study of German Red Cross hospitals in 1907. Adding to the German Nurses' Association estimate that the careers of 24 percent of German nurses ended in suicide was the estimated 30 percent of nurses and 53 percent of probationers whose careers ended in invalidism.[79] Though illness and injury among nurses was a longstanding problem, the more recent boom in hospital training schools, private duty nurses, and unaffiliated nurses had highlighted the vast social problems that grew out of unregulated and exploited nursing labor. Overwork was recognized by physicians, nurses, and social reformers as a particularly important challenge requiring state intervention and alleviation. But the terms of such intervention were highly contested, and the debates reflected fundamental disagreements among nurses as to what a profession of nursing should be.

By 1912, nurses were looking for wide-reaching protection of their health and livelihood. On the one hand was the urgent recognition that the state must intervene in the exploitation of nurses in training schools, public hospitals, and private duty. Nursing organizations such as the German Association of Male and Female Nurses (Deutscher Verband der Krankenpfleger und -Pflegerinnen) called for collective organizing under the umbrella of one national nursing organization, which would demand social welfare provisions provided to wage laborers. Women's organizations were wary of this plan, although aspects of it were widely promoted in various nursing journals. Female nurses saw the mixed-gender unification of nursing under a working-class ideology as giving up their two strongest tools in the professionalization movement—class superiority and gender autonomy. Middle-class nursing reformers had worked hard for generations to create a clear distinction between nursing and waged labor. Accepting inclusion in the expanding social welfare programs for the working classes undermined national and international nursing leaders' professionalization agenda.

The foray of European states into national social welfare and insurance plans had an especially charged effect on the class-based tensions within nursing. The social insurance provisions of the 1880s offered by the German state offered working men economic security as a means of stifling working-class insurgency. Nurses saw these benefits as inherently linked to the privileges of citizenship, because they were as women deprived of both. British efforts to implement social insurance in the early twentieth century were in many ways quite similar, but held no such appeal to British nurses, who were much more self-conscious about demeaning their class position and saw citizenship to be as much a privilege of class as of gender.

In Dock's "Nursing Organizations in Germany and England" and later journal columns she details her view of the differences between the German example of social insurance legislation from the late nineteenth century and the English Pension Fund and subsequent National Insurance Act. The Pension Fund was a charitable endowment rather than a governmental program and required contributions from its potential recipients that Dock deemed less effective than private insurance policies or savings accounts.[80] The National Insurance Act of 1911 attempted to remedy the major shortfalls of the Pension Fund system, but nursing leaders continued to be skeptical of qualifying recipients on the basis of wage earnings (excluding married women and private duty nurses and midwives), not recognizing midwives and nurses as approved practitioners for insurance payments, and failing to recognize health and welfare insurance as a privilege of citizenship.[81] After the act passed, Dock called it "a powerful argument for woman suffrage" and "a terrifying example of the present unchecked power of men to legislate for women."[82] Whereas in Germany Karll had advocated for many years to see nurses included in an insurance plan to protect them from the illness, injury, and disability that often arose from nursing work, the British plan incited the ire of British and international nursing leaders primarily because of its perceived association with charity and wage labor.[83] Whereas German nursing leaders saw an insurance and pension plan controlled and earned by nurses, the British plan was seen to degrade the status of nursing to that of the pauper class and as contrary to the centrality of a respectable middle-class identity in the professional nursing movement.

Class stratifications among nurses were clear, but they were perhaps a well-kept secret of the International Council of Nurses. British and American nursing delegations had enough superintendents or matrons of economic means who could afford to attend international conferences at three-year intervals. This was clearly not the case for German nurses, who Karll feared would not even be able to afford the train fare across Germany for the Cologne Congress.[84] Of course, it was also common for American and British nurses to have their trips sponsored by an association, hospital, or private benefactor. German associations such as the Kaiserswerth Administration had made clear that they would not support or finance the attendance of deaconesses at the Cologne Congress, and by its charter, the German Nurses' Association represented nurses who had by definition no such associational support.

Still, in all three countries, hospitals and nursing organizations lamented the shortage of "probationers of the well-educated type," while housemaids flocked to fill the void. American hospitals blamed the shortages on state registration laws, but Dock points out a similar phenomenon in Great Britain, where no such laws yet existed.[85] Whatever the cause, class stratifications clearly continued to play a defining role in the organization of nursing, but, as Dock challenged her colleagues to consider, "If we acknowledge our relation to the working world and fulfill the obligation that this relation brings, we shall live and become ever more useful and respected."[86] This shift away from class-based professionalization and toward a gendered sense of professional unity based on the attainment of full citizenship was the characteristic marker of the new path in nursing before the war.

Professionalization for a New Generation

By the end of 1912, the landscape of nursing reform had undergone significant changes, and the new path would call on nursing leaders to move on from the unity of purpose offered by nineteenth-century gender ideologies of social motherhood, bourgeois respectability, and the paternalistic protection of the state. The new generation of nursing leaders gravitated toward political citizenship and suffrage as a strategy for becoming active participants in the nation-state to which they had entrusted the regulation of their profession. However, the growth of citizenship as a modern framework for understanding the privileges and exclusions based in older socioeconomic identities did not displace the role of class in defining nurses' values and agendas, but added new dimensions to the discourses of inclusion and exclusion that helped define their own professional identity through models of middle-class professionalization and political citizenship for women.[87]

As this article has argued, the uneven attainment of state registration and regulation of nursing ushered in a new phase of transnational collaboration among nurses in Germany, Great Britain, and the United States. This moment also marked a polarization of national nursing identities, in which German nursing would be almost exclusively characterized by dependence on the state whereas American nursing became tied to the higher-status ranks of university-educated women. Though the new era introduced various educational and organizational innovations that brought the professionalization movement to the height of its success, the increasing institutionalization of these geographic and class-based variations also hampered further collaboration and advancement. The reality of European and American nursing professionalization in 1912 was that the masculine model of middle-class professionalization became increasingly impossible for middle-class women to emulate without the privilege of political citizenship and equal educational opportunities, and with the burden of quelling working-class exploitation. As these nursing leaders attempted to make the best of their circumstances with the familiar strategy of compromise, they triumphed in the short term but also set the foundation for future challenges against the ongoing project of nursing professionalization in the long term.

AELEAH SOINE
University of Minnesota
Department of History
1110 Heller Hall
271 19th Avenue South
Minneapolis, MN 55455

Notes

1. Lavinia Dock, "The Status of the Nurse in the Working World," in "Proceedings of the Sixteenth Annual Convention of the American Nurses' Association," *American Journal of Nursing* 13, no. 12 (September 1913): 971 (hereafter *AJN*). Dock suggested in her address that the paper should more accurately be called "The Relation of the Nurse to the Working World," capturing the ambiguity that characterized nurses as workers and professionals.

2. Ibid.: 972–75.

3. Henry Bonham-Carter, *Is a General Register for Nurses Desirable?* (London: Blades, East and Blades, 1888), 1. Bonham-Carter quotes the BNA, representing the nursing position, as claiming "that nursing is a profession as Medicine and Law are professions; but that it is not acknowledged as such; and that the legal registration of Nurses is the only means by which Nursing can be established as an acknowledged and legally constituted profession."

4. Agnes Karll, "The Results of State Registration for Nurses in Germany," address to Third Regular Meeting of the International Council of Nurses at Gürzenich in Cologne, Germany, August 5, 1912, 42; Agnes Karll Archive, Berlin (hereafter AKA). The Imperial Registration Act of 1909–10 called for nursing registration throughout the German Empire, but its implementation was still being stalled by the states of Bavaria, Baden, Oldenburg, and Mecklenburg as of 1912.

5. "Proceedings of the Fifteenth Annual Convention of the American Nurses' Association (June 5–7, 1912)," reprinted in *AJN* 12, no. 11 (August 1912), 890.

6. Hester Viney, "The State in Relation to the British Nurse," *AJN* 30, no. 8 (August 1930): 1019. The British Parliament first implemented a system of nursing registration in 1919.

7. Barbara L. Brush and Meryn Stuart, "Unity Amidst Difference: The ICN Project and Writing International Nursing History," *Nursing History Review* 2 (1994): 198–99 (hereafter *NHR*). Brush and Stuart argue that professional ideology neutralized political and demographic differences among nurses in the ICN and quote Ethel Fenwick as claiming that nurses were "happily untroubled by national considerations." Though they rightly depict the role of professionalization as a foundation for ideological unity in the ICN, the period between the attainment of state registration and the outbreak of World War I was

also characterized by increasing recognition of the central role of the nation-state in nursing professionalization.

8. Canada was also a charter member; at the time it was represented by the same organization as the U.S. nurses, which Canadian nurses later left to form their own association.

9. Susan McGann, "Collaboration and Conflict in International Nursing, 1920–1939," *NHR* 16 (2008): 29–57. McGann takes up a similar analytical task in the interwar period, which provides an interesting overview of transnational nursing associations and projects after World War I.

10. For more on the relationship between nurses and the state, politics, and feminism, see Cynthia Anne Connelly, "Beyond Social History: New Approaches to Understanding the State of and the State in Nursing History," *NHR* 12 (2004): 5–24; and Sandra Lewenson, "Of Logical Necessity . . . They Hang Together": Nursing and the Woman's Movement, 1901–1912," *NHR* 2 (1994): 99–117.

11. This is the central argument of the classic text, David Blackbourn and Geoff Eley, *The Peculiarities of German History: Bourgeois Society and Politics in Nineteenth-Century Germany* (Oxford: Oxford University Press, 1984). See pages 75–90 for Eley's explicit discussion of how the German bourgeoisie was able to meet its goals within a semiauthoritarian state and without the particularly British constellation of bourgeois revolution, liberalism, and democracy.

12. See classic work of George Dangerfield, *The Strange Death of Liberal England* (1935; Stanford, Calif.: Stanford University Press, 1997); or a more contemporary analysis from Jose Harris, *Private Lives, Public Spirit: Britain: 1870–1914* (Oxford: Oxford University Press, 1993).

13. Robert Dingwall, Anne Marie Rafferty, and Charles Webster; *An Introduction to the Social History of Nursing* (London: Routledge, 1988), 83.

14. *Report from the Select Committee on Registration of Nurses; together with the Proceedings of the Committee, Minutes of Evidence, and Appendix* (July 26, 1904) (London: Wyman & Sons, 1904); Royal British Nurses' Association collection 9: General Letters and Papers, King's College Archives, London, 28. See also Lavinia Dock, "The London Meeting of the International Council and Congress of Nurses," *AJN* 10, no. 1 (October 1909); reprinted in *The Lavinia Dock Reader*, ed. Janet Wilson James (New York: Garland, 1985), 19, in which Sydney Holland disrupted the proceedings to object to what he saw as the "unrepresentative" nature of the International Council of Nurses.

15. See David Blackbourn, *History of Germany, 1780–1918: The Long Nineteenth Century*, 2nd ed. (Malden, Mass.: Blackwell, 2003), 200.

16. Kaiserliches Gesundheits-Amt. Abteilung II. Akten betreffend: Krankenpflege (vom Anfang September 1904 bis Dezember 1907), Band 4 siehe Fortsetzung Band 5, Medizinalwesen XV, No. 1, German Federal Archives, Berlin. These archival records include an ongoing dialogue among bureaucrats in the Imperial Health Ministry and physicians interested in the cause of nursing registration, but reflect little input from the German Nurses' Association or other nurses as individuals or groups.

17. See Ann Taylor Allen, *Feminism and Motherhood in Germany, 1800–1914* (New Brunswick, N.J.: Rutgers University Press, 1991); and Kathleen Canning, *Gender History in Practice: Historical Perspectives on Bodies, Class, and Citizenship* (Ithaca, N.Y.: Cornell University Press, 2006).

18. Kathryn Kish Sklar, Anja Schüler, and Susan Strasser, *Social Justice Feminists of the United States and Germany: A Dialogue in Documents, 1885–1933* (Ithaca, N.Y.: Cornell University Press, 1998), 23.

19. For comparative analyses of the relationship between women and the emerging welfare state and related strategies of maternalism, see Seth Koven and Sonya Michel, *Mothers of a New World: Maternalist Politics and the Origins of the Welfare States* (London: Routledge, 1993); and Gisela Bock and Pat Thane, *Maternity and Gender Policies: Women and the Rise of the European Welfare States, 1880s–1950s* (London: Routledge, 1994).

20. Sandra Beth Lewenson, *Taking Charge: Nursing, Suffrage, and Feminism in America, 1873–1920* (New York: National League for Nursing Press, 1996), 29–33.

21. See Sklar et al., *Social Justice Feminists*, for a full-length study focused on the relationship of American and German social justice feminists.

22. See Robyn Muncy, *Creating a Female Dominion in American Reform, 1890–1935* (New York: Oxford University Press, 1991).

23. Alice Saloman, "II. Women's Professions." For the Adoption in the Four Congress Sections (1904 International Congress of Women in Berlin), Helene-Lange Archive, State Archive of Berlin, League of German Women's Associations collection: B Rep 235–321–23, Karton 81/Abt 17, IV, Film 3219.

24. For example, nurses had to complete a three-year course of nursing—far beyond the time required by law—to participate in ICN functions. This was a rule Karll disagreed with, because she would have been happy to have any registered nurses join the organization, especially since three-year programs were still rare in Germany.

25. I have translated "Berufsorganisation der Krankenpflegerinnen Deutschlands" as "German Nurses' Association" rather than the more literal "Professional Organization of German Nurses" for consistency with contemporary British and American documents.

26. Margaret Breay and Ethel Gordon Fenwick, *History of the International Council of Nurses, 1899–1925* (Geneva: ICN, 1929), 52–53.

27. Ibid., 90.

28. Ethel Fenwick, "Editorial. Nurses and the New Year," *British Journal of Nursing* 48, no. 1240 (January 6, 1912): 1 (hereafter *BJN*).

29. Agnes Karll to Lavinia Dock, February 7, 1912, AKA.

30. Mrs. Bedford Fenwick, "A Plea for the Higher Education of Nurses," Address to the International Congress of Nurses, Buffalo, N.Y., September 21, 1901.

31. "Teachers College, Columbia University, New York," *AJN* 3, no. 6 (March 1903): 33.

32. James Gray, *Education for Nursing: A History of the University of Minnesota School* (Minneapolis: University of Minnesota Press, 1960), 15–16.

33. Ibid., 19–20.

34. Ibid., 22.

35. Agnes Karll, Jahresbericht der B.O.K.D.,*Unterm Lazaruskreuz: Mitteilungen der Berufsorganisation der Krankenpflegerinnen Deutschlands* (*Under the Cross of Lazarus: Notes from the German Nurses' Association*) 8, no. 6 (March 15, 1913): 1 (hereafter UL).

36. Agnes Karll, "Ausbildung von Krankenpflegerinnen zu Oberschwestern und Oberinnen und für soziale Arbeit an der Frauen-Hochschule Leipzig (Entwurf)" ("Training of Nurses as Ward Supervisors and Superintendents and for Social Work at the Women's College of Leipzig"), 1912, AKA, 1.

37. Though a college or university degree does have greater prestige than one from other postsecondary educational institutions, many technical occupations, like nursing, are offered in other institutions.

38. Karll, "Ausbildung von Krankenpflegerinnen," 1.

39. Ibid., 2–3.

40. For a more extensive discussion of these debates within the medical community, see Anne Marie Rafferty, *The Politics of Nursing Knowledge* (London: Routledge, 1996), 48–67.

41. Ethel Fenwick, "Speech About the Founding of the British Nurses' Association" (c. 1887), Royal British Nurses' Association Collection 9/GL 8, King's College London Archives.

42. "British Nurses' Association. Draft Bye-Laws" (*to be confirmed at General Meeting on Friday February 24, 1888*), General Council Minutes, Royal British Nurses' Association Collection 1/1, King's College London Archives.

43. "Outside the Gates," *BJN* 48, no. 1242 (January 20, 1912): 51; this example expresses a suffragist's response to an antisuffrage press statement belittling women's ability to contribute to victory in war. "Outside the Gates," *BJN* 48, no. 1244 (February 3, 1912): 94, includes several events reported for their association with the cause of women's suffrage and advice was given for dealing with antisuffrage methods.

44. Fenwick and Breay, *History of the International Council of Nurses*, 55.

45. Agnes Karll to Lavinia Dock, September 14, 1911, AKA.

46. Lavinia Dock, "Foreign Department," *AJN* 12, no. 8 (May 1912): 656.

47. Ibid., 657.

48. Lavinia Dock, "Foreign Department," *AJN* 13, no. 1 (October 1912): 49.

49. Agnes Karll, "Der deutsche Frauenkongreß in Berlin (The German Women's Congress in Berlin)," *UL* 7, no. 2 (January 15, 1912): 15.

50. Herman Hecker, "Ueberbürdung der Krankenpflegerinnen," speech at the International Council of Nurses Third Regular Meeting, Cologne, Germany; reprinted in *UL* 7, no. 19 (October 1, 1912) and published in English as "The Overstrain of Nurses: An Address Delivered by Dr. H. Hecker, Regierungs und Geheimer Medizinalrat in Strasbourg-Alsace to ICN Cologne, 1912," trans. Gain Praetorius and Anita Becker, Adelaide Nutting Historical Nursing Collection (hereafter ANHNC), 24–26. Hecker explains that, despite impressive provisions for religious-affiliated and Red Cross nurses in Germany, the high entrance fees and lack of wages paid to them during their working time inhibit them from saving money in case illness or injury occurs before they reach the mandated number of years to qualify for such retirement or invalid pensions. In one motherhouse, Hecker found that only 12 of 120 nurses had reached the ten years of service required to qualify for a pension.

51. See Allen, *Feminism and Motherhood in Germany, 1800–1914*.

52. See Leila J. Rupp, *Worlds of Women: The Making of an International Women's Movement* (Princeton, N.J.: Princeton University Press, 1997); or Sklar et al., *Social Justice Feminists*, for the historical, political, and economic context from which these women's transnational collaborative relationships arose.

53. Dr. C. W. Saleeby, *Modern Surgery and Its Making* (London: Herbert & Daniel, 1912); quote reprinted in M.B., "Professional Review. Modern Surgery and Its Making: A Tribute to Listerism," *BJN* 48, no. 1247 (February 24, 1912): 154.

54. Carole Adams argues that the "rewards of professionalization favored class solidarity over feminist collaboration." As evidence, Adams illustrates the collusion of

bourgeois women with male clerks against working-class women. This was yet another example of "respectable" women consciously distinguishing themselves from their working-class counterparts and the more radical feminist commitments of socialist women. Quoted in Jean H. Quataert, "Introduction 2: Writing the History of Women and Gender in Imperial Germany," in *Society, Culture, and the State in Germany 1870–1930*, ed. Geoff Eley (Ann Arbor: University of Michigan Press, 1996), 57.

55. A superintendent (American), matron (British), or Oberin (German) is a nursing manager for a hospital or institution. They are higher in rank than an Oberschwester or ward sister, which more closely approximates a department manager. I will attempt to use the term that fits geographically with the reference, or superintendent as the generic.

56. A.C.F., "The Cologne Congress" (Letter to the Editor), *BJN* 48, no. 1241 (January 13, 1912): 37.

57. "The Cologne Congress" (Response to Letter to the Editor), ibid.

58. One Who Loves Unity, "The Cologne Congress" (Letter to the Editor), *BJN* 48, no. 1243 (January 27, 1912): 78.

59. Lavinia L. Dock, "Foreign Department," *AJN* 12, no. 6 (March 1912): 490–91.

60. Susan Reverby, *Ordered to Care: The Dilemma of American Nursing, 1850–1945* (Cambridge: Cambridge University Press, 1987), 123.

61. The British Nurses' Association became the Royal British Nurses' Association to correspond with the royal charter it received in 1893.

62. Dock, "Status of the Nurse in the Working World," 971.

63. Lavinia Dock, "Nursing Organizations in Germany and England," in "Short Papers on Nursing Subjects" (1900), reprinted in *A Lavinia Dock Reader*, ed. James, 23–24.

64. Reverby, *Ordered to Care*, 124.

65. Agnes Karll, "Der Weltbund der Krankenpflegerinnen," *UL* 7, no. 14 (July 15, 1912): 160.

66. Claudia Bischoff, *Frauen in der Krankenpflege: Zur Entwicklung von Frauenrolle und Frauenberufstätigkeit im 19. und 20. Jahrhundert* (*Women in Nursing: Toward the Development of Women's Roles and Professional Activities in the Nineteenth and Twentieth Century*) (Frankfurt: Campus, 1997), 103.

67. Karll, "Der Weltbund der Krankenpflegerinnen," 160. Karll notes that the Red Cross took eighteen years to assemble 4,500 members, while the German Nurses' Association recruited 3,000 in only nine years.

68. Reverby, *Ordered to Care*, 123–24.

69. "Proceedings of the Fifteenth Annual Convention of the American Nurses' Association," 882.

70. Ibid., 862.

71. Joan I. Roberts and Thetis M. Group, *Feminism and Nursing: An Historical Perspective on Power, Status, and Political Activism in the Nursing Profession* (Westport, Conn.: Praeger, 1995), 90.

72. Lavinia L. Dock, "Foreign Department," *AJN* 13, no. 7 (October 1912): 48. Miss Samuels and Mrs. Williams attended as fraternal delegates representing the colored nurses' national association of the United States. They were received at events (unlike nurses who were eligible for membership but did not join) but could not vote and usually represented national associations not yet fulfilling the requirements for affiliation as national association members or countries without such an association.

73. Hecker, "The Overstrain of Nurses," 17.
74. Lavinia Dock, "Foreign Department," *AJN* 13, no. 1 (October 1912): 48.
75. Reverby, *Ordered to Care*, 95–105.
76. Hecker, "The Overstrain of Nurses," 34.
77. Anna Sticker, *Agnes Karll: Die Reformerin der deutschen Krankenpflege* (Stuttgart: Kohlhammer, 1984), 89, 102–4.
78. Hecker, "The Overstrain of Nurses," 20–22, 27–28.
79. Ibid., 28.
80. Dock, "Nursing Organizations in Germany and England," 24–25.
81. "The National Insurance Bill," *The Midwife, BJN Supplement* (June 17, 1911): 483–84.
82. Lavinia Dock, "Foreign Department," *AJN* 12, no. 9 (June 1912), 733.
83. Dock, "Nursing Organizations in Germany and England," 24–25.
84. Agnes Karll to Lavinia Dock, January 7, 1911, AKA.
85. Lavinia Dock, "Foreign Department," *AJN* 12, no. 8 (May 1912): 657–58.
86. Dock, "Status of the Nurse in the Working World," 975.
87. Canning, *Gender History in Practice*, 194.

REFRAMING ACTIVISM: NURSING AND SOCIAL ACTION IN THE UNITED STATES

Guest Editor's Note

In April 2008, the members of the Sigerist Circle invited a group of historians of nursing to present their ideas about nursing and activism at its annual meeting, held in conjunction with that of the American Association for the History of Medicine. We were all challenged with writing about what "activism" meant, and as Patricia D'Antonio wrote in her 2009 editorial of *Nursing History Review*, "We tried to unpack the trope of *activism* by wondering about the ways in which more ordinary nurses we studied thought about the social and political implications of their own actions."[1]

One of the questions I asked, as the panel's commentator, was: Is activism a religion? Are those who worked actively for social change in health care akin to evangelicals, religiously focused and tenacious until the goal is met? For example, Margaret Sanger, the early twentieth-century nurse and fervent birth control activist, was jailed for her illegal activity promoting and providing birth control, calling it "her religion."[2] I asked also: Are there distinctions to be made between radicalism and reformism, between revolutionaries and activists? Is this even important? Many of the nurses in the following articles would have been called radicals and revolutionaries *because* they worked with marginalized and vulnerable populations and individuals. Indeed, in a recent Canadian textbook on community health nursing, becoming an activist with and for stigmatized, vulnerable people at risk for health problems is seen as a key nursing role.[3] Whether one calls it social action, political intervention, or activism, this is the same role that nurses undertook in the early to late twentieth century in their communities.

In Cynthia Connolly's article, "'I am a Trained Nurse': The Nursing Identity of Anarchist and Radical Emma Goldman," we similarly see that the *very act* of public health nursing was radical on the Lower East Side of New York City for Emma Goldman and Lillian Wald in the late 1890s and early 1900s. Connolly quotes Emma Goldman, who wrote that coming "face to face [as a nurse] with the living conditions of workers in their squalid surroundings" made her realize how much the anticapitalist movement needed to change social conditions. Nursing seemed almost clandestine. Goldman even used a pseudonym when she took private-duty nursing cases because she had been imprisoned for her anarchism and was well known in New York. The act of nursing was also a cause for them, a religion even. For example, in the early twentieth century, Goldman visited Wald at Henry Street and described Wald and her nurses as having "consecrated" themselves to their cause. Although Wald did not see herself as a radical, believing herself to be more a reformer, Connolly questions the difference between the two terms because Wald was able to agitate for social change inside the system with her powerful network. Goldman was outside, but Wald still supported her financially and emotionally.

In Barbra Mann Wall's "Conflict and Compromise: Catholic and Public Hospital Partnerships," Daughters of Charity nuns, many of whom nurses, *risked their religious careers* in taking over the administration of a Protestant city hospital in Austin, Texas, that cared for the indigent, especially women and children. Worse yet for the nuns, the hospital performed abortions and gave birth control advice, strictly outside of Vatican policies. The nuns persevered and were able to keep free, public reproductive services (although not abortion) against the considerable male power of the bishop of Austin, conservative Austin Catholics, the pope, and Vatican officials. This action was taken to reach the most vulnerable and provide free care to women and children. This was in the 1990s. As Mann Wall tells us, the sisters experienced a "conflict of conscience" over the field of reproductive services because they were committed to care for the poor, but Vatican directives prevented the kind of services the protestant hospital provided. Working with other groups in the community led to their success.

Julie Fairman's "'Go to Ruth's House': The Social Activism of Ruth Lubic and the Family Health and Birth Center" is the final article in this section. Fairman reveals a nurse midwife—now eighty years old—literally turning around the high infant mortality rate in Washington, D.C.'s poorest area because of her tenacity, lobbying skills, passion, and ability to work with larger activist organizations in medicine, feminism, and others. She was not always successful in keeping two earlier birthing centers open, but according to the American College of Obstetricians and Gynecologists, she advocated "radical" birthing outside of hospitals. And the care that Lubic facilitated was free to poor people in 2000 in Washington, D.C. Perhaps this is why many doctors did not support Lubic over her forty-year career, which is still ongoing. She may have been perceived as taking business away from physicians. Fairman describes the atmosphere of social support in an all-female birthing environment that was unique in the 1970s when the first birthing centers opened.

The nurses we meet in these articles could certainly be called fervent activists and radicals, women whose solutions to the lack of health care for vulnerable, disadvantaged people were a religion to them. They created their own independent systems and were not "employees." Throughout the twentieth century, the injustice of the health care system in the United States bred nurses who had to do something to fix their small piece of the world, no matter the risk. Perhaps this is a history lesson for nurses today?

MERYN STUART, RN, PhD
Associate Professor and Director
Associated Medical Services Nursing History Research Unit
Unité de recherche sur l'histoire des sciences infirmières de l'AMS
School of Nursing
University of Ottawa
Ottawa, Canada

Notes

1. Editorial, *Nursing History Review* 17 (2009): 11–12.
2. Rebecca Tuhus-Dubrow, "Sanger vs. Sanger," *Nation,* July 30, 2007, 38.
3. Dave Holmes and Amélie Perron, "Les groupes vulnerables: Comprendre la vulnerabilité et agir," in *Pratiques en santé communautaire,* ed. Gisele Carroll (Montreal, Quebec: Chenelière Éducation, 2006), 195–203.

"I Am a Trained Nurse": The Nursing Identity of Anarchist and Radical Emma Goldman

Cynthia Anne Connolly
University of Pennsylvania

Abstract. For more than a century, scholars have analyzed the many dimensions of Emma Goldman. Remembered as an agent of revolution, feminism, sexual freedom, anarchy, and atheism, Goldman's motives, personality, and actions have generated an entire subgenre of historical scholarship. But although Goldman practiced nursing in New York City for ten years, one facet of her life that has been neglected is her nursing identity. Goldman's autobiography, *Living My Life*, reveals the way her nursing experiences informed her evolving anarchist political philosophy and international activism. She valued nursing for many reasons—for the economic independence it offered, identity it provided, and sense of community and connectivity she believed it encouraged. Finally, for Goldman, nursing represented was a vehicle to understand people's struggles and as a way of translating political philosophy into meaningful, practical solutions.

Iconic paragon of revolution, feminism, sexual freedom, anarchy, and atheism, Emma Goldman's motives, personality, and work have generated substantial interest for more than a century.[1] Although Goldman practiced nursing both before and after formal training, one facet of her life that has been underexplored is her nursing career. Alice Wexler's magisterial two-volume biography of Goldman's American years, for example, deemphasized her ten years as a private duty nurse in New York City's poorest neighborhoods, characterizing her work primarily as a "grim round of drudgery."[2] For Goldman herself, however, nursing was a key component to her identity. This article resurrects Emma Goldman's years as a nurse with an emphasis on the period between 1893 and 1906. It also connects her nursing work to her political activism, arguing that her nursing practice helped shape her utopian anarchist vision.

Born in Lithuania in 1869, Goldman's Jewish birth meant that she and her family faced state-sanctioned anti-Semitism and few prospects for a better

Nursing History Review 18 (2010): 84–99. A Publication of the American Association for the History of Nursing. Copyright © 2010 Springer Publishing Company.
DOI: 10.1891/1062–8061.18.84

life. She later remembered her early years with an unhappiness attributed to lack of parental nurturing and even physical abuse from her father on at least one occasion. Her family's relocation to St. Petersburg, Russia, in 1881 came at an inauspicious time. Just after the Goldmans arrived, resentment toward the Czarist autocracy boiled over, resulting in a cadre of radicals' successful assassination of Alexander II. The government of Alexander III responded by targeting Jews through pogroms and restrictive new anti-Jewish legislation. In 1886, seventeen-year-old Emma, dispirited by prospects for life in Russia, decided to accompany her sister Helene to Rochester, New York, to join their sister Lena.[3]

Life in America was not the utopia she sought. Goldman worked long hours in one of Rochester's garment industry sweatshops and soon entered into an unhappy marriage to fellow Russian Jewish immigrant Jacob Kershner. Looking for intellectual escape, she grew interested in the trial of anarchist labor organizers in Chicago. Having romanticized the Russian revolutionary movement, Goldman dreamed that American labor unrest might result in an anarchist paradise defined by communalism, opposition to a structured wage system, and rejection of governmental authority.[4] Her hope was grounded in the profound changes reshaping the United States during the last two decades of the nineteenth century. No longer was the American economy characterized primarily by small specialized family-owned and -operated firms the way it had been before the Civil War. By the 1880s, the number of large, more impersonal, bureaucratically organized companies was growing. As an agrarian economy of small producers evolved into a more industrialized one of large corporations, tensions between workers and the managerial classes escalated.[5]

The demand on the part of newly organized unions to improve working conditions stimulated laborer protest. Tensions boiled over into violence on numerous occasions. One of this era's most memorable incidents of labor strife occurred in Chicago in May 1886, when union sympathizers, agitating to reduce the standard twelve-hour work day to eight, joined strikers locked out of the McCormick Reaper plant. When nonunion replacement workers attempted to enter the plant, a fight broke out between the two groups and police. During the confusion, police fired into the crowd of demonstrators, killing four people. That night, during a meeting at Haymarket Square to denounce police actions, a bomb exploded, taking the lives of eight officers. The resulting battle between police and protesters killed or injured fifty-eight people, and eight anarchists were charged with the bombing. The trial that followed riveted the nation, radicalizing Emma Goldman, who decided to leave her marriage and Rochester and join the battle aimed at reshaping the United States into an anarchist utopia.[6]

Becoming "Red Emma"

Goldman arrived in New York during the summer of 1889. Immediately drawn to the city's radical community, she began crafting her anarchist vision for a "new social order," one that stressed mutual aid and voluntary association and believed that "all forms of government rest on violence, and are therefore wrong and harmful, as well as unnecessary."[7] Like one of her political mentors and lover, Alexander Berkman, she advocated boycotts and acts of civil disobedience. In 1892, with Goldman's knowledge, Berkman attempted to murder Henry Clay Frick. Frick, a wealthy businessman, was locked in a bitter labor dispute with members of the Amalgamated Association of Iron, Steel, and Tin Workers at a plant he co-owned in Homestead, Pennsylvania, with one of the world's richest industrialist capitalists, Andrew Carnegie.[8]

Frick survived, but Berkman was captured, convicted, and sent to jail for the next fourteen years. Police suspected Goldman of complicity in the crime but did not have evidence to charge her as an accomplice. Harassed by police and unable to rent an apartment because of her infamy, a series of late night experiences made her realize how easily nurses moved around the city and how little suspicion their travels attracted:

> Often I would sit in a café on Second Avenue until three in the morning, or I would ride back and forth to the Bronx in a street-car. . . . I wore a blue and white striped dress and a long, grey coat that resembled a nurse's uniform. Soon I found that it gave me considerable protection. Conductors and policemen would often ask me whether I had just come off duty and was taking a breath of air. One young policeman on Tompkins Square was particularly solicitous about me. He frequently entertained me with stories in his luscious Irish brogue, or he would tell me just to snooze off, that he would be near enough to protect me. "You look all in, kid," he would say; "you're working too hard, ain't you?" I had told him that I was on day and night duty with only a few hours' respite. I could not help laughing inwardly over the humour of my being protected by a policeman! I wondered how my cop would act if he knew who the demure-looking nurse was.[9]

While laboring to secure Berkman's release in 1893, Goldman entered into a romantic relationship with Austrian-born anarchist Edward Brady.[10] Galvanized by the worst economic depression in decades and hoping to capitalize on public anger over the escalating unemployment rate and what she and her colleagues saw as the excesses of "Gilded Age" industrialists such as Frick, Carnegie, Cornelius Vanderbilt, John D. Rockefeller, and J. P. Morgan, Goldman accepted an invitation to speak at a rally in New York's Union Square.

Standing in front of several thousand people on Monday, August 21, Goldman sought to stoke the anger of the "starved and fettered" at the greed of the ruling class as well as governmental complicity in sustaining their actions: "Do you not realize that the State is the worst enemy you have? . . . The State is the pillar of capitalism, and it is ridiculous to expect any redress from it." But it was Goldman's explosive last words that got her arrested and convicted for inciting to riot. She told the audience that the poor should feel free to "demonstrate before the palaces of the rich," and if denied sustenance it was their "sacred right" to "take bread."[11]

Goldman was sentenced to a year in prison at New York's notorious Blackwell's Island Penitentiary on a strip of land in the East River. The jail was part of a complex that housed 8,000 patients including the 1,000-bed Charity Hospital, Smallpox Hospital with accommodations for 500 patients, Fever Hospital for contagious diseases, and facilities for "incurables" as well as "lunatics, epileptics, and paralytics." It also served as New York City's center for the indigent suffering from venereal disease. At times it was estimated that as many as 20 percent of Charity Hospital's patients were included in this category.[12]

Goldman clashed with the prison matron, first for declaring her atheism and later for refusing to pressure the women under her charge in the sewing shop to work like "slaves."[13] After serving three weeks in the prison's "Tombs" as punishment, Goldman became so ill she entered a Charity Hospital ward as a patient. During her recovery, one of the physicians invited her to stay on as a nurse. Blackwell's Island hospitals faced a chronic and severe shortage of nurses. Its formal nurses' training program, opened in 1875, strove to build on the success of New York's first nursing school, founded two years earlier at the city's largest public hospital, Bellevue. But unlike Bellevue, Charity Hospital found it impossible to find enough young women from "good families" to staff the hospital, and a trained nurse could only be spared for operations and "grave" cases.[14] As a result of the nursing shortage, Blackwell's Island prisoners were sometimes pressed into service as nurses. Intrigued by the physician's offer, Goldman hoped that working as a nurse might reduce the power that her enemy, the prison matron, held over her daily life. But she also wanted to be clear that she knew little about the work. "I should indeed," she replied to his query, "but I know nothing about nursing."[15] Promising to teach her everything she needed to know, the prison physician placed her in charge of a sixteen-bed women's ward. Goldman faced a diverse group of challenging patients. Some were acutely ill with infectious diseases; others were giving birth, withdrawing from narcotics, or recuperating from surgery.

Jail on Blackwell's Island completed Goldman's radicalization. Thrilled at the breadth and depth of the prison library, she devoured the works of John Stuart Mill, Walt Whitman, Ralph Waldo Emerson, and others. Goldman forever after referred to her time in jail as a "school of experience" and the "crucible" that completed her revolutionary transformation. She also found that she loved nursing. Her experience among the other women prisoners—and as their nurse—provided an education in what she saw as a major injustice; women were jailed for having "ministered" to men's sexual demands while the men themselves went free. Abused, often afflicted with venereal disease and other illnesses, "they were victims, links in an endless chain of injustice and inequality," an experience to which Goldman could relate, having written about the violence that accompanied her own first sexual experience before leaving Russia. As a fifteen-year-old working at a corset factory, she met a handsome young man who worked as a hotel clerk. When he offered her a tour of the luxurious building, she readily agreed, only to find herself overpowered in an isolated part of the hotel.[16]

Released from prison in 1894, Goldman began supporting her political activities by working in the office of a sympathetic physician at Beth Israel Hospital and serving as what she called a "practical nurse." Taking private duty cases referred to her by the physicians she had gotten to know at Charity Hospital, she "loved her profession." Goldman hoped to undertake formal nurse training in the near future, not only because she wanted to gain additional knowledge, but because she believed that "practical nurses were paid and treated like servants."[17]

It was at this time that Goldman met Lillian Wald, cofounder of the Henry Street Settlement. Wald, two years older, also hailed from Rochester, although she was raised in a loving and much more prosperous German Jewish family. Wald had arrived in New York City the same summer as Goldman, entering nurse training at New York Hospital in 1889.

In many respects, Goldman's and Wald's shared future was forged in the summer of 1893. It was then that Goldman led the rally in Union Square and was subsequently imprisoned. At almost exactly the same time, Wald had experienced an epiphany. During a visit to a sick woman's tenement apartment, she had been shocked by the weak social safety net for the poor and became determined to invent a humane and effective community- and home-based nursing care model. After philosophically framing her idea for a nursing settlement, in the late summer of 1893 she prevailed on wealthy banker Jacob Schiff to donate funds for her cause and had been busy making her ideas a reality in one of Manhattan's poorest neighborhoods, the Lower East Side's Henry Street.[18]

Similar in age and having found their voice at almost exactly the same moment, Goldman and Wald also shared a passion for the overthrow of the Russian Czarist regime. Wald's support for the advocacy group known as "Friends of Russian Freedom" deeply impressed Goldman and cemented her respect for Wald.

Although their views on international affairs may have been similar and they identified many of the same societal problems within the United States, their solutions differed substantively.[19] Goldman believed in revolution and the absence of any formal state. Wald, a realist, believed that government action could improve people's lives. When she acted subversively, she preferred to do so quietly, unlike Goldman, who aggressively sought out opportunities for provocation.[20]

Goldman conferred high praise on Wald, emphasizing that the Henry Street nurses were the "first American women I met who felt an interest in the economic conditions of the masses" and who had "consecrated themselves to what they considered a great cause." She complained, however, that Wald's approach seemed "palliative," arguing that "teaching the poor to eat with a fork is all very well, but what good does it do if they have not the food?" Goldman concluded that "sincere as the settlement workers were, their ministrations did "more harm than good," because they provided enough support to dampen people's revolutionary spirit but not enough for them to really thrive.[21] Wald later made clear that she had little patience for such ideas. Although she did not mention Goldman by name, it is reasonable to assume that she had Goldman and her friends in mind when she lamented that "in some quarters mere radicalism has become perilously popular," mentioning their "naivete" and suggesting that because radicals' "spirit of adventure . . . [is] . . . not always balanced with knowledge of definite issues or the constructive processes that are underway, [they] deflect forces that might be employed for immediate advances in social welfare."[22]

Despite her concern that public health nurses' efforts had the potential to derail the societal change she sought, Goldman wanted to acquire a formal nursing education. She contemplated enrolling at the training school at New York's St. Mark's Hospital. One of the physicians she had worked with at Charity Hospital assured her not only that St. Mark's would admit her, but that he could make sure she received credit for her practical nursing work. But Brady's descriptions of Vienna captivated her, and when a benefactor offered her funds to attend nursing school at the prestigious Allegemeines Krankenhaus she accepted with alacrity. She later informed a reporter that although she believed the United States possessed the world's premier nursing schools, she wanted to study midwifery and massage in addition to nursing, courses of study not available to her in America.[23] Although public health nurses provided pre- and postpartum care, the European style midwifery model met with resistance from physicians in the United States.[24]

In 1895, only nine years after emigrating to the United States, unknown and penniless, Goldman returned to Europe to study nursing as a sophisticated political leader. Fluent in German, she had little trouble settling into the routine at Allegemeines Krankenhaus. She especially enjoyed her pediatric nursing course and she preferred caring for children throughout her nursing career. As she later recounted:

> In my short experience as nurse I had seen how ill-fitted most graduate nurses were to take care of children. They were harsh and domineering and lacked understanding. My own childhood had been made hideous by these things, but it had also filled me with sympathy for children. I had much more patience with them than with grown-ups. Their dependence, aggravated by illness, always moved me deeply. I wanted not merely to give them affection, but to equip myself for their care.[25]

In addition to enjoying her nursing program, Goldman also delighted in Vienna's cultural offerings, reading Nietzsche and attending lectures by the young Sigmund Freud. But she later gave conflicting accounts as to whether she had graduated from Allegemeines Krankenhaus. In her 1931 autobiography, she reported that in 1896 she became the "proud holder of two diplomas, one for midwifery and one for nursing." She later confided to Lillian Wald, however, that she had been arrested and unable to graduate, but there is no evidence she experienced legal difficulties in Vienna.[26]

On her return to New York in 1896, Goldman practiced nursing on the Lower East Side of Manhattan for the next ten years. In the late 1890s she briefly tried to fulfill a childhood dream of becoming a physician. She enrolled in medical school in Switzerland, but she found that her program of study interfered too much with her political work. Because Goldman attended class irregularly, the patron paying her tuition stopped sending her funds and she dropped out and returned to the United States.[27]

"E. G. Smith, Trained Nurse"

Goldman settled into a routine, accepting cases as a midwife, private duty nurse, and surgical assistant on call to the physician who had mentored her at Blackwell's Island. But she made no effort to participate in the growing nurses' professionalization movement, probably because of her antistatist beliefs. Nursing provided Goldman with important rewards. First, like the workers and disenfranchised with whom she identified, she made sure that others knew that she, too, needed to labor to support herself. Second, nursing provided a way to earn a living without compromising her anarchist philosophical beliefs. This represented a significant dilemma for many anarchists. Unless they came to anarchism independently wealthy, they were forced to seek employment. Yet if they wanted to remain true to their anarchist principles, they needed to avoid exploiting workers or directly participating in a capitalistic economic system. Nursing allowed Goldman to sidestep this ideological predicament.[28]

Goldman took her profession seriously, and her nursing identity suffuses her autobiography *Living My Life*. In this memoir she mentioned how on at least one occasion she postponed an important political engagement to care for a patient she felt she could not leave.[29] She wrote poignantly of the challenges of tuberculosis nursing and of caring for a morphine-addicted madam who operated a notorious brothel. She accepted the latter case reluctantly, but out of necessity. The irregular employment that all private duty nurses faced during this period frustrated Goldman.[30] But Goldman was at an even greater disadvantage than many of her colleagues when it came to procuring work. Private duty nurses often relied on contacts from their training schools for cases. Having trained abroad, Goldman's only referral base came from physicians sympathetic to her cause.

The high maternal mortality she observed in her midwifery practice made the most memorable impression on Goldman during her nursing years. It also contributed to her growing feminist impulse: "In a two-room flat on Houston Street, on the sixth floor of a tenement-house, I found three children asleep and the woman writhing in labour pains. There was no gas-jet, only a kerosene lamp, over which I had to heat the water. . . . Incredible poverty oozed from every corner."[31]

Disheartened that physicians increasingly controlled obstetrical services in the United States, Goldman lamented: "My profession of midwife was not very lucrative, only the poorest of the foreign element resorting to such services. Those who had risen in the scale of material Americanism lost their native diffidence together with many other original traits. Like the American women they, too, would be confined only by doctors."[32] The problems encountered by indigent women struggling through repeated pregnancies frustrated her: "After such confinements I would return home sick and distressed, hating the men responsible for the frightful condition of their wives and children, hating myself most of all because I did not know how to help them." But she hesitated to perform abortions no matter how much she sympathized with their plight:

> I could not prevail upon myself to perform the much-coveted operation. I lacked faith in my skill and I remembered my Vienna professor who had often demonstrated to us the terrible results of abortion. He held that even when such practices prove successful, they undermine the health of the patient. I would not undertake the task. It was not any moral consideration for the sanctity of life; a life unwanted and forced into abject poverty did not seem sacred to me. But my interests embraced the entire social problem, not merely a single aspect of it, and I would not jeopardize my freedom for that one part of the human struggle. I refused to perform abortions and I knew no methods to prevent conception.[33]

Like other nurses, Goldman sometimes grew annoyed when families interfered with her nursing judgment, especially when their cultural practices clashed with her own beliefs and professional education grounded in the germ theory. In order to mitigate family members' influence, work as steadily as possible, and perhaps have more time for her political activities, she preferred night duty:

> The presence of relatives and their constant interference, much talking and weeping, and, above all, their horror of fresh air made day work most trying for me. "You wicked one!" an old lady once berated me for opening a window in the sick-room; "do you want to kill my child?" At night I had a free hand to give my patients the attention they needed. With the help of a book and a large pot of coffee, brewed by myself, the night hours passed quickly.[34]

That so few people could afford professional nursing care spurred Goldman's radical convictions. In her experience, the care of a trained nurse, no matter how sick or disabled the person, was usually not available to the indigent. For those people who could not afford to hire nurses, they constituted "luxuries indulged only in very serious illness," and as such, she believed she "had to find other ways of helping those poor people than by merely taking care of their sick."[35] But her nursing and midwifery practice grounded her in the day-to-day struggles of the impoverished and laboring classes. She credited her practice with furnishing an "excellent field for experience":

> It put me into intimate contact with the very people my ideal strove to help and emancipate. It brought me face to face with the living conditions of the workers, about which, until then, I had talked and written mostly from theory. Their squalid surroundings, the dull and inert submission to their lot, made me realize the

colossal work yet to be done to bring about the change our movement was struggling to achieve.³⁶

But Goldman's ability to earn her living as a professional nurse grew much more difficult after September 1901. Leon Czolgosz, a twenty-nine-year-old Polish immigrant and anarchy sympathizer, shot President William McKinley, claiming that Goldman inspired his actions. Goldman and other radicals came under extreme pressure to disavow Czolgosz's actions, and many did so.³⁷ Goldman not only refused to impugn his violent act, she stridently defended him. But she also confused and shocked a reporter when she professed that because the president was a "human being in need of assistance: in my professional capacity I would take care of McKinley if I were called upon to nurse him, though my sympathies were with Czolgosz." The juxtaposition of the caring nature of nursing and support for violence was so incongruent to the journalist that Goldman claimed it led to the following headline in a Chicago newspaper: "EMMA GOLDMAN WANTS TO NURSE PRESIDENT; SYMPATHIES ARE WITH SLAYER."³⁸

McKinley lingered for eight days before his death, after which authorities arrested a defiant Goldman and many other anarchist sympathizers. Although she was later released because there was insufficient evidence to charge her with complicity in McKinley's assassination, she felt her notoriety made it necessary for her to again use an alias, E. G. Smith³⁹:

> I gained one more proof that I had become a pariah. Several doctors I visited, men who had known me for years and who had always been entirely satisfied with my work as a nurse, were indignant that I had dared to call on them. Did I want to get their names in the papers or cause them trouble with the police? I was being shadowed by the authorities; how could I expect them to recommend me? Dr. White was more humane. He had never credited the stories connecting me with Czolgosz, he assured me; he was certain that I was incapable of murder. Still he could not employ me in his office. "Smith is an ordinary enough name," he said, "but how long do you suppose it will be before you are discovered? I cannot take the chance; it would mean my ruin."⁴⁰

Neighbors in her New York City apartment building reported that some knew the woman who lived on the fifth floor by the sign that hung outside the door, which read "E. G. Smith, Trained Nurse." Others called her Emma Goldman but believed she was a teacher.⁴¹ Goldman found it humorous and flattering when patients realized her true identity. For example, one young man she met through her political activities begged her to nurse his mother, who was very ill with pneumonia. Although he confided to Goldman that his mother was "violently antagonistic" to her political beliefs, Goldman accepted the case. After nursing the woman for three weeks, Goldman's care so impressed her patient that the woman fired her other nurses, retaining Goldman only. After the patient exclaimed to her son, "Miss Smith is a wonderful nurse," he reluctantly told her the truth about her nurse's identity: "Do you know who she really is? . . . it's the terrible Emma Goldman!" Shocked, the young man's mother exclaimed, "My God. . . . I hope you have not told her what I said about her." When the boy admitted that he had informed Goldman about her remarks, his mother burst out, "and she nursed me so fine? Oi, a wonderful nurse!"[42]

By 1905, however, Goldman admitted that she increasingly struggled with the "hard work, responsibility, and anxiety" of nursing.[43] She later acknowledged that "every rise in the temperature of my charges used to alarm me, and a death would upset me for weeks. In all my years of nursing I had never learned detachment or indifference to suffering."[44] When a manicurist friend offered to refer to her women who sought "facial and scalp massage," Goldman jumped at the opportunity. Not only was it less stressful, the work allowed her to devote more time to her latest enterprise, creating a magazine devoted to anarchist struggles. The first issue of *Mother Earth* debuted in March 1906. Successfully launching the magazine was the culmination of a dream, and Goldman left nursing to devote herself full time to its success.[45]

"I Am a Trained Nurse"

Although Goldman no longer actively practiced nursing, she still retained her nursing identity. In 1909 a train she was riding in California ran over a man, severing his legs. The *Los Angeles Times* reported that the "Queen of the anarchists" raced to the man's side. Using her petticoat to bind his stumps, she stopped his bleeding. Although he later died, hospital authorities publicly thanked her for her quick response and decisive action. When informed of hospital officials' gratitude, she linked nursing's caring features to her political philosophy: "That is my work. I believe in doing all in my power for my fellowman, that's all anarchy is."[46]

In the ensuing years Goldman continued writing and promoting her political beliefs. She was regularly arrested for engaging in political theater, which was sometimes linked to health activism, particularly on behalf of women and children. Remembering the women she cared for during her years as a midwife in New York, for example, she published birth control-related literature in *Mother Earth*. She lent support to nurse Margaret Sanger's crusade for women's control over procreation and was arrested in 1916 for distributing birth control literature.[47] In 1917, she and her old friend Alexander Berkman, who had been released from prison in 1906, were arrested for conspiring to obstruct the World War I draft effort. Goldman and Berkman came under suspicion at an inopportune moment. Fears that radicals might conspire to overthrow the government reduced any tolerance American leaders felt for anarchy. The profound xenophobia and a hunt for agitators was soon to be remembered as the "Red Scare."[48] Charged and convicted for antiwar activities under the newly enacted Espionage Act, Goldman and Berkman spent two years in prison and were deported to Russia in 1919.[49]

Goldman found Russia a bitter disappointment, arriving during a very turbulent period in the nation's history.[50] After the army forced Czar Nicholas II to abdicate, its leaders established a provisional government. Its authority was soon challenged by the Bolsheviks, a Marxist labor party faction. The year before Goldman and Berkman arrived, Vladimir Lenin dissolved the formal structures underpinning the provisional government and ushered in the Soviet era. Until 1923, however, when the Civil War ended, Bolshevik and anti-Bolshevik continued to fight one another for dominance.[51]

Although the new state was anticapitalist, Russia's formal autocratic structure offended her anarchist sensibilities. Shocked by the nation's repressiveness, many of her reactions were viewed through her American nurse's eyes. She expressed dismay, for example, that officials cared so little about the health of the nation's own people that she was not allowed to work as a nurse despite Russia's "ghastly hospitals, lack of medical supplies, [and] no adequate care of patients." The commissar of the Petrograd Board of Health, at first thrilled to learn of her availability because he believed he needed "several hundred American nurses," refused her services when she made her distaste for Soviet communism known.[52] Goldman left Russia after only a few years. Except for a brief trip to the United States in the 1930s to promote her autobiography, a visit Lillian Wald helped arrange because the U.S. government was reluctant to admit Goldman, she spent the rest of her life traveling and lecturing in Europe and Canada.[53] She died in Toronto in 1940 and was buried, at her request, in a cemetery in Chicago adjacent to the graves of the Haymarket defendants.

Over the subsequent generations, Goldman-related historical research abounded. Yet her nursing years are usually mentioned cursorily, and even her most thorough biographers tend to isolate Goldman's nursing and midwifery identity from her political persona.[54] But there is clear evidence in newspaper reports, letters, and *Living My Life* that Goldman herself did not.

It is important to remember that autobiographies are flawed historical documents. Often written long after particular occurrences, the past is usually analyzed reconstructed in ways that make them cohere logically into a narrative structure. Illogical or less than appealing impulses and actions can also be suppressed. But it is one of the few ways historical figures can speak for themselves, and thus, autobiographies do yield insight into the writer's motivations and thoughts.

It was important to Goldman that no one question her motives for her many public lectures and political actions. She wanted it to be clear that she was an anarchist because of her principles, not because of any monetary rewards her activities may have yielded. Until 1906, when the *Mother Earth* editorship became Goldman's full-time occupation, nursing allowed her to respond proudly to those who leveled the charge that she profited financially from anarchy: "I am a trained nurse. I support myself by my work."[55]

Goldman's words confirm that she linked her nursing experiences to the ongoing development of her political philosophy, activism, and sense of self. Not only was she proud that she could earn a living outside what she saw as the evils of capitalism, she valued nursing for the sense of community and connectivity she believed it encouraged, for helping her understand real world problems, and as a vehicle to translate political philosophy into meaningful, practical activism.

It is perhaps this interconnectedness of her personal and professional life that made Emma Goldman most similar to other nurses of her era. Although historians have tended to divide women's work into unpaid labor women performed in their roles as wives and mothers and that for which they received remuneration, recent scholarship suggests that women themselves did not necessarily sharply distinguish between these endeavors.[56] Neither did Goldman, who blurred the personal, professional, and political domains of her life. Her efforts to reshape the political and social context in which nurses' caregiving practices were situated both informed and were informed by her years as a practicing nurse and midwife in New York City and her lifelong self-definition as a nurse.

Cynthia Anne Connolly, PhD, RN
Associate Professor
University of Pennsylvania School of Nursing
427 Claire M. Fagin Hall
418 Curie Boulevard
Philadelphia, PA 19104–6096

Acknowledgments

I am very grateful to Karen Buhler-Wilkerson, PhD, RN, FAAN, professor emerita, University of Pennsylvania School of Nursing, and director emerita, Barbara Bates Center for the Study of the History of Nursing, for piquing my curiosity about Goldman and setting me on a path that resulted in uncovering this story.

Notes

1. Oz Frankel, "Whatever Happened to 'Red Emma'? Emma Goldman from Alien Rebel to American Icon?" *Journal of American History* 83 (December 1996): 903–42. Biographies of Goldman include Richard Drinnan, *Rebel in Paradise: A Biography of Emma Goldman* (Chicago: University of Chicago Press, 1961). A more recent biography is Alice Wexler's two-volume *Emma Goldman: An Intimate Life* (New York: Pantheon, 1984) and *Emma Goldman in Exile: From the Russian Revolution to the Spanish Civil War* (Boston: Beacon Press, 1989).

2. Wexler, *An Intimate Life*, 112.

3. Ibid., 27.

4. Ibid., 25, 33.

5. Walter Licht, *Industrializing America: The Nineteenth Century* (Baltimore: Johns Hopkins University Press, 1995), 133, 168–69 .

6. Ibid., 169; Bruce Nelson, *Beyond the Martyrs: A Social History of Chicago's Anarchists, 1870–1900* (New Brunswick, N.J.: Rutgers University Press, 1988).

7. Emma Goldman, "Anarchism: What It Really Stands For," in Goldman, *Anarchism and Other Essays* (Port Washington, N.Y.: Kennikat Press, 1910), 56.

8. Wexler, *An Intimate Life*, 10–13, 18–19; Emma Goldman, *Living My Life* (1934; reprint New York: AMS Press, 1970), 11, 59–60.

9. Goldman, *Living My Life*, 103–4.

10. Wexler, *An Intimate Life*, 72–73.

11. Goldman, *Living My Life*, 122–23; Wexler, *An Intimate Life*, 76.

12. John Duffy, *A History of Public Health in New York City, 1866–1966* (New York: Russell Sage), 182–83.

13. Goldman, *Living My Life*, 135–36.

14. *Daily Tribune*, September 4, 1875, *Docs of Bd. of Aldermen* 1 (January 3, 1876), part 1, 42–45, quoted in Duffy, *History of Public Health*, 187–88; Goldman, *Living My Life*, 137.

15. Goldman, *Living My Life*, 137.

16. Ibid., 22–23, 136, 143.

17. Ibid., 157, 161. In this era most nurses left hospital work after training and provided care for hire to people in their homes. The work was hard and employment irregular. Susan Reverby, *Ordered to Care: The Dilemma of American Nursing, 1850–1945* (Cambridge: Cambridge University Press, 1987), 95–103.

18. Lillian Wald, *The House on Henry Street* (New York: Henry Holt, 1915).

19. Doris Groshen Daniels, *Always a Sister: The Feminism of Lillian Wald* (New York: Feminist Press at City University of New York, 1989); Karen Buhler-Wilkerson, "Bringing Care to the People: Lillian Wald's Legacy to Public Health Nursing," *American Journal of Public Health* 83 (December 1993): 1778–86, Karen Buhler-Wilkerson, *No Place like Home: A History of Nursing and Home Care in the United States* (Baltimore: John Hopkins University Press, 2001).

20. Daniels, *Always a Sister*, 71; Blanche Wcisen Cook, "Female Support Networks and Political Activism: Lillian Wald, Crystal Eastman, Emma Goldman," *Chrysalis* 3 (1977): 43–61.

21. Goldman, *Living My Life*, 160.

22. Wald, *House on Henry Street*, 276.

23. Wexler, *An Intimate Life*, 84.

24. Goldman, *Living My Life*, 162; Katy Dawley, "Ideology and Self-Interest: Nursing, Medicine, and the Campaign to Eliminate the Midwife," *Nursing History Review* 9 (2001): 99–127.

25. Goldman, *Living My Life*, 170.

26. Ibid., 174; Emma Goldman to Lillian Wald, November 12, 1904, Goldman Collection, University of California, Berkeley, Reel 1.

27. Candace Falk, *Love, Anarchy, and Emma Goldman* (New York: Holt, Rinehart, 1984), 31–33; Goldman, *Living My Life*, 268–69.

28. Blaine McKinley, "'The Quagmires of Necessity': American Anarchists and Dilemmas of Vocation," *American Quarterly* 34 (Winter 1982): 505–23.

29. Goldman, *Living My Life*, 286.

30. Reverby, *Ordered to Care*, 95–103; Goldman, *Living My Life*, 283–86, 319.

31. Goldman, *Living My Life*, 184.

32. Ibid., 185.

33. Ibid., 186.

34. Ibid., 326–27.

35. Ibid., 326.

36. Ibid., 185.

37. Wexler, *An Intimate Life*, 104–9.

38. Goldman, *Living My Life*, 305–6.

39. Ibid., 318.

40. Ibid., 319.

41. "Berkman Will Lead New York Anarchists," *New York Times*, May 20, 1906, 2.

42. Goldman, *Living My Life*, 327. For another example of Goldman's reaction when a patient recognized her, see 284.

43. Ibid., 364.

44. Ibid., 365. For other instances in which Goldman comments on how emotionally taxing she found nursing, see 327, 337.

45. Wexler, *An Intimate Life*, 121–25; Falk, *Love, Anarchy and Emma Goldman*, 37.

46. "Uses Petticoat for Bandages: Woman Anarchist Plays Nurse at Santa Barbara," *Los Angeles Times*, March 4, 1909, II11.

47. The alliance between Goldman and Sanger became strained, partly because Goldman believed Sanger strayed from her radical roots and perhaps because neither was willing to cede leadership of the movement to the other. Wexler, *An Intimate Life*, 211–13.

48. William Preston, Jr., *Aliens and Dissenters: Federal Suppression of Radicals, 1903–1933* (Cambridge, Mass.: Harvard University Press, 1963).

49. Marriage to Kershner had offered no respite because he had been denaturalized in 1908. Wexler, *An Intimate Life*, 247–76.

50. Emma Goldman, *My Disillusionment in Russia* (New York: Doubleday, 1923); Emma Goldman, *My Further Disillusionment in Russia, by Emma Goldman; Being a Continuation of Miss Goldman's Experiences in Russia as given in "My Disillusionment in Russia"* (Garden City, N.Y.: Doubleday, 1924); Alice Wexler, *Emma Goldman in Exile: From the Russian Revolution to the Spanish Civil War* (Boston: Beacon Press, 1989).

51. Beryl Williams, *The Russian Revolution, 1917–1921* (Oxford: Blackwell, 1987).

52. Goldman, *Living My Life*, 778–79.

53. Emma Goldman to Lillian Wald, June 5, 1935, Goldman Collection, University of California, Berkeley, Reel 1.

54. Wexler, *An Intimate Life*, 112.

55. Miriam Michelson, "A Character Study of Emma Goldman," *Philadelphia North American*, April 11, 1901, reprinted in *Emma Goldman: A Documentary History of the American Years*, vol. 1, *Made for America, 1890–1901*, ed. Candace Falk, Barry Pateman, and Jessica M. Moran (Berkeley: University of California Press, 2003), 444.

56. Patricia D'Antonio, "Nurses—And Wives and Mothers," *Journal of Women's History* 19 (2007): 112–36.

Conflict and Compromise: Catholic and Public Hospital Partnerships

Barbra Mann Wall
University of Pennsylvania School of Nursing

Abstract. This article analyzes the tensions and uneasy negotiations, based on a case study, that occurred among Catholic sisters, administrators, bishops, physicians, and the Vatican for more than seven years at a hospital in Austin, Texas. Here, the largest health care system in the city, which was Catholic, joined with the local public, tax-supported hospital that provided the majority of reproductive health care services in the region. A clash resulted over whether the hospital could continue providing sterilization and contraceptive services to its primarily poor patients. This article examines the fierce debates that occurred, especially over emergency contraception and attempts to develop creative solutions after a hierarchical crackdown from the Vatican. The end result was a compromise that included the creation of a "hospital within a hospital."

On May 4, 1995, Charles J. Barnett, president and CEO of Seton Medical Center in Austin, Texas, announced an agreement between Seton, a Catholic facility owned and operated by the Daughters of Charity of St. Vincent DePaul, and the city manager of Austin, which owned Brackenridge Hospital. Seton would take full management and control of Brackenridge, a public facility that had primary responsibility to care for the medically indigent and that had accumulated a $61 million debt. The declared purpose of the transaction was to "ensure the continuation of essential health care services, including trauma, women's and reproductive services, and children' services, for all citizens of Austin and Travis County, regardless of their financial means."[1]

Under the agreement, Seton committed itself to pay $10 million up front and $2.2 million annually to lease Brackenridge buildings and consolidate services, which would result in Seton becoming the city's largest hospital system.[2] In turn, the city would pay Seton $5.6 million dollars annually for charity care provided at Brackenridge. This public/private partnership was not unusual; it was part of a trend toward overall consolidation in the hospital marketplace. What complicated it was that Seton had to adhere to the *Ethical and Religious Directives for Catholic Health Care Services*, developed by the U.S. Conference of Catholic Bishops (USCCB) in 1994, which banned direct involvement in reproductive services to which the Catholic Church morally objected. These services included contraception, sterilization, abortion, and infertility services such as in vitro fertilization and artificial insemination. The *Ethical and Religious Directives* did permit an indirect role in the delivery of some of these services, should a Catholic hospital affiliate with a non-Catholic institution.[3]

As a condition of the lease, Brackenridge insisted that its reproductive services be maintained, except for abortions, which had not been done in Brackenridge and were referred to an outside provider. Key to this agreement was that Brackenridge retain ownership of its facility and that Seton not identify Brackenridge as a Catholic institution. Because of this important stipulation, and after consultation with Catholic ethicists and theologians, the Daughters of Charity announced that, "in recognition of the community's need for reproductive services, those . . . that are currently available at Brackenridge will be retained." Seton Leader Letter, May 4, 2005.

The compromise agreement between Seton and Brackenridge served as a model for other consolidation efforts between religious and public hospitals. Between 1994 and 1999, 93 percent of mergers involving Catholic institutions were with secular partners. In 1998 alone, the Catholic Hospital Association (CHA) reported thirty-two such mergers and affiliations; other sources said the number was as high as forty-three.[4] The partnership between Seton and Brackenridge was a lease arrangement rather than a merger, but its saga can be viewed as a microcosm of the longstanding and complex debate over Catholic hospitals' involvement in reproductive health care services in the United States in the latter half of the twentieth century.[5] This article explores how activists from Seton and Brackenridge hospitals managed a controversy that ensued over the provision of reproductive services as a result of their partnership. The conflict of views and values involved all the aspects of the national debate, including the Vatican's direct involvement, intense deliberation over the provision of emergency contraception, and compromising attempts at solutions.

The Vatican Context

The Catholic Church was and is a major stakeholder in the health care field and exerts enormous influence on the shape of American health care. More than 600 Catholic hospitals function in forty-seven states, with one in six hospital patients cared for in a Catholic hospital.[6] Seton Medical Center was part of the Daughters of Charity National Health System (DCNHS),[7] which had a long history of nursing and managing successful hospitals in Austin and throughout the nation. Indeed, a unique characteristic of Catholic health care in the United States was its establishment, administration, and nursing by dedicated and talented religious women.[8] Yet Catholic sister nurses faced new challenges over the course of the twentieth century as a result of greater restrictions from Rome and increasing secularization of society.

The Daughters of Charity were profoundly influenced by the Second Vatican Council (Vatican II), which met from 1962 to 1965 and emphasized social justice and human dignity.[9] The Daughters held meetings during which they redefined their governance and ministry and renewed their commitment to the poor and oppressed. An essay by James L. Connor, S.J., described the change in the sisters' ministry emphasis: They no longer saw themselves as bringing students and patients into the nuns' world but saw themselves rather as "entering into *their* world, to share *their* experience" (emphasis original). Yet this change in ministry focus was not easy to achieve.[10] After Pope John Paul II was elected in 1978, the hierarchical model of the church made a comeback and replaced the more collegial model that had emerged after Vatican II.[11] By the 1970s, vocations to women's religious congregations were rapidly declining, and the Catholic Church increasingly relied on lay participation. Secular influences at Seton grew through the appointment of lay administrators, nursing supervisors, and trustees. These lay leaders, along with the Daughters of Charity, played a significant part in the Seton-Brackenridge partnership debates.

In addition, in cases where a Catholic facility sought affiliation with a non-Catholic institution, it had to ask the local bishop for approval. Thus, the Daughters of Charity had to consult with the bishop in Austin, who usually was not involved in hospital policy decisions in the independently owned and operated DCNHS. As a bishop, it was his responsibility to communicate directly with the Vatican's Congregation for the Doctrine of the Faith, which was responsible for ensuring that Catholic teachings were implemented in all church facilities. The USCCB also stepped into the fray. Initially founded as the National Conference of Catholic Bishops in 1966 as a church policy-making body in the United States, it is composed of all members of the Roman Catholic hierarchy; its work includes rulings on the issues of abortion and reproductive services in Catholic hospitals.

It is important to note that three decades had passed since Pope Paul VI's 1968 encyclical, *Humanae Vitae*, reiterated the Catholic Church's stance against birth control. The encyclical caused a serious divide between church hierarchy and laity and split the Catholic clergy.[12] By the early 1990s, abortion, which had always been a divisive issue, again became politicized as President Bill Clinton included reproductive care in his health plan. Opponents and the small but powerful Christian Coalition came out against the health plan and included family planning in the abortion debate. Particularly disconcerting to supporters of family planning was the growing elimination of reproductive health services when Catholic hospitals merged or partnered with secular hospitals.[13] This was especially important because the Catholic Church was the nation's largest group of not-for-profit health care sponsors, systems, and facilities. Thus, women's rights activists in Austin joined the Brackenridge discussion and insisted on being part of the decision-making process.

Austin Health Care Context

The Daughters of Charity established Seton Hospital in 1902 with a special concern for the sick and poor. Their history began in 1633, when the order was founded in France by Vincent de Paul and Louise de Marillac to serve those most in need and abandoned. Brackenridge, too, had a commitment of community service to the poor. Established in 1884, it was the oldest public hospital in Texas, and in 1995 it had the city's only trauma center and only graduate medical education program. The city also owned Children's Hospital of Austin. Losing all these services would mean a significant loss to the community.

Brackenridge Hospital's longstanding financial problems came to a head in 1995.[14] Realizing that it could not survive as a stand-alone hospital, its administrator asked the Daughters of Charity to submit a proposal describing how Seton might assist the city's operation of Brackenridge and Children's Hospital to place these facilities in a better position to compete in the Austin marketplace. The active involvement of the huge Columbia/Hospital Corporation of America (HCA) chain, the nation's largest for-profit hospital group in the country, had changed the health care landscape in Austin when it took over four of the other previously independent full-service hospitals in the area. Columbia/HCA owned nearby Round Rock Hospital and South Austin Medical Center; it partnered with the Austin Diagnostic Medical Center that was under construction; and it was in the process of solidifying a partnership with St. David's Medical Center, originally affiliated with the Episcopal Church. In the face of these changes, the Daughters of Charity and the City of Austin as owner of Brackenridge agreed that some form of consolidation was mandatory for the survival of both hospitals. Indeed, it was projected that Seton's payments to Brackenridge more than thirty years would allow the city to pay its hospital debts and leave a $38 million balance.[15]

Two national studies gave reason for concern should Brackenridge close its doors. One reported that eighty-six hospitals in twenty-two states had been cited by the government for refusing to treat emergency indigent patients for nonmedical reasons in 1993 and early 1994.[16] The other examined the impact of a public hospital's closing on access to health care in California. A significant number of uninsured patients were denied access to care at other facilities, and the closing was associated with a decline in their health status.[17] Most important, then, the partnership between Seton and Brackenridge would continue the safety net function to the medically indigent, a function long embraced by both institutions.

Still, some citizens were concerned that a private hospital's management of Brackenridge would remove it from public scrutiny. One member of Brackenridge's Advisory Board lamented, "When you can do things behind closed doors—you can decide who gets care and who doesn't—I assume the worst is going to happen." In addition, 520 Brackenridge employees had signed a petition opposing the lease. They wanted to remain city employees, and they believed that the city had not sufficiently explored alternative funding. City Manager Jesus Garza admitted that Seton's management of Brackenridge would remove it from public accountability. To solve this problem, the city council appointed a board to oversee Seton's responsibility for the city's indigent health care programs.[18]

Material Cooperation

After the city council approved the lease in May 1995, final acceptance had to come from the Seton Board of Trustees and its parent organization, the DCNHS, to whom Seton's religious and lay administrators and trustees were ultimately responsible. Prior to any final decision and public announcement, however, the Daughters of Charity, Seton's lay leaders, and the bishop consulted with four medical ethicists and Monsignor William Broussard, executive director of the Texas Conference of Catholic Health Facilities and vicar general for the Diocese of Austin, to ensure that the lease arrangement was in compliance with the *Ethical and Religious Directives*.[19] The Daughters in St. Louis questioned Monsignor Broussard about the challenges an agreement between a Catholic and non-Catholic hospital would bring. Noting his consultation with canon and civil lawyers, he replied, "First, they felt that a lease arrangement would not mean ownership in the strict sense." Instead, ownership would remain with Brackenridge. Second, "a lease arrangement does not give the facility a Catholic identity, but rather gives the lessee certain rights and privileges."[20]

Broussard and Rev. Gerard Magill, a theology professor and ethicist at St. Louis University, prepared a position paper analyzing the Seton/Brackenridge partnership from the perspective of church teachings and ethical principles. The paper circulated among area clergy and other interested persons to help prevent the possibility of scandal. It built on the Catholic tradition of social justice and the *Ethical and Religious Directives*. Specifically, Directive 69 stated that Catholic institutions could participate in networking arrangements that included cooperating, in a limited way, with the provision of services such as sterilization that Catholic teaching prohibited, although this did not include abortion (Directive 45).[21] The *Ethical and Religious Directives* justified the principle of "material cooperation," and this principle was used to clarify Seton's position. Material cooperation "permits a person to cooperate in some way in a wrong procedure," ethicist David F. Kelly argues. It does not excuse wrongdoing but enables limited cooperation with other parties who engage in wrongful acts as long as certain conditions are met. Had the Daughters of Charity at Seton agreed with the idea of reproductive services as morally right, and had they intended to be active in providing them, then they would be guilty of formal cooperation. Formal cooperation, which was always wrong, involved the cooperator desiring that the wrong act be performed. Kelly continues, "But all of us are at one time or another caught up in some form of cooperation with actions we consider morally wrong." Catholic tradition says that "material cooperation is morally right . . . if the good effects to be realized . . . outweigh the bad effects."[22] Thus, when Magill wrote about Seton's situation, he argued, "The act of cooperation is justified when it occurs to achieve *a greater good or to avoid a more serious evil*" (emphasis original). In Seton's case, the more serious evil was the closing of the hospital and the resulting lack of health care to the poor. Specifically, "not doing good could be a serious dereliction of moral duty" by "forfeiting the valuable contribution of Brackenridge's health care to the community." The greater good was that Seton could "extend its mission and values in the community . . . , continue its provision of indigent care," protect "its witness to pro-life values . . . and maintain and strengthen its position in the health care market."[23]

Magill emphasized that because the Daughters of Charity and Seton Medical Center did not approve of the illicit procedures or want them to take place, "there is no formal cooperation." This was also where Brackenridge's designation as a non-Catholic facility was emphasized, in that the lease agreement stated that the city retained "reserved powers over Brackenridge." As Magill pointed out, it was very important to "clearly establish that Brackenridge is a non-Catholic hospital." Furthermore, those performing the services considered illicit would not be Seton employees.[24]

The Controversy

It was the responsibility of Austin's Bishop John McCarthy to approve the partnership because it involved a Catholic and non-Catholic partnership in his diocese. Considered one of the nation's more moderate bishops, McCarthy had long been an activist for working men and women, dating back to the 1950s and 1960s when he became involved in the labor movement. As part of his fight for social justice, he participated in the Civil Rights march in Selma, Alabama, in 1965.[25] When faced with the problem of whether the poor in Austin would receive care, his and the Daughters' stance was predictable. They believed that the hospital could not survive alone against the growing power of the four Columbia/HCA hospitals, which would underbid Seton for services. Seton would then lose patients and would be forced to close.[26] A partnership with Brackenridge was especially needed; otherwise, the for-profit Columbia/HCA group would become the major player in the Austin hospital marketplace. To Bishop McCarthy and the Daughters of Charity, this meant that the poor would not get the care they needed, because one could not assume that Columbia/HCA would be willing to provide the kind of care Seton did. The St. David's contract with Columbia/HCA retained the right to make some provisions for the poor, but that area was still under negotiation at the time. In May 1995, Bishop McCarthy wrote Sister Patricia Elder, D.C., Chair of Seton's Board of Trustees, that pending final review of the document, he supported the lease arrangement, justifying it on the principle of material cooperation. This would maintain the church's commitment to the poverty-stricken people of central Texas and ensure the survival of Seton Hospital.[27]

Despite consultation with ethicists, Catholic theologians, and other health care providers, the Seton/Brackenridge partnership was the beginning of a long battle between the Daughters of Charity, lay Seton leaders, and Bishop McCarthy on the one hand, and the Vatican and conservative Austin laity on the other. On May 17, 1995, before the agreement was finalized by the regional and national boards of the Daughters of Charity, a group calling itself Concerned Catholics of Austin wrote to the Vatican. Using the conservative Saint Joseph Foundation in San Antonio as intermediary, the group complained that the Daughters were cooperating in abortions in their hospital.[28] Specifically, the group sent a letter to Cardinal Joseph Ratzinger, head of the Vatican's Congregation for the Doctrine of the Faith. This agency's role included investigating any action or publication that seemed contradictory to the faith, asking the authors of such acts or writings for an explanation and reproving them if satisfaction was not reached.[29] In June 1995, Archbishop Tarcisio Bertone, representative of the Congregation for the Doctrine of the Faith, wrote Bishop McCarthy, challenging the proposed agreement and asking the bishop not to sign the contract. In July, McCarthy aggressively defended Seton's position and provided the Vatican with background information on the proposed lease. But several months elapsed between his letter and the Vatican's response in March 1996. The bishop "assumed that silence meant consent" and signed the lease in October 1995.[30]

On at least two occasions in 1997, the Vatican instructed the bishop and the Daughters to stop all sterilizations and contraceptive programs at Brackenridge. McCarthy and the Daughters again commissioned canon lawyers, ethicists, and health care representatives and asked for more time to study the situation. In all his correspondence with the Vatican, McCarthy was unsuccessful in convincing it that the city of Austin owned Brackenridge and that it was not a Catholic hospital. City officials had reserved this right and placed conditions in the agreement that reproductive services would be continued. Any breach of the contract would subject Seton to a multimillion-dollar fine. But the Vatican argued that the lease agreement did not meet the tenets of Catholic moral teaching and that formal rather than material cooperation existed.[31] In June 1998, Bishop McCarthy went to Rome, where Cardinal Ratzinger asked for more detailed information about the lease. By then, the controversy was making front-page headlines in Austin.

On July 30 a story appeared in the *Austin American Statesman* that discussed the issues over the past three years. In it, Bishop McCarthy asserted that helping the poor was a "cornerstone of the Catholic faith. . . . We are not trying to expand our hospital empire. We don't think of health care as a business. . . . We are trying to protect health care for the poor." In the same article, Patricia Hayes, Seton's chief operating officer, highlighted Seton's commitment to the Austin community. The Daughters of Charity had hired Hayes in the late 1990s after she had served as the first woman and second lay president of St. Edward's University for fourteen years. With a doctorate in philosophy from Georgetown University, this powerful woman had vast experience in dealing with the public, including having been chair of Austin's United Way and the Greater

Austin Chamber of Commerce. In the article, she compared the amount of charity care Seton was able to provide both before and after the lease agreement with Brackenridge. In the fiscal year ending June 30, 1998, Seton had delivered $17 million in charity health care, while the projection for fiscal 1999 was $50 million. Thus, she asserted, "Seton would never break the lease."[32]

On the day this newspaper article was published, Hayes wrote to Seton's Board of Trustees that the hospital remained in compliance with the lease agreement, and all services, including reproductive, remained available at Brackenridge. She clarified that the dialogue between Bishop McCarthy and the Vatican "was a private, internal discussion within the Church, to which Seton was not a party."[33] Still, it was an example of similar dialogues going on in many communities, and bishops nationwide closely watched the Austin case. The outcome could determine how much discretion they would have in matters as more Catholic hospitals allied with secular facilities. A DCNHS official noted that failure to maintain their position would influence their work with public hospitals throughout the country.[34]

The language used in an article in *The Wanderer*, a conservative Catholic publication, was scathing. It accused the bishop of deceiving the Vatican and presenting "a dismal portrait of episcopal solicitude for the poor and the degeneration of Catholic social teaching." Furthermore, "McCarthy showed that his view of the poor is apparently Sangerite," referring to Margaret Sanger's advocacy for birth control.[35]

To counter this criticism, an *Austin American Statesman* editorial on July 31, 1998, called for community support for Bishop McCarthy. It provided further insight into his standoff with the Vatican:

> One of the highlights of the tenure of McCarthy, a warmly regarded local leader, has been his insistence that diocesan social programs be managed at the parish level. Were the Vatican willing to confer a comparable amount of local autonomy and cease micromanaging operations at a distant hospital, a local crisis would subside.[36]

"A Wall of Separation"

If the Vatican determined that Seton did not conform to Catholic moral teaching, the hospital would be at risk of losing church sponsorship for its facilities. Thus, through 1998 the Daughters of Charity, Bishop McCarthy, lay Seton officials, and the city of Austin worked on a deal to amend the contract. In August, Patricia Hayes was quoted in the *Austin American Statesman* that a new agreement for sterilizations and reproductive services had been negotiated that created "a wall of separation" between Seton and the services the church deemed sinful.[37] This involved employees of the city-county health department providing family planning and counseling services and independent practitioners, rather than Seton employees, performing surgical sterilizations. Hayes noted, "We feel this firewall that is important to us—and has been important from the beginning—is even stronger." To pay for the outside services, the city reduced its annual payment to Seton for indigent care at Brackenridge. This deduction from the indigent care money made it clear that Seton was not paying for city offices and services inside the hospital.

Although reproductive services continued at Brackenridge, women's activists from Planned Parenthood and the Texas Family Planning Association, who had been consulted in the original agreement, were angry because they were not informed of the renegotiations. "I know there is pressure from the Vatican," said the executive director of Planned Parenthood, "but once again it is this stuff behind closed doors that makes you feel very uneasy."[38] The executive director of the Texas Family Planning Association stated, "I have a huge problem with the separation of church and state in this particular arrangement."[39]

The new compromise to allow city employees to do the proscribed practices remained in effect until 2001, when the USCCB revised the *Ethical and Religious Directives* to prohibit the very solution created at Brackenridge. This move began in 2000, when, with Seton's situation in the forefront, the Vatican's Congregation for the Doctrine of the Faith ordered American bishops to change the *Ethical and Religious Directives* concerning mergers and partnerships with non-Catholic facilities. Material cooperation could not be used as justification for sterilization and other procedures. Because Seton had implemented its lease, five other similar collaborations involving Catholic hospitals had taken place in the United States. Under Vatican pressure, two such alliances had ended their agreements, one in New Jersey and one in Arkansas.[40] Seton officials remained optimistic, however. Hayes thought it premature to speculate on what changes might occur at Seton. But Frances Kissling of Catholics for a Free Choice (CFFC), a group based in Washington, D.C., that worked to decriminalize abortion and contraception, was more pessimistic. The *Austin American Statesman* quoted her: "As long as sterilizations take place in that building . . . it is not going to pass muster with the Vatican."[41]

In 2000, Pope John Paul II appointed a new bishop, Gregory Aymond, to succeed McCarthy on his retirement. The more conservative Aymond was known for his support of Vatican teachings, and he was the representative to the USCCB meeting in 2001 when the bishops developed new *Ethical and Religious Directives*. They voted overwhelmingly to tighten the reins on Catholic hospitals; their main focus was Part Six, "Forming New Partnerships with Health Care Organizations and Providers." Specifically, a new Directive 70 forbade Catholic health care organizations from engaging "in immediate material cooperation in actions that are intrinsically immoral, such as abortion, euthanasia, assisted suicide, and direct sterilization."[42] Some theologians and ethicists objected to the new *Ethical and Religious Directives*. According to Kelly, this ecclesiastical decree usurped any "right use of reason" in applying principles of moral teaching. "Perhaps the intention here is to enforce a disciplinary rule in Catholic hospitals," he asserted, "rather than to suggest a change in the underlying moral teaching about material cooperation."[43] Bishop Aymond had a different view. To him, the new *Ethical and Religious Directives* provided "an opportunity to teach strongly about the respect for human life and also our belief in the sacredness of marriage and sexuality. I feel very positive that the *Directives* have been clarified."[44]

Not "*If* Reproductive Services Remain Available, But *How*"

The new *Directives* forced the Daughters of Charity to renegotiate again with the city of Austin. On June 8, 2001, Seton announced that, to comply with church teachings, it could no longer allow sterilizations and other contraceptive services to be provided at Brackenridge, even by city employees. In a press conference that day, Mayor Kirk Watson was adamant that reproductive services would still be available to Austin citizens, regardless of ability to pay. "The question isn't *if* reproductive services remain available, but *how*," he said (emphasis original).[45] After considering several options, the city proposed to create "a hospital within a hospital" system, whereby the city would operate a separately licensed hospital on Brackenridge's fifth floor. A second entity, either the city or another health organization, would be licensed to handle the reproductive services.[46] The separate floor would handle all sterilization and contraceptive services. It also would house a labor and delivery area for low-income women who wanted to have their babies there for ready access to sterilization, rather than in Brackenridge's labor and delivery department.

Women's health activists did not want to see sterilizations moved from Brackenridge, preferring a seamless transition between delivery and the sterilization option. Rosemary Mirriam, a spokeswoman for the Women's Health and Family Planning Association of Texas, saw this as "a discrimination issue. We're talking about low-income, uninsured women. They don't have a choice."

To further complicate matters, Seton announced that emergency contraception (EC) would be allowed, either in its own emergency room or on the fifth floor, but only if a test proved that the woman was not ovulating at the time. Advocates for women's health wanted Brackenridge to provide the medicine to women on request. They viewed Seton's restrictions as placing the services out of reach of the women who most needed them.[47]

Seton's actions regarding EC were in compliance with the 2001 Directive 36, which permitted Catholic hospitals to provide EC after a woman was sexually assaulted "if, after appropriate testing, there is no evidence that conception has occurred already."[48] But Seton was in the minority in providing EC, even with restrictions, compared to other Catholic facilities. In a 1999 CFFC national survey of 589 such institutions, 82 percent said they did not provide EC at all, even if a woman had been sexually assaulted. And only 22 percent of those providing no EC made any referrals for such.[49]

Four more months of negotiation brought a coalition of community groups together. A compromise resulted on the "hospital within a hospital" plan that involved Seton paying for remodeling the fifth floor, which would have its own pharmacy, medical records area, nursing unit, housekeeping, and separate elevator. Seton also agreed to pay approximately $500,000 less a year on its annual lease to Brackenridge, and it allowed EC to be provided on the fifth floor, but only to women who were sexually assaulted. It agreed to refer to a city clinic any woman requesting EC without being raped, but that meant that indigent women seeking this service would have to go elsewhere rather than the public hospital.[50] The city council approved the measure, and the Vatican had no problem with the "hospital within a hospital" system.[51]

Still, women's rights activists protested. Lesley Ramsey, vice president of Austin's National Organization for Women chapter, had concerns but believed that "realistically, it's the best offer we're going to get." Just before the final agreement was announced in 2001, her organization and another women's advocacy group, the Democracy Coalition, had sponsored a town hall meeting on the Brackenridge issue. Many attendees objected to a church organization running a public hospital. They planned a protest march that would start at Brackenridge and end at the Catholic Diocesan Office a few blocks away. A member of the Democracy Coalition noted that "moving reproductive services to a separate floor suggests something is wrong. . . . Seamlessness works great in a bra, but it does not work well in a hospital situation."[52] One letter in a local newspaper, however, defended the Daughters of Charity, stating, "Without Seton and its Catholic values, low-income citizens of Austin would have nowhere to turn for emergency medical treatment. . . . No organization should be condemned for following its conscience."[53]

The DCNHS succeeded in putting Brackenridge in the black, largely because of its many resources and its level of philanthropy. It was easier to absorb charity care across a large system. And Brackenridge provided most of the city's care to the poor. According to one newspaper account, Seton and Brackenridge together accounted for more than 60 percent of the entire system's charitable care and 80 percent of its Medicaid billings. "Seton gave 10 cents of every dollar it took in to charity last year and will report more than $41 million in charity care for 1998, significantly more than its rival, St. David's." In return, millions of Medicare reimbursements went to Seton, as well as money from the city's medical assistance programs for the indigent, which St. David's did not get.[54] Activists for women's reproductive rights called the 2001 *Ethical and Religious Directives* "just another example of the challenges of allowing faith-based institutions—especially the Catholic Church—to deal with public medicine."[55] Frances Kissling from CFFC questioned Catholic hospitals' acceptance of federal Medicaid reimbursements and then denying legal and publicly supported reproductive services.[56] In the end, however, Seton became the region's largest community service organization, including the home of a Level II Trauma Center, pediatric facility, and teaching hospital.

Conclusion

This study illustrates the growing influence of the Catholic Church in the hospital marketplace and the increased centralization of power in the Vatican that is a legacy of Pope John Paul II, with all its rulings on the provision of reproductive services. Important to this discussion is that Cardinal Joseph Ratzinger, who played such a large role in the Seton/Brackenridge controversy, is now Pope Benedict XVI. As the Daughters of Charity attempted to be a safety net provider to residents in Austin, they were challenged to succeed in an increasingly competitive and performance-oriented environment. The decision to create a "hospital within a hospital" system was not easy for them or for the other church and hospital officials who took criticism from both sides of the reproductive question. Reflecting on the issue in a recent interview, Bishop McCarthy, who had battled the Vatican for six years, stated, "When the right wing Catholics and the left wing pro-choicers are both against you—then you know you're doing something right!"[57]

The Daughters of Charity experienced a conflict of conscience over the field of reproductive services. They were committed to care of the poor, but like all Catholic hospitals they had to base their actions on the *Ethical and Religious Directives*, developed by U.S. bishops with approval from the Vatican. Indeed, adherence to them was a matter of survival, as the Daughters could not afford to lose Catholic sponsorship. In the end, they responded to a hardening of the Vatican's opposition to reproductive services with an innovative compromise. It was not a case of Catholic sister nurses alone confronting hierarchical authority; rather, it involved multiple stakeholders. What the Daughters of Charity and the city of Austin especially needed to maintain their partnership while adhering to Catholic Church policies was strong leadership at the board and management levels of each hospital, a clear understanding of the benefits of the partnership, and an aggressive pursuit of key goals, especially the provision of health care to all Austin's people, including the indigent.[58]

In closing, half the mergers or partnerships between Catholic and non-Catholic facilities resulted in the limitation or discontinuation of reproductive health services, and more than 80 percent denied emergency contraception even to women who had been sexually assaulted.[59] These figures highlight the importance of the compromise between the Daughters of Charity and the city of Austin, because the "hospital within a hospital" solution was not what most Catholic hospitals were doing. Still, the issue of provision of reproductive services caused conflict among many groups. Whereas the Daughters found themselves at odds with the Catholic Church's newest directives proscribing such services, women's activists thought the compromise was too limited, and they accused Catholic bishops of politicizing their hospitals. Conservative Catholic advocates were unhappy that the services were offered at all. The Vatican thought the Daughters were bending church doctrine too far and initially ordered them to cease the services altogether. The outcome, however, did permit some reproductive services to continue, and it allowed the Daughters of Charity to claim that they did not abandon their mission to the poor. To them, this served as an example of their willingness to work on compromise solutions.[60] Yet, the Daughters' delicate balancing of the Vatican's demands with their own social and religious mission continues.

BARBRA MANN WALL, PHD, RN
Associate Professor and Associate Director
Barbara Bates Center for the Study of the History of Nursing
University of Pennsylvania School of Nursing
418 Curie Blvd.
Fagin Hall, #2016
Philadelphia, PA 19146

Acknowledgments

The author thanks the Daughters of Charity, West Central Province, St. Louis, Missouri, for the use of their archives, and Carol Prietto, archivist; Bishop John McCarthy; the Catholic Archives of Texas; and the Austin History Center. The author also acknowledges the following sources of funding: a University of Pennsylvania University Research Foundation Grant; the Trustee Council for Penn Women Award; a Fichter Grant from the Association for the Sociology of Religion; and an American Association for the History of Nursing H15 Grant for Historical Research. Funding for this "Scholarly Works" project also was made possible by grant 1G13 IM009691–01 from the National Library of Medicine, NIH, DHHS. The views expressed in any written publication or other media do not necessarily reflect the official policies of the Department of Health and Human Services; nor does mention by trade names, commercial practices, or organizations imply endorsement by the U.S. government.

Notes

1. Charles J. Barnett, Memo, May 4, 1995; *Seton Leader Letter*, Seton Network Special Issue, May 4, 1995, Austin History Center, Austin, Texas (hereafter AHC).

2. Charles J. Barnett to David B. Coats, January 13, 1995; Memo, January 19, 1995; Charles J. Barnett to David B. Coats and Jesus Garza, January 31, 1995; Memorandum to Mayor and Council Members from Jesus Garza, City Manager, May 3, 1995, AHC.

3. United States Conference of Catholic Bishops (USCCB), *Ethical and Religious Directives for Catholic Health Care Services* (Washington, D.C.: USCCB, 1994). See also Kevin O'Rourke, Thomas Kopfensteiner, and Ron Hamel, "A Brief History," *Health Progress* 82, no. 6 (November–December 2001): n.p.; Rachel Benson Gold, "Hierarchy Crackdown Clouds Future of Sterilization, EC Provision at Catholic Hospitals," *Guttmacher Report on Public Policy* 5, no. 2 (May 2002), accessed December 30, 2007, at http://www.guttmacher.org/pubs/tgr/05/2/gr050211.html. The Alan Guttmacher Institute is a New York-based think tank on reproductive issues.

4. Liz Bucar, "Caution: Catholic Health Restrictions May Be Hazardous to Your Health" (Washington, D.C.: Catholics for a Free Choice, 1999); Deanna Bellandi, "CHA Counterattacks Study on Mergers," *Modern Healthcare* 29, no. 19 (May 10, 1999): 14; "Report of the Task Force on Ethical and Religious Directives," *Linacre Quarterly* (May 2005): 174.

5. Gold, "Hierarchy Crackdown."

6. Catholic Health Association, 2007, accessed December 30, 2007, at http://www.chausa.org/Pub/MainNav/AboutCHA/whoweare/

7. In 1998, the DCNHS ranked among the top five hospital systems nationally.

8. Barbra Mann Wall, *Unlikely Entrepreneurs: Catholic Sisters and the Hospital Marketplace, 1865–1925* (Columbus: Ohio State University Press, 2005).

9. *Gaudium et Spes*, the Pastoral Constitution on the Church in the Modern World, renewed Catholic commitment to social justice. See R. Scott Appleby, "Priesthood Reformed: Experiments in Parochial Presence, 1962–1972," in *Transforming Parish Ministry: The Changing Roles of Catholic Clergy, Laity, and Women Religious*, eds. Jay P. Dolan, R. Scott Appleby, Patricia Byrne, and Debra Campbell (New York: Crossroad, 1990).

10. Quotation noted in Patricia Byrne, "A Tumultuous Decade, 1960–1979," in ibid., 182.

11. Jay P. Dolan, *In Search of An American Catholicism: A History of Religion and Culture in Tension* (New York: Oxford University Press, 2002).

12. Leslie Woodcock Tentler, *Catholics and Contraception: An American History* (Ithaca, N.Y.: Cornell University Press, 2004). See also *Humanae Vitae*, Encyclical of Pope Paul VI on the Regulation of Birth (1968), accessed January 15, 2008, at http://www.vatican.va/holy_father/paul_vi/encyclicals/documents/hf_p-vi_enc_25071968_humanae-vitae_en.html; and *Casti Connubii*, Encyclical of Pope Pius XI on Christian Marriage (1930) at http://www.vatican.va/holy_father/pius_xi/encyclicals/documents/hf_p-xi_enc_31121930_casti-connubii_en.html

13. Rachel Benson Gold, "Contraceptive Coverage: Toward Ensuring Access While Respecting Conscience," *Guttmacher Report on Public Policy* 1, no. 6 (December 1998), accessed August 23, 2007, at http://www.guttmacher.org/pubs/tgr/01/6/gr010601.html; Gloria Feldt, "Congress Is Foiling Americans' Desire for Reproductive Choice," *USA Today* (May 1999); "Baby Boom: American Anti-Abortion Politics Blocks Family Planning Funding Around the World," *emagazine.com*. 9, no. 6 (November–December 1998). Accessed August 23, 2007 at http://www.emagazine.com/view/?822&src=; Rosemary Radford Ruether, "Women, Reproductive Rights and the Catholic Church," *Catholics for a Free Choice* (May 2006), accessed August 24, 2007, at http://www.catholicsforchoice.org/print.asp

14. Memo re. Brackenridge Hospital Governance/Austin Hospital Authority; John Nuveen and Co., Inc., "Nuveen Mergers and Acquisitions, Introduction to Services for Seton Medical Center," AHC.

15. *Seton Leader Letter*, May 4, 1995.

16. "Hospitals Are Still Deflecting Emergency Patients, Group Says," *New York Times*, October 30, 1994. The study was done by the Public Citizen Health Research Group.

17. Andrew B. Bindman, Dennis Keane, and Nicole Lurie, "A Public Hospital Closes: Impact on Patients' Access to Care and Health Status," *Journal of the American Medical Association* 264, no. 22 (December 12, 1990), accessed January 1, 2008, at http://jama.ama-assn.org/cgi/content/abstract/264/22/2899

18. Louisa C. Brinsmade, "Brack Gets Religion," AHC, n.d.; Mike Todd, "City Council Approves Brackenridge Lease," *Austin American Statesman*, May 26, 1995, B1.

19. In addition to Monsignor Broussard, ethicists included Rev. Gerard Magill, Ph.D., associate professor of theology at St. Louis University; Rev. Dennis Brodeur, senior vice president for stewardship for the Franciscan Sisters of Mary Health Systems in St. Louis; and the Dominican fathers, Rev. Kevin O'Rourke and Rev. Benedict Ashley, who coauthored a two-volume theological analysis of health care ethics.

20. Monsignor William L. Broussard to Mr. James Kramer, April 24, 1995, AHC.

21. The principle of cooperation in the 1994 *Directives* was in line with the Congregation for the Defense of the Faith's statement on sterilization, *Quaecumque Sterilizatio*.

22. Kelly, *Contemporary Catholic Health Care Ethics* (Washington, DC: Georgetown University Press, 2004), 256.

23. Gerard Magill, "Seton/Brackenridge Lease Agreement and the Principle of Material Cooperation," June 28, 1995, 13–14, AHC.

24. Ibid., 19–20.

25. Richard Daly, "John McCarthy," in *Brief Biographies of the First Two Directors: The Texas Catholic Conference, 1963–1979* (Austin: Texas Catholic Conference, 1979); interview with Bishop John McCarthy by Barbra Mann Wall, December 5, 2007.

26. McCarthy interview.

27. Ibid.; John McCarthy, bishop of Austin, to Sister Patricia Elder, D.C., chair Seton Medical Center Board of Trustees, May 18, 1995, AHC.

28. Charles M. Wilson to His Eminence Joseph Cardinal Ratzinger, May 17, 1995, AHC; McCarthy interview. A later letter from Concerned Catholics of Austin to Charles J. Barnett, May 27, 1997, also asserted these charges.

29. Richard P. McBrien, ed., *Encyclopedia of Catholicism* (San Francisco: HarperCollins, 1995), 354.

30. McCarthy interview; Memo to Seton Board of Trustees, July 30, 1998; Kim Sue Lia Perkes, "Vatican Questions Austin Bishop over Brackenridge," and "Chronology of a Controversy," *Austin American Statesman*, July 30, 1998, A1, A6.

31. McCarthy interview.

32. Perkes, "Vatican Questions Austin Bishop."

33. Memo, Pat Hayes to Seton Board of Trustees, July 30, 1998, AHC.

34. Dennis J. Eike to Sister Marie Therese Sedgwick, July 7, 1997, AHC.

35. Paul Likoudis, "Chancery Documents Indicate Bishop Deceived Vatican," *The Wanderer*, n.d.

36. Editorial, "Bishop Needs Support," *Austin American Statesman*, July 31, 1998. According to Jay P. Dolan, the hierarchical nature of the church versus its communal character has been a contentious issue for American Catholics since the early 1800s. See Jay P. Dolan, *The American Catholic Experience: A History from Colonial Times to the Present* (Notre Dame, Ind.: University of Notre Dame Press, 1992).

37. Kim Sue Lia Perkes, "Seton, Austin, Working on Brackenridge Lease," *Austin American Statesman*, August 20, 1998.

38. Ibid.

39. Kim Sue Lia Perkes and Mary Ann Roser, "For Seton, a Debate of Church vs. Choice," *Austin American Statesman*, December 31, 2000, A1.

40. Ibid.; Perkes, "Vatican Questions Austin Bishop."

41. Kim Sue Lia Perkes, "Bishops to Weigh Hospital Services," *Austin American Statesman*, October 26, 2000, A1. See also Frances Kissling, "Is There Life After *Roe*? How to Think About the Fetus," *Conscience: The News Journal of Catholic Opinion* (Winter 2004–5), accessed January 2, 2008, at http://www.catholicsforchoice.org/print/asp

42. USCCB, *Ethical and Religious Directives for Catholic Health Care Services* (4th ed.), June 15, 2001. See also Kevin O'Rourke, "A Brief History," *Health Progress* 82, no. 6, accessed January 2, 2008, at http://findarticles.com/p/articles/mi_qa3859/is_200111/ai_n9007144/print

43. Kelly, *Contemporary Catholic Health Care Ethics*, 121.

44. Gayle White and Mary Ann Roser, "Catholic Bishops Adopt Policies That Reinforce Beliefs," *Austin American Statesman*, June 16, 2001, A11.

45. *Austin Chronicle*, June 8, 2001, accessed August 23, 2007, at http://www.austinchronicle.com/gyrobase/BeaderComments/?ContainerID=82161

46. Mary Ann Roser and Kim Sue Lia Perkes, "Seton to Limit Some Services at Brack," *Austin American Statesman*, June 8, 2001, A1.

47. Gold, "Hierarchy Crackdown." Before September 1998, no EC product had been approved, labeled, and marketed in the United States, and emergency hormonal contraception was available only through "off-label" use of oral contraceptive pills. Off-label use of approved medications was legal, and some hospital emergency rooms and family planning clinics provided women with EC this way. In September 1998, the FDA approved the first EC product, the PREVEN™ Emergency Contraceptive Kit. After several clinical trials, Mifepristone (RU-486) went on approvable status in the United States in 1996. The FDA approved it for abortion in September 2000. It is a steroidal abortifacient also referred to as the "Abortion Pill." The Abortion Pill is not the same as the "Morning after Pill," or Plan B, which prevents or delays ovulation and thus prevents pregnancy. The FDA approved Plan B in 1999. See also "Emergency Contraception Use Up—New ECP Arrives," *Contraceptive Technology Update* 20, no. 9 (1999): 108–9.

48. USCCB, *Ethical and Religious Directives*, 2001.

49. Catholics for a Free Choice, "Second Chance Denied: Emergency Contraception in Catholic Hospital Emergency Rooms," 2002; http://www.catholicsforchoice.org/topics/healthcare/documents/2002secondchancedenied_001.pdf, accessed August 23, 2007; idem, "The Facts About Catholic Health Care in the United States," *Catholic Health Care Update* (September 2005): 4.

50. Gold, "Hierarchy Crackdown"; Suzanne Batchelor, "Clash and Compromise: Ethics at Issue When Public Hospital Is Put into Catholic Hands," *National Catholic Reporter* (July 4, 2003), accessed August 23, 2007, at www.findarticles.com/p/articles/mi_m1141/is_33_39/ai_105480211/

51. Had Brackenridge existed only to provide reproductive care, the Daughters could not have kept the partnership; instead, it offered many services to the poor.

52. Quoted in Mary Ann Roser and Kim Sue Lia Perkes, "City May Run Birth Control at Brack," *Austin American Statesman*, August 22, 2001, News Section.

53. "Letters," *Austin American Statesman*, December 21, 2001.

54. Andrew Park, "Seton Extending Health-Care Reach," *Austin American Statesman*, October 6, 1998, A1.

55. Quoted in *Austin Chronicle*, June 8, 2001.

56. "Baby Boom."

57. McCarthy interview.

58. Alan M. Zukerman, "A Promising Form of Consolidation: Joint Operating Agreements Are Gaining Popularity," *Health Progress* 81 (July–August 2000): 14–16.

59. Rachel Benson Gold, "Advocates Work to Preserve Reproductive Health Care Access When Hospitals Merge," *Guttmacher Report on Public Policy* 3, no. 2 (April 2000), accessed September 23, 2008, at http://www.guttmacher.org/pubs/tgr/03/2/gr030203.html; Catholics for a Free Choice, "Second Chance Denied."

60. *Austin Chronicle*, June 8, 2001.

"Go to Ruth's House": The Social Activism of Ruth Lubic and the Family Health and Birth Center

JULIE FAIRMAN
University of Pennsylvania

Abstract. This case of the work of Ruth Watson Lubic, an internationally known nurse midwife and women's and children's health care activist, provides a modern-day example of the intersection of forceful individual personalities, nursing as a type of activism in itself, and grassroots and local actions that produce larger movement-based activist organizations. Her work as a nurse midwife, in partnership with other nurse midwives, physicians, and community members, illustrates how the efforts of individual actors at a grassroots community level can be as significant as larger traditionally situated activist movements on the lives of everyday citizens.

> If I could leave you with the single most important prescription to address the tragic and seemingly intransigent phenomenon known as infant mortality it would be this: Go to Ruth's House.[1]

So testified physician Ronald David in his address to congressional staffers in 2007. David, a neonatologist, was cochair of the 2005 National Commission on Infant Mortality of the Joint Center for Political and Economic Studies.[2] "Ruth" is Ruth Lubic, an eighty-year-old (in 2009) internationally known nurse-midwife who has over decades worked on issues of social justice, and in particular for the improvement of women's and children's health across all races, ethnic groups, and classes.

"Ruth's House" is the freestanding Family Health and Birth Center Lubic opened in northeast Washington, D.C., in 2000, an area with one of the highest infant mortality rates in the country. The center is, as Ruth calls it, "the glue that holds together social support and child care services" that were long inadequate in this area populated by immigrant and low-income families.[3] Lubic is the glue that holds together the whole enterprise—the center's philosophy and its services—and she provides a modern-day example of the intersection of forceful individual personalities, nursing as a type of activism in itself, and grassroots and local actions that produce larger movement-based activist organizations. Her work as a nurse midwife, in partnership with other nurse midwives, physicians, and community members, illustrates how the efforts of individual actors at a grassroots community level can be as significant as larger traditionally situated activist movements on the lives of everyday citizens.[4]

Nursing, as a female-gendered profession with social and cultural mandates to provide a broadly defined array of care services, is situated at the fulcrum where health disparities and social justice movements intertwine. Its history illustrates this nexus through its long tradition of focusing on the issues of children's and women's health, and interceding between the dominant power of local and national governments and medical men and women, and disenfranchised groups and populations. We see this in examples such as the settlement house movement and Lillian Wald's work with others to establish the Children's Bureau in the early twentieth century, midwife Mary Breckinridge and the Frontier Nursing midwifery service and school, the clinics and nurse midwifery programs of the Maternity Center Association in New York City, as well as the later school nurse movement.[5] There are, of course, other professions that work from a foundation of social justice, and other areas of focus for nursing activism, but nursing's involvement with children and women represents a century-long continuity for practice and policy.

Until the early twentieth century, women traditionally gave birth in their home surrounded by friends and family.[6] But in the late nineteenth and early twentieth centuries, as childbirth became medicalized and paternalized and pregnancy was reconceptualized as a kind of pathologic state, childbearing women gradually lost control of the process, birthing in institutions controlled by medical practitioners and characterized by a rising caesarean section rate. The unique contribution of women's social support before, during, and after births was deprioritized in favor of scientific methods, technology, and institutionalization of medical expertise.[7] Women, especially those who were poor, lower class, or non-White, were sometimes seen by the medical profession as incompetent participants in the role of bearing and raising children, despite historical evidence harkening from slavery. Women gave birth in sterile delivery rooms, under sedation, without the encouragement of familiar faces, and even fathers were banned from many delivery rooms until the late 1960s.[8]

The women's health movement of the late 1960s and 1970s along with the forces surrounding the women's, civil rights, and peace movements supported the questioning of traditional narratives of normal birth and women's ability to control their bodies.⁹ Freestanding birth centers, emerging in the rugged social terrain of the 1970s, were products of the ideas of women like Ruth Lubic, who questioned the male-dominated medical childbirth paradigm that denormatized out-of-hospital births, and who wondered why infant mortality and caesarean section rates in the United States were so high despite the surrounding affluence and medical capabilities.[10] The birthing center model situated birth as a normal process and women and their bodies as trustworthy to birth infants with minimal intervention and in places other than hospitals. In fact, from this perspective childbearing women of all races and ethnic groups became socially active community members themselves who defied the traditional label "patient" and its implications of dependency because they and their friends and families were actively involved before, during, and after the infant's birth. Additionally, although the birthing center concept values the health of both the fetus and the mother, it is more targeted to the process of birth than the medical model. The outcome of a healthy baby is key, but how mothers get to this outcome is equally important to healthy births, mothering, and the woman's postnatal health.

In 1975, Lubic and her midwifery colleagues from the New York-based Maternity Center Association (MCA), where she was general director, opened the Childbearing Center in a private home in affluent East Manhattan.[11] The center was a response to several issues. First, the MCA heard from middle-class women activists who wanted more dynamic participation in their own experiences in health care and childbirth in particular and could not find a place to operationalize this role. The freestanding birth concept was a way to reduce in-home births and to bring these women to a place that provided birthing without the medicalization and with the support of expert women providers.[12] There were a few other freestanding centers operating at the time, although not in New York; most of them served poor or communities without access to health services.[13] Second, the MCA nurse midwives were stimulated in part by their feminist beliefs and the opportunity the social climate of the 1970s offered them as women to gain control over their place of practice. And third, the MCA was receiving numerous complaints from the public about unnecessary medical intervention during childbirth in hospitals.[14] The center founders wanted to create a place where women could help manage their birthing event, make informed decisions about medical intervention, and feel more at home in an environment controlled by clinically competent women practitioners who shared their ideals.[15]

The center opened during a period when nursing roles in general were expanding and moving into new types of practices, including that of the nurse practitioner.[16] Nurse midwives were, of course, one of the earliest models of expanded nursing practice, and they have a long history of meshing practice and social issues such as the MCA. The history of activism and the changing context of social issues surrounding disparities of race, gender, and class supported nurse midwives' growing efforts to provide models of obstetric care during a time when many women were discouraged with traditional medicalized childbirth. These efforts also came in the 1970s when the local and national birth rate was dropping as more and safer birth control became available and the number of women entering the workplace increased.

Similar to the experiences of nurse practitioners, collaboration with physicians supported new childbirth practice models that expanded choices for childbearing women and increased access to services.[17] Nurse midwives relied on physician colleagues to support their childbirth services and gain hospital privileges and coverage during emergencies. But in some instances physicians threw up barriers to freestanding centers, citing the dangers of childbirth outside hospitals despite the lack of concrete evidence. In the case of the MCA and Childbearing Center, some physicians and hospitals provided support and backup during emergencies. But the declining birth rate and maternity ward closures in New York City during that time, coupled with middle-class flight from the city and a large number of practicing obstetricians in the area, created an environment of competition and conflict. In the center's later development phase, more than half its physician advisory board members resigned in protest or because of professional pressure.[18] The center also experienced difficulties obtaining a facility license that, as later noted in a Federal Trade Commission Report, was due more to medical organizations' and the city public health department's attempts to restrict competition than to quality of care concerns.[19] Some of the physicians' alarm over competition was probably not misplaced, as the patients served by the center were typically seen in obstetricians' offices—White, middle-class, and able to pay. These patients saw the birth center as an attractive alternative to in-hospital deliveries and the culture of medical intervention.

Couples who went to the Upper East Side Center "felt like pioneers, braving grandparents' nervous admonitions and doctors' doomsday scenarios."[20] Their choices were "radical" as they opted for delivery supervised by nurse midwives (rather than physicians) outside a hospital and went home within twelve hours of delivery. Besides a more homelike and natural setting for delivery, economics also factored into patient choices. This early center charged $550 for a complete package of prenatal and postnatal care, delivery in a homelike environment, and educational services, compared to the $2,000–3,000 charge for typical inpatient deliveries. At first, families paid their expenses out of pocket, but soon most major insurance plans contained some provision for service reimbursement for out-of-hospital deliveries, as did state-supported entitlement programs.[21]

Lubic's work with women, particularly those who were marginalized by poverty and race, sprang from an overwhelming sense of altruism and voluntarism translated by her parents. Living during the Great Depression, she remembered that her father, a pharmacist, frequently provided free services to his neediest customers, and her mother pawned her jewelry to buy medicine for the poor. They advocated the principle: "Always try to help people who were worse off than you."[22] These values guided Lubic and her MCA colleagues, who opened a second birth center in 1988 in the Bronx, deliberately choosing one of the poorest areas of the city, with one of the highest infant mortality and preterm birth rates in the country. These women were different from the clientele at the first Childbearing Center—they were poor, typically Black and Hispanic women. But they also shared with women in the earlier center the aim to regain control over their bodies during and after delivery.

Many of these women had histories of "bad outcomes," not because they were high risk but because they lacked access to prenatal care, proper nutrition, or consistent social support—all of which contributed to preterm and low birth weight deliveries and their accompanying high rate of infant complications. The response to the birth center approach was remarkable; Bronx women came to the center for services with their families and friends and delivered their infants in their company. One woman brought members of her church choir, who welcomed the infant with gospel songs and encouragement.[23]

Many others followed Lubic's and the MCA's lead. By 1980 there were 45 similar centers; by 1984 there were 120 centers with more than 300 in development.[24] Several studies, including one published by the *New England Journal of Medicine* (*NEJM*) and another by the Federal Trade Commission, showed that the birth centers could claim rates of infant mortality and infant Apgar scores similar to those of hospitals for low-risk deliveries. Perhaps most critically, the studies revealed that the childbearing services provided by freestanding birth centers led to relatively few caesarean sections and stimulated New York City hospitals to humanize their obstetric services through birthing rooms and expanded nurse midwife services.[25] The support for birth centers was also demonstrated across disciplines, as the American Public Health Association endorsed them in 1979 and developed suggestions for guidelines in 1983.[26] On the other hand, the American Academy of Pediatrics, a group that typically did not support the unsupervised practice of nurse practitioners, and the American College of Obstetricians and Gynecologists (ACOG) issued a joint statement opposing out-of-hospital births in 1983 (after ACOG issued a similar statement in 1976).[27]

In 1993, Lubic received a MacArthur Foundation Fellowship and supplemented this funding with additional money to open a new freestanding birth center in Washington, D.C., a city with infant mortality twice the national average.[28] By 2000, she converted a former supermarket into the Family Health and Birth Center in northeast Washington. Following nursing tradition, Lubic developed the center in collaboration with community leaders to offer an innovative array of health care services for women and children provided by a team of expert health providers and supervised by nurse midwives. But Lubic's unique vision also entailed intertwining nursing and health as a form of social justice, a sort of "social health care movement."[29] She offered women—particularly those who lacked access to high quality care or who were marginalized through poverty and race—a package of services including prenatal care, childbirth education, and child care services more similar to women's traditional birthing experiences before the medicalization of childbirth.

The freestanding childbirth center model that frames the Family Health and Birth Center operates from a foundation of social support—women interacting with other women who will give birth at the same time, have their children play together in the child care centers, and receive life skills services together. The center program also offers choices to women who usually have only a few. They may opt for in-center birth, but they can also deliver in a hospital still attended by the midwife they have come to know and who supports having friends and families with them.[30] The center provides continuity of service as its resources cover the entire pre- and postdelivery period and beyond, providing educational programs on child care, jobs skills for mothers, and nutrition counseling.

Strands That Mark the Intersection of Individual Activism, Social Justice, and Larger Movements

At least five strands run through Ruth Lubic's story; they mark both the success and difficulties of the birthing center concept, nursing as kind of activism, and the opportunities and limits of individual actions. They include continued focus on the health of women and children, physician support and opposition, federal support and lack thereof, the economic nightmare of malpractice costs, and shifting weight of cost-saving and clinical outcomes. The strands coalesced to threaten birth centers despite the individual and organizational efforts of their supporters or the rightness of their cause.

Lubic acknowledges the important role physician collaboration played in the success of the birth centers. Similar to nurse practitioners, nurse midwives can practice without direct physician supervision. But, as Lubic notes, nurse midwives "can't function without physicians."[31] They need to have a place—an institution—to send their mothers and babies for consultation, midwife-supervised deliveries, and emergencies. Although Lubic was able to form collaborative relationships for all her centers, this process was very difficult. In the Family Health and Birth Center's first year, the midwives negotiated practice agreements with Howard Medical Center. Although some obstetricians at Howard indeed formed partnerships with them, they lacked support from other key obstetricians who were not as collaborative, made the midwives and patients feel unwelcome, and at times were not available when the midwives needed help or consultation.[32] New arrangements had to be renegotiated and relocated more than once.

When physicians did not collaborate with the center, typical arguments about patient safety when delivering outside a hospital—lack of fetal monitors and inability to predict complications—were fairly characteristic and still pervasive despite the evidence of good outcomes with freestanding birth centers.[33] These arguments are institutionalized in the ACOG patient education materials. The text of one pamphlet published in 2000 (still live on its Web site) reads: "There are also freestanding birth centers that are not in a hospital. These centers may not offer all the services you may need if an emergency arises. Because of this, the safest places to give birth are thought to be a hospital or birthing center within the hospital complex."[34] The language of safety, risk, and fear ("emergency") is used to shed doubt on the quality of care offered by freestanding centers. In contrast, in February 2008 the same organization issued a statement on home births that supported freestanding birth centers meeting the standards of the Accreditation Association for Ambulatory Health Care, the Joint Commission, or the American Association of Birth Centers, as legitimate places for childbirth (vs. home birth).[35]

Besides the difficulties of establishing physician and hospital support, the unreliable and inadequate funding stream also threatens the centers. The Family Health and Birth Center in Washington, D.C., exists on a flow of Medicaid payments, District of Columbia funding allocations, and private donations. The sustainability of these sources rests on the individual and enormous political and social lobbying skills of Ruth Lubic. She has powerful advocates in Supreme Court justice Ruth Bader Ginsburg, former Secretary for Health and Human Services Donna Shalala, physician and former Assistant Secretary for Health and Human Services Philip Randolph Lee, and Alma Powell, philanthropist and wife of General Colin Powell. But, as the center's director noted, "Unfortunately our model works on an [80-year-old woman] bringing in $500,000 a year [in grants and donations]."[36] Medicaid reimbursements are declining and pay only approximately 55 percent of the charges for a delivery, which makes Lubic's ability to raise private funds a key piece of her activism.

The Family Health and Birth Center relies on the District of Columbia Council for financial support and to cover its increasingly costly malpractice premiums. Malpractice insurance rates have increased phenomenally (not only for the center but for obstetricians as well), from $90,000 in 2005 to almost $300,000 in 2008. Lubic lobbied vociferously for the district to cover the premiums of all safety net clinics; the legislation stalled not for lack of will but for lack of resources. Malpractice insurance cost was the major reason the earliest New York center closed. So Lubic regularly lobbies legislators, staffers, and policy strategists on Capitol Hill. In one week in January 2007 alone, she met with the health staffers of two powerful senators, gave tours of the centers, attended several lectures where she might interact with powerful legislators or policy advocates, and went to numerous dinners and community meetings to keep the center and its needs illuminated.

The fight for funding in some ways obscures the successes of the center. One of the important things accomplished by birth centers in general, including the Family Health and Birth Center, has been the decreased rate of preterm births (less than thirty-seven weeks) and low birth weight infants, and an impressive decrease in caesarean sections compared to District of Columbia and national rates. The center serves primarily low-income Black women (although Lubic has seen a recent increase in the number of middle-income women, mainly due to closure of suburban birth centers) and their infants, those documented to have the worst outcomes. "Infant mortality," David recounted, "is a direct consequence of social injustices—racism, misogyny and its attendant sexism, and income inequality that is itself a pale proxy for social inequalities more generally."[37]

Data compiled by Lubic for 2002–5 illustrate some of the disparities and the success of the center's efforts to address them. The proportion of preterm births for the Black population in the District of Columbia rests at 14.2 percent compared to 9 percent at the Family Health and Birth Center; 14.6 percent of all Black births in the district resulted in low birth weight babies (less than 2,500 grams), compared to 7 percent at the center (comparable to the national rate), and the caesarean section rate in the District was 29 percent compared to 15.3 percent at the center.[38]

In this cost-conscious health environment, better outcomes and social justice alone are not reason enough for service support from local and national government sources. Cost savings have become the standard of therapeutic success. The Family Health and Birth Center is well positioned, having both good outcomes and cost-effective services. Lubic's data show that the center saved the health care system (federal and district) more money than it cost to run the facility for 2005. According to the Institute of Medicine, preterm births cost our society at least $26 billion in 2005, $51,600 per infant.[39] The center also estimates that the reductions actualized in preterm births saved the health care system over a half a million dollars in 2005.[40]

Through their work, Lubic and the nurse midwives at the Family Health and Birth Center actualized cost savings and quality in a low-tech, high-touch environment that provided social support, careful monitoring during pregnancy and delivery, nutrition and health education, and community outreach.[41] Lubic's individual activism—her search for funding, consciousness raising, and operationalizing her ideas—challenges the primacy of larger institutional movements and positions her work as essential to supporting broader social change. Her work, to be sure, is supported by larger social movements, and broader institutional change has happened as an outgrowth of the work of the MCA, as evidenced by a substantial and well-recognized accreditation process in place for birth centers. Yet only 1 percent of United States births occur outside hospitals, and birth in general is still highly medicalized.[42]

For individual women in this center, some of the country's most vulnerable, Lubic's work makes a difference. Women can consider their childbirth choices in the company of expert and primarily women practitioners, family, and friends if they so choose. Their outcomes are better, their children healthier. They see their experience as positive and enriching and learn skills that will take them and their children to a different level of coping and existence. And these important things are accomplished in a system of nursing care, in a highly cost-effective way without corporatization and with minimal technical intervention. Although birthing in a freestanding birth center supported by nurse midwives has not yet been established as a cultural ideal, Lubic and the women she serves have contributed to the rewriting of the cultural narrative surrounding birth. Their successes and their stories show the promise of individual activism, be it as a provider or patient, that can in fact provide an alternative account of normal birthing and reframe it within the promise of social justice.

Ronald David, author of the opening passage, effectively illustrates the intertwining of Ruth Lubic's individual activism with larger social justice movements, as she maintains her joy in the original mission, pushing and prodding for women, both with resources and those less fortunate. He ends his remarks with following admonitions:

If you want to see children survive to see their first birthday in an otherwise toxic social milieu, go to Ruth's House. Go there and break bread with Ruth and her sisters. Listen to them. Talk with them. Learn of their hopes and fears, their plans and practices. Learn from the stories they tell about themselves firsthand. Do not begin or end your quest to address the tragedy of infant mortality in a university or for-profit health care system. Go to Ruth's House.[43]

JULIE FAIRMAN, PHD, RN, FAAN
217 Glenn Rd
Ardmore, PA 19003

Notes

1. Ronald David, M.D., "Go to Ruth's House: A Response to Infant Mortality," address to staff of Rep. Steve Cohen (D-Tenn.), Washington, D.C., October 16, 2007.

2. Joint Center for Political and Economic Studies, http://www.jointcenter.org/, accessed December 2007. The Joint Center is a nonprofit research and public policy think tank focused solely on issues concerning African Americans and people of color.

3. Ruth Lubic, telephone interview with author, February 18, 2007.

4. For example, Eunice "Kitty" Ernest is another leader in the birthing center movement who was influential both as an individual and as part of organizations such as the MCA. See Katherine Louise Dawley, "Leaving the Nest: Nurse-Midwifery in the United States, 1940–1980," Ph.D. dissertation, University of Pennsylvania, 2001.

5. See Karen Buhler-Wilkerson, *No Place like Home: A History of Nursing and Home Care in the United* States (Baltimore: Johns Hopkins University Press, 2001); Cynthia Connolly, *Saving Sickly Children: The Tuberculosis Preventorium in American Life, 1909–1970* (New Brunswick, N.J.: Rutgers University Press, 2008); Arlene W. Keeling, *Nursing and the Privilege of Prescription, 1893–2000* (Columbus: Ohio State University Press, 2007); Dawley, "Leaving the Nest." The MCA changed its name in 2005 to the Childbirth Connection.

6. Judith Leavitt, *Brought to Bed: Childbearing in America, 1750–1950* (New York: Oxford University Press, 1986).

7. Robbie Davis-Floyd, *Birth As an American Rite of Passage* (Berkeley: University of California Press, 1992).

8. Kathy Davis, *The Making of Our Bodies, Ourselves* (Durham, N.C.: Duke University Press, 2007); Rima Apple, "Constructing Mothers: Scientific Motherhood in the Nineteenth and Twentieth Centuries," *Social History of Medicine* 8 (1995): 161–78; Sandra Morgan, *Into Our Own Hands: The Women's Health Movement in the United States, 1969–1990* (New Brunswick, N.J.: Rutgers University Press, 2002).

9. Davis, *The Making of Our Bodies, Ourselves*; Apple, "Constructing Mothers"; Morgan, *Into Our Own Hands*.

10. This rise was documented in many studies, for example, Judith P. Rooks, Norman L. Weatherby, Eunice K. M. Ernst, Susan Stapleton, David Rosen, and Allan

Rosenfield, "Outcomes of Care in Birth Centers: The National Birth Center Study," *New England Journal of Medicine* 321 (December 28, 1989): 1804–11, and was attributed to physician and patient convenience as well as falling pregnancy rates in insured patients and a lower patient pool. Caesarean sections brought higher reimbursement rates.

11. The MCA was founded in 1918 by a collection of philanthropists and health professionals as a nonprofit organization to care for poor women in New York City. The association has a long history of advocacy and support for education programs for women and providers, founding the first New York City nurse midwifery school in 1931.

12. Lubic, interview.

13. Pamela S. Eakins, "The Rise of the Free Standing Birth Center: Principles and Practice," *Women and Health* 9 (1984): 49–64.

14. Michael deCourcy Hinds, "Study Lauds Midwife Center," *New York Times*, July 17, 1982, Late City Final Edition.

15. Ibid. The study referred to was a 1981 Federal Trade Commission study; see Wendy Lazarus, E. S. Levine, and L. S. Lewin, *Competition Among Health Practitioners: The Influence of the Medical Profession on the Health Manpower Market* (Washington, D.C.: Federal Trade Commission, 1981).

16. Julie Fairman, *Making Room in the Clinic: Nurse Practitioners and the Evolution of Modern Health Care* (New Brunswick, N.J.: Rutgers University Press, 2008).

17. Fairman, *Making Room in the Clinic*.

18. deCourcy Hinds, "Study Lauds Midwife Center"; Ruth Watson Lubic, "Nurse Midwifery: A Specialty Comes of Age," *Journal of the New York State Nurses Association* 26 (1995): 34–36. This discord is also noted in Lazarus et al., *Competition Among Health Practitioners*, 17, which cites Lubic's dissertation, "Barriers and Conflict in Maternity Care Innovation," Ph.D. dissertation, Department of Education, Columbia University, 1979.

19. Lazarus et al., *Competition Among Health Practitioners*.

20. Dorothy J. Gaiter, "Center Finding a Boom in Non-Hospital Births," *New York Times*, December 18, 1981, Late City Final Edition, Section B.

21. Jane Brody, *New York Times*, September 15, 1975; John Carey with Susan Katz, "The Comforts of Home," *Newsweek*, November 26, 1984, 96. State Medicaid payment came only after political conflict and two years after opening. See Dawley, "Leaving the Nest," 310.

22. Lubic, interview.

23. "Entering the World on Wings of Song," *International Herald Tribune*, October 21, 1996 (Neuilly-sur-Seine, France).

24. Carey with Katz, "The Comforts of Home."

25. Rooks et al., "Outcomes of Care in Birth Centers"; Lazarus et al., *Competition Among Health Practitioners*.

26. American Public Health Association, "Guidelines for Licensing and Regulating Birth Centers," *American Journal of Public Health* 73 (1983): 331–34.

27. Joan Matthews and Kathleen Zadak, "The Alternative Birth Movement in the United States: History and Current Status," *Women and Health* 17 (1991): 39–54; ACOG, District II, "Position Paper on Out-of-Hospital Births," January 1976, from Lazarus et al., *Competition Among Health Practitioners*, Appendix 2.

28. The MacArthur Foundation, one of the largest independent foundations in the nation, is known for its "genius" fellowships, given to recipients who show exceptional promise and creativity toward achieving the goals of the foundation, including

world peace. See http://www.macfound.org/site/c.lkLXJ8MQKrH/b.860781/k.D616/Overview.htm

29. Lubic cites the term in an interview with Catherine Spader in "Changing Our World," *Nursing Spectrum*, May 5, 2008, Philadelphia Tri-State Edition.

30. By 2008, the program included the Family Health and Birthing Center, the Developing Families Center, Partners United Planning Organization, and the Healthy Babies Project. Together, these offerings provide a spectrum of services from prenatal care to child development services.

31. Lubic, interview.

32. Ibid.

33. Sandra Boodman, "Giving Birth, More Women Choose Free-Standing Centers," *Washington Post*, January 9, 1990, Final Edition.

34. American College of Obstetricians and Gynecologists, "Planning Your Pregnancy," http://www.acog.org/publications/patient_education/ab012.cfm, 2000 (accessed January 22, 2008).

35. The text from the 2000 pamphlet still stands. See ACOG News Release, "Statement on Home Births," http://www.acog.org/from_home/publications/press_releases/nr02-06-08-2.cfm, February 6, 2008 (accessed December 21, 2008).

36. Phuong Ly, "Labor Without End," *Washington Post Magazine*, May 27, 2007, 24.

37. David, "Go to Ruth's House"; Joint Center for Political and Economic Studies, "The Courage to Love: Implications for Care, Research, and Public Policy to Reduce Infant Mortality Rates Commission," http://www.jointcenter.org/new_site/infantmortality.htm (accessed March 30, 2008).

38. Family Health and Birthing Center, "Outcome Data," unpublished data sheet used with permission from Ruth Lubic. The Washington, D.C., data are for 2002, the Birthing Center for 2005. Lubic had the data certified by Vijava Hogan, Lloyd Edwards, and Christian Douglas from the University of North Carolina at Chapel Hill, School of Public Health. See letter from above to Ruth Lubic, May 5, 2006. Used with permission from Ruth Lubic. Lubic's data are consistent with other national data sets; see also "Best Evidence for Choosing a Place for Birth," http://www.childbirthconnection.org/article.asp?ck=10142, accessed January 12, 2009; Judith Rooks, Norman Weatherby, and Eunice Ernst, "The National Birth Center Study: Part III," *Journal of Nurse Midwifery* 37 (1992): 361–97.

39. Richard E. Behrman and Adrienne S. Butler, eds., Committee on Understanding Premature Birth and Assuring Healthy Outcomes, *Preterm Birth: Causes, Consequences, and Prevention* (Washington, D.C.: National Academies Press, 2007), 325.

40. Family Health and Birthing Center, "Outcome Data."

41. Ibid.

42. Eugene R. Declercq, "Changing Childbirth in England: Lessons for U.S. Health Reform," *Journal of Health Politics, Policy, and Law* 23, no. 5 (1998): 833–59.

43. David, "Go to Ruth's House."

THE PLACE OF RELIGION AS AN INTERPRETIVE TOOL IN NURSING HISTORY

Guest Editor's Note

Often historiography keeps religion at arm's length. In writing about the place of religion within history, David Gary Shaw discusses the challenges this brings, including rearranging "our conceptualizations of the religious and the secular, of our own vision, and the paradigms that organize our knowledge, so that we can see our way to a more productive and less anxious relationship between secular eyes and religious topics." As important are the ways we write about people whose beliefs differ from ours. Indeed, historians may need to revise their methods "if they are to cope productively with believers past and present, even if we can disregard what historians themselves believe."[1]

In this issue, we feature two essays that open paths for historians of nursing to rethink the relationship between religion and nursing history. One is a local study by Anne Z. Cockerham and Arlene W. Keeling, who examine the Catholic Medical Mission Sisters as nurse-midwives in Santa Fe, New Mexico. They are interested in the relationship between the sisters' religious practices and beliefs and the economics involved in their work with Spanish American clients. The other is an international comparative study by Susanne Kreutzer about deaconesses in Germany and the United States. She answers the question of why the German concept of the parish deaconess failed in the United States compared to its success in Germany.

Women and religion is a relatively new topic in historical research, and interest is growing in international circles. An important milestone was Sioban Nelson's *Say Little, Do Much*, which first corrected the historical "blind spot" in nursing history. She argued that long before Florence Nightingale came on the scene, Catholic sisters were organizing home care, creating and administering hospitals, and volunteering their work in military and epidemic nursing.[2] Though she studied religious nursing orders in Australia, the United States, Germany, England, and Ireland, there has been little scholarship on women religious in the Nordic countries. Theologian and Dominican Sister Else-Britt Nilsen is an exception, and she has published a number of studies on Catholic sisters' nursing in Norway. Then the publication in 1998 of Susanne Malchau's innovative study of the Danish-born Catholic Sister Benedictine Ramsing was the beginning of serious scholarly interest in this research field in Denmark and in other areas of Scandinavia.[3]

Other scholars of religious nursing bear mentioning. Katrin Schultheiss's examination of the professionalization of nursing in France integrates social, political, and religious issues in the evolution of nursing. It links themes of nursing and the state by showing how nurses forged a feminine citizen during the Third Republic. And it reveals continuities with nursing histories in other Western countries in class and gender struggles and the rise of the medical profession.[4]

The two articles in this issue build on these works. They also support other social and cultural histories of nursing, ethnicity, and religion. For example, studies of Catholic sisters by Mary Tarbox, Bernadette McCauley, and Jean Richardson have shown particular influences of geographic region on hospital development and nursing.[5] However, they have mainly focused on the nineteenth and early twentieth centuries. Cockerham and Keeling expand these studies by focusing on a heretofore unstudied region, New Mexico, in the mid-twentieth century. Kreutzer shows the power of place as she analyzes distinct differences in parish nursing in the United States and Germany.

My own research on the work of Catholic nursing sisters in the United States examines the construction of gender, religious, and economic roles as sisters successfully established large American hospitals. They ran their acute-care institutions with support from substantial Catholic immigrant communities.[6] But comparative studies are important, and Cockerham and Keeling's essay shows a very different picture of religious nurses in home care and a small clinic in the American Southwest. They had to rely on their own funding when most of their patients could not pay for the services. The essay also builds on the work of Sonya Grypma on missionary nurses, who argues for understanding the women nurses on their own terms.[7] Kreutzer's essay helps us understand why, unlike Catholic sisters, Protestant deaconesses did not proliferate in the United States. As parish nursing is becoming more prominent today, she suggests that often history is reinvented without knowledge of historical predecessors.

Returning to the theme of religion and history, Shaw argues that methodologically, historians pay attention to both written and oral past sources, and as long as they are willing to follow their skeptical methods, they can remain alive to the power that religious traditions, beliefs, and practices have.[8] Brad Gregory believes that historians can expand their range of study to include the significance of the religious past for the ones who lived it. If scholars want to understand religious persons so that the actors will recognize what is being written about them, then historians should put aside their own secular biases and ask, "What did it mean to them?"[9] An intriguing aspect of both articles in this issue is their interest in the significance of the past for the Catholic and Protestant women themselves. What did their experiences mean to them? What were the consequences of the decisions they made? In addition, both articles speak to the power that women would have if they were able to work relatively independently of male church leaders.

These essays prompt us to ponder what such a methodology of determining what individuals' experiences meant to them can have for multiple religious traditions. What would a focus on India or Egypt tell us about religious beliefs and nursing practice? Historiography on nursing is growing in Ireland.[10] But think about the mixed religious communities there. What would nursing histories look like that take these differences into account? Through *Nursing History Review*, we have a great venue to rethink issues such as the intersections of religion, history, and power in a globalized context.

BARBRA MANN WALL, PHD, RN
Associate Professor and Associate Director
Barbara Bates Center for the Study of the History of Nursing
University of Pennsylvania
Philadelphia, PA 19104

Notes

1. David Gary Shaw, "Modernity Between Us and Them: The Place of Religion Within History," *History and Theory* 45 (December 2006): 4.
2. Sioban Nelson, *Say Little, Do Much: Nursing, Nuns, and Hospitals in the Nineteenth Century* (Philadelphia: University of Pennsylvania Press, 2001). Quotation is on page 6. See also ibid., "Entering the Professional Domain: The Making of the Modern Nurse in 17th Century France," *Nursing History Review* 7 (1999): 171–87.
3. Else-Britt Nilsen, "Religious Identity and National Loyalty: Women Religious in Norway during the Second World War," in *Nuns and Sisters in the Nordic Countries after the Reformation: A Female Counter-Culture in Modern Society*, ed. Yvonne Maria Werner (Uppsala, Sweden: Swedish Institute of Mission Research, 2004), 213–53; Susanne Malchau, "Women Religious and Protestant Welfare: The Sisters of Saint Joseph's Empire of Catholic Hospitals in Denmark," in ibid., 107–48; and Susanne Malchau, *Love Is to Serve. Sister Benedicte Ramsing – A Biography* (Dissertation from the Faculty of Health Sciences at Aarhus University, Denmark, 1998). See also Asa Andersson, "To Work in the Garden

of God: The Swedish Nursing Association and the Concept of the Calling, 1909–1933," *Nursing History Review* 10 (2002): 3–19.

4. Katrin Schulththeiss, *Bodies and Souls: Politics and the Professionalization of Nursing in France, 1880–1922* (Cambridge, Mass., and London, England: Harvard University Press, 2001).

5. Mary P. Tarbox, "The Origins of Nursing by the Sisters of Mercy in the United States: 1843–1910" (Ed.D. diss., Columbia University Teachers College, 1986); Bernadette McCauley, *Who Shall Take Care of Our Sick? Roman Catholic Sisters and the Development of Catholic Hospitals in New York City* (Baltimore: Johns Hopkins University Press, 2005); Jean Richardson, *A History of the Sisters of Charity Hospital, Buffalo, New York, 1848–1900* (Lewiston, N.Y.: The Edwin Mellen Press, 2005).

6. Barbra Mann Wall, *Unlikely Entrepreneurs: Catholic Sisters and the Hospital Marketplace, 1865–1925* (Columbus: Ohio State University Press, 2005).

7. Sonya J. Grypma, *Healing Henan: Canadian Nurses at the North China Mission, 1888–1947* (Vancouver: University of British Columbia Press, 2008).

8. Shaw, "Modernity Between Us and Them," 6–7.

9. Brad S. Gregory, "The Other Confessional History: On Secular Bias in the Study of Religion," in *History and Theory* 45 (December 2006): 132.

10. Gerard M. Fealy, *Care to Remember: Nursing and Midwifery in Ireland* (Douglas Village, Cork, Ireland: Mercier Press); Ann Wickham, "The Nursing Radicalism of the Honourable Alvinia Brodrick, 1861–1955," *Nursing History Review* 15 (2007): 51–64.

Nursing Body and Soul in the Parish: Lutheran Deaconess Motherhouses in Germany and the United States

Susanne Kreutzer
Department for Humanities/Nursing Science, University of Osnabrück

Abstract. In Lutheran Germany, parish nursing traditionally constituted the deaconesses' principal work. As "Christian mothers of the parish" they were charged with a wide spectrum of tasks, including nursing, social service, and pastoral care. At the center of the Christian understanding of nursing was the idea of nursing body and soul as a unity.

This article analyzes the conception and transformation of Protestant parish nursing in the nineteenth and twentieth centuries in Germany and the United States, which developed very differently. In West Germany, parish nursing proved surprisingly resistant to modernization even in the face of upheavals of the 1960s, and in some places this traditional model survived as late as the 1980s and 1990s. In the United States, by contrast, an understanding of nursing rooted in the division of labor between care for body and care for soul had come to prevail by the 1920s and '30s, pushing out the German model of the parish deaconess altogether.

When the first German Lutheran deaconess motherhouse was founded in Kaiserswerth near Düsseldorf in 1836, its focus was not on hospital work but on sending nurses to work in parishes. The parish deaconess was regarded as the "crown of the Female Diaconate."[1] As a "Christian mother of the parish," she was charged with a wide spectrum of tasks, including nursing, social service work, and pastoral care. The pastoral care she provided, however, as opposed to the work of the parish pastors, was called "care of the soul." At the center of the Christian understanding of nursing was the idea of nursing body and soul as a unity.[2]

Modeled on the Kaiserswerth example, deaconess institutions were founded not only in German-speaking areas but in many other countries. Some of them sprang from the initiative of German motherhouses and some were established by local women who followed the Kaiserswerth model. Founding activities in Scandinavia were particularly successful. In the United States as well, German, Swedish, and Norwegian immigrant communities established deaconess institutions. The focus of this article is on German deaconess establishments in the United States as they compare to such establishments in Germany. These Protestant motherhouses, like the Catholic model they followed, were based on a simple principle of exchange: The sisters were promised training and lifelong care and support with their pledge to service in the sisterhood. Still, the idea of the motherhouse and the role of the deaconess could not be simply transplanted but had to be adapted to the American social context. It is this process of adaptation that makes the deaconess motherhouses an excellent focus for an international comparative history study.[3]

Two very different traditions of nursing in Germany and the United States are central in this study. During the nineteenth century in Germany and continuing into the 1960s, the motherhouse system was the dominant organizational form in nursing. Foundationally, nursing in West Germany was based on the Christian model of caring, combining both physical and spiritual care. Later the occupational field was fundamentally restructured: The formerly celibate "labor of love" devoted to the sick became a female profession brought in line with labor law provisions and scientific standards.[4] In the United States, by contrast, a professional strategy emphasizing efficiency, standardization, and scientific management began to characterize the development of nursing as early as the nineteenth century, and deaconess institutions remained marginal.[5]

In this article, I investigate the factors responsible for the differences in how well deaconess motherhouses in the two countries were able to establish themselves and take a closer look at one traditional area of nursing that constituted the deaconesses' principal work: parish nursing. I examine two deaconess motherhouses in particular: first, the Henriettenstiftung, which was founded in Hannover, Germany, in 1860 and, alongside parish nursing, was active in a number of other areas of nursing and social work; and second, the German American Lutheran deaconess motherhouse established in Baltimore in 1895, which specialized in parish nursing and teaching deaconesses. As the following account will show, Protestant parish nursing in the two countries developed very differently. In West Germany, parish nursing proved surprisingly resistant to modernization even in the face of the upheavals of the 1960s, and in some places this traditional model of nursing was even able to survive as late as the 1980s and 1990s. In the United States, by contrast, an understanding of nursing rooted in the division of labor between care for body and care for soul had come to prevail by the 1920s and 1930s, pushing out the German model of the parish deaconess altogether.

In a first step, I sketch out the origins and establishment of deaconess motherhouses in the context of German nineteenth-century society. A more detailed description of the work of the Henriettenstiftung's parish nurses will focus on developments after 1945. In a second step, I will briefly introduce the history of U.S. deaconess motherhouses. Finally, I will examine the conception and transformation of parish nursing in the United States, drawing on the example of the motherhouse in Baltimore, and compare and contrast the findings to parish nursing in Germany.

Information on the West German deaconess motherhouse was obtained from biographical interviews (conducted in 2004 and 2005) and from the Henriettenstiftung's extensive archive. The personal files of parish nurses were particularly valuable as some of them include elaborate correspondence between nurses and the motherhouse. Unfortunately, most of the earliest archival material dates from 1944 and 1945 because the Hannover motherhouse was destroyed by bombs during World War II (October 1943). As for the motherhouse in Baltimore, few ego-documents like personal letters of nurses have been preserved after 1900. The majority of the available material primarily consisted of minutes from various committee meetings at the motherhouse and at the United Lutheran Church in America, which address questions of education, employment of labor, and organization of the sisterhood. These sources allow for a sound reconstruction of the conception of parish nursing and its changes over time. A history of everyday life and of personal experience comparable to that of the Henriettenstiftung, however, cannot be written on the basis of these sources.

Deaconess Motherhouses in Germany: A Successful Model for the Nineteenth Century

The first German Lutheran deaconess motherhouse was founded by Protestant pastor Theodor Fliedner in 1836, with the aim of training as nurses daughters from the bourgeoisie who had Christian ambitions, and then sending them as "missionaries within the country" in the struggle against illness, poverty, and faithlessness, particularly in poor communities. This concept of an "inner mission" was based on the underlying assumption that material and spiritual impoverishment were closely related. For this reason, the deaconesses were charged with spiritual care of the poor, as well as physical nursing and social care. It was hoped that deaconesses, because their training was nonacademic, would have more immediate contact with the poor than pastors.[6] The sisters were trained at the deaconess hospital in Kaiserswerth and then sent out to fulfill various practical tasks in parishes, hospitals, private settings, schools, and foreign missions.

The deaconess institutions emerged in the context of the so-called German Awakening, a movement that aimed at a renewal of religious life and put personal faith experience—awakening—at the center of its religious understanding. By enhancing the status of personal belief vis-à-vis university education, the movement opened up entirely new fields of activity to women—including religious charity work in the public sphere.[7] Indeed it can be said that the idea of the deaconess institution, as developed in Kaiserswerth, was more or less in the air at the time and was accordingly taken up in many places such as, in 1860, Hannover, where the Henriettenstiftung was founded. Furthermore, Fliedner was able to base his work on that of several precursors such as the Catholic Sisters of Mercy. In contrast to the Catholic model, however, deaconesses did not make binding vows. They were permitted to leave the motherhouse and marry thereafter.[8]

If at first—contrary to the original intention—only daughters from the lower middle classes and from farming families were successfully recruited, the second half of the nineteenth century saw an increased interest in deaconess institutions among middle-class circles as well.[9] After all, with their training programs and the room and board they offered, the motherhouses were among the few institutions in nineteenth-century Germany that enabled women to acquire sound training and have a respected life and livelihood outside marriage.[10] However, the power of the motherhouses over the lives of individual sisters was formidable. For example, the sisters could be relocated at any time and were not able to establish an independent personal social security net. Though the benefits of nineteenth-century motherhouses were certainly attractive, they were attended by a substantial degree of dependence.

During the late nineteenth century, the concept of the deaconess institution, confronted by the emerging middle-class women's movement, became increasingly subject to criticism. At the turn of the century, new forms of sisterhoods developed that allowed their members more independence. These "free" nurses did not establish a lasting relationship to their sisterhood, and they received a salary for their work.[11] Compared to sisters who were connected to motherhouses, however, they were few in number until the late 1950s.[12] Particularly in times of economic crisis—most notably following the Second World War—deaconess institutions even experienced a renewed influx of students. With the tremendous need that accompanied the postwar years, the training and boarding programs offered by motherhouses appealed greatly to women. This was especially true for many young female refugees from the former eastern territories of the German Reich.

As the example of parish nursing shows, the deaconess model opened up interesting prospects for women even independently of economic considerations. It is in this light that I will take a closer look at the work and life circumstances of parish deaconesses. I will start by juxtaposing rural and urban parish nurse stations as contexts of activity and then present the nurses' work itself in more detail. The effect of the fundamental social change of the 1960s on parish nursing will be discussed in the section thereafter.

Urban and Rural Parish Nurse Stations: Two Different Contexts of Activity

In contrast to work in hospitals, parish nursing in general was organized in such a way to allow more independence. In rural parish nurse stations, in particular, where usually only one sister was in charge of several villages, women could rely only on themselves for the work. Sister Ella,[13] who worked as a parish nurse in remote villages in the Harz mountains into the 1980s and 1990s, recalled her work in an interview:

> I enjoyed that, coming into the church village. Aunt Emma, the walking newspaper, would be looking out of her window and would tell me what was going on in the village and whom, she thought, I absolutely had to visit. For example, someone had hurt himself chopping wood, and I should go take a look at him: he must have to go to the hospital. So I had a look and sure enough, it was quite the wound. I told him: "You'll actually need to be stitched up, sir." "Nonsense," he said, "I don't want any stitches. Just put a new bandage over it and it'll heal by itself." . . . They were pretty tough, those people, and not as whiny as the town folk. That was really nice work.[14]

Particularly in the rural nursing stations, the parish nurse was often the first contact person in cases of illness and other emergencies, because the next doctor was usually far away. The reticence about going to a hospital felt by the men and women living in the villages probably contributed to a widening of the scope of tasks parish nurses would take on. On top of this, the motherhouse had little access to individual sisters because of the geographical distance. The means of control available to the sisterhood, then, were very limited.

Service at the rural parish nurse stations hence suited women who enjoyed self-sufficiency at work and who wanted to live more or less independently of the sisterhood. The high degree of independence enjoyed by parish nurses fundamentally challenges the prevalent image of the "barracked" deaconess. And biographies of parish deaconesses indeed show that a motherhouse was able to offer women considerable room for maneuver. Many parish nurses were trained at the motherhouse hospital. But following their training they would spend decades working in far-away parishes and usually only visit Hannover once a year for the annual gathering at the Henriettenstiftung. They even spent their evening years—as retirement is called among deaconesses—in "their" parish, to which they usually felt very connected after working there for many years.

But not all sisters sought the independence of the rural nursing stations. Many deaconesses were apprehensive about the seclusion and physically demanding work. Especially in the rural parishes, long bicycle rides were part of the sisters' daily life. In the winter, letters from sisters to the motherhouse would pile up—letters reporting cases of frostbite or bicycle accidents due to ice and snow.[15] Many parish nurses thus preferred working in urban stations, where generally two to five sisters would live and work together. They shared an apartment and ran the household together. The nurses were each assigned a different district in which to work. The work itself was carried out with a degree of independence similar to that of the rural parish stations. The city women, however, were more integrated into the sisterhood. In cases where the Henriettenstiftung was involved in a city's local hospital, a relatively large group of sisters resided locally. If they maintained a good rapport, parish nurses in the city were able to obtain various kinds of support through talks and activities with other sisters, effectively benefiting from a network of mutually caring relationships. Above all, it was easier to live a religious life together and also easier to get help from one another and arrange stand-ins. It is not surprising, then, that the well-being of the women working at city parish stations depended largely on how well the sisters cooperated as a group.

Yet living in close quarters and running the household together also harbored an enormous potential for conflict. The personal difficulties among parish nurses thus became a subject that continually kept the directors of a motherhouse on their toes.[16] The responses of the directing sister and the directing pastor ranged from hope that things would somehow be sorted out, to counseling, to the relocation of individual women. Sister Frederike, for instance, following prolonged conflict at a parish station, was able to effect her recall from the station. The directing sister accommodated Sister Frederike's wish for more independence and relocated her to a "*very* free"[17] parish station in the countryside.

Many similar decisions are documented, proving that the motherhouse was indeed interested in the well-being of the women. Although the deaconesses, at their consecration, promised to be loyal and dutiful daughters to the motherhouse and attend to its orders, the deployment practice also shows that with the image of the "good" daughter came that of the "good" parents, whose responsibility was to care for the physical and spiritual well-being of the nurses. The command to obey, on the side of the sisters, corresponded with a paternalist command to provide for the sisters on the side of the motherhouse directors. Depending on available alternative positions, it was certainly possible for sisters to resist a deployment with some chance of success and to assert their interests. As long as more than 600 sisters belonged to the motherhouse and fulfilled a broad range of duties, as was the case in the early postwar years, the conditions were right for flexible dispatching practices that respected the wishes of the sisters.[18] There were often, however, intense struggles over where exactly the line was to be drawn between tolerable and intolerable conditions and whether a relocation was justified.

The Practice of Protestant Parish Nursing in West Germany

Having considered rural and urban nurse stations as different contexts of activity, let us now look at the parish nurses' work itself. Sister Marianne recalled in an interview her work as a parish nurse in the 1950s:

> I liked being in the parish. From the moment you were with the patient, you were there for him; nobody rang the doorbell. You got to know the surroundings, the family. Somehow, that's a more natural life. We didn't simply look after the sick but also paid many visits, got the stove going, cooked a little soup or brought food over. That's the kind of thing that was possible back then. Time wasn't a concern yet. I always felt that whatever I do, it's never in vain.[19]

Unlike in the hospital setting, parish nurses got to know patients in their personal family settings. When they paid a visit to a sick woman or man, they were primarily in charge of this one person and not subject to conflict with the other demands that typically arise in a hospital setting. This allowed the nurses to act according to what the situation and the sick person required and could mean visiting for a chat or making soup.[20] In addition, the nurses in the parishes were responsible not only for the sick but also for the elderly, for the "sad and hard-done-bys,"[21] as an obituary issued by the motherhouse for a deceased deaconess put it. This tells us that the directorship of the motherhouse had a broad understanding of need, which encompassed both physical and spiritual suffering. It would have been this engagement with people and response to their needs that convinced Sister Marianne of the meaning of her occupation, contributing significantly to her deep professional satisfaction.

The sisters themselves often related in interviews and letters that the broad range of responsibilities was something about parish nursing they found very satisfying. They took pleasure in reporting that, in many communities, holding the children's service was among the deaconesses' responsibilities.[22] In March 1944, Sister Josephine wrote to pastor Otto Meyer, directing pastor of the Henriettenstiftung:

> I am so grateful to God that I may do this service to the children. It is probably one of the most beautiful things for a deaconess to be standing in front of a group of children and announcing the word of our Savior. . . . For myself, this is always a blessing of our God and I have become very satisfied and happy deep inside—I might almost say happy for the first time as a deaconess in this service to the children.[23]

The assignment to do the children's service constituted an important counterbalance to the demanding aspects of nursing. It enabled the deaconesses to do something other than caring for elderly, diseased, or needy individuals. Here they worked with young, healthy children, singing with them and announcing the Word of God. In addition, when doing the children's service they were able to apply their theological knowledge in a way that was visible to the church and gained them recognition. When the nurses succeeded in fulfilling their various tasks and integrating themselves into parish life, they acquired a prominent position locally, one that went with a high social standing. It seems to be the case—and this is hardly surprising—that parish nurses in particular were able to recruit new members to the motherhouse. After all it was they who, through their children's services and home visits, demonstrated to girls and young women what motherhouse deaconry achieved in practical terms, and that it could gain high regard in the community.[24]

Parish Nursing in West Germany During the Upheavals of the 1960s

As opposed to hospital work, which saw a fundamental reorganization as early as the 1960s, parish nursing proved remarkably resistant to modernization for a long time. This can be seen in the above example of Sister Ella, working in Harz mountain villages, where the old structures of Protestant parish nursing stayed intact into the 1980s. Unlike in the 1950s, however, Sister Ella eventually no longer used a bicycle but had a car to get around. For a long time, motorization remained the most significant innovation in parish nursing: Mopeds for sisters were introduced in the 1950s and cars in the 1960s.

The reason behind the endurance of the nineteenth-century understanding of nursing in the parish compared to hospitals can likely be seen in the fact that ambulant care retained a relatively strong independence from technology. Compared to care in a hospital, the pressure to adapt to the rules of a scientific and technological understanding of medicine was considerably less pronounced in parish nursing. Moreover, parish nurses enjoyed relative freedom in organizing their work. When the motherhouse was no longer able to run a parish nurse station exclusively with nurses from the Henriettenstiftung, the parish could be subdivided into several different assignment areas. The deaconesses could continue their work as they always had in their own areas, whereas secular nurses would serve one or more other areas, working under their respective conditions. In this way, the traditional nursing stations could coexist with the newly developing diaconal and welfare centers, which were based on a division of labor and employed qualified workers specializing in sick-nursing, geriatric care, and family nursing to serve the area.[25] As opposed to work in the parishes, deaconesses at hospitals worked closely with secular personnel and were thus confronted to a much greater degree with the coming generation's modern image of nursing and needed to make compromises.[26]

Even if the traditional structures of parish nursing remained intact for a remarkably long time, we can assume that the focus of the work changed. With an increasing number of people who suffered from more severe diseases checking themselves into hospitals, the field would have shifted ever more toward care for the elderly.[27] The active involvement of deaconesses in church life seems to have become more problematic as well. The lifestyle of religiousness represented by the deaconesses increasingly seemed antiquated, even within the church. The deaconess role came to look like a phased-out model, not only in hospitals but in the church itself. Finding themselves confronted with this situation, the deaconesses presumably turned to work at the sickbed and the deathbed, where their services and the certainties of religion were still in demand.

Deaconess Motherhouses in the United States: A Model of Failure

Whereas in nineteenth-century Germany the motherhouse became the dominant organizational form, making its mark on the vocational field in West

Germany into the 1960s, deaconess institutions in the United States met with little success.[28] The first attempt at establishing a Protestant motherhouse, in Pittsburgh in the late 1840s, failed because not enough new sisters were coming in.[29] It was not until the late 1880s that a successful, if modest, wave of founding activity arose, resulting in ten deaconess institutions.[30] Among them was the Lutheran deaconess motherhouse in Baltimore, which was founded in 1895 and became the third-largest deaconess motherhouse in the United States. In 1946, it counted sixty-seven members—a tenth of the Henriettenstiftung's membership.[31]

Considering the low numbers, it is not surprising that a discussion of the reasons behind difficulties in recruiting new members is found throughout the history of U.S. deaconess motherhouses. The relatively independent status of women in American society compared to Germany was seen as the main reason why becoming a deaconess had so little appeal for women. In the United States, women grew so accustomed to earning their living that occupational work without salary became an impossibility. Moreover, the greater number of male than female settlers in late nineteenth-century America meant that women had better chances for marriage in the New World. With a wider range of personal and professional opportunities, employers needed to come up with attractive offers to interest women in working as nurses. It only makes sense that, in this context, the deaconess motherhouse with its concept of organized honorary posts for women had only a slim chance of success.[32]

To complicate matters further, the deaconess motherhouses were only partially funded by the church due to the fragmentation of the Protestant environment in the United States into a large number of denominations. Thus, the general circumstances of American deaconess institutions were fundamentally different not only from the German situation, which was characterized by the large, unified Protestant church supporting the concept of deaconess institutions. There was also a considerable difference from the situation of the Catholic orders in the United States, which had been able to establish themselves quite successfully.[33] More to the point, in the United States there were Episcopal, Methodist, Evangelical, and Mennonite deaconesses. And the few existing deaconess institutions were not only divided into different Protestant churches but further divided into German, Swedish, and Norwegian motherhouses. Such conditions, created by society and church history, were hardly helpful to furthering deaconess institutions. As the example of the motherhouse in Baltimore will show, another important reason for the failure in transferring the German deaconess model was the lack of support in local communities. Because few ego-documents have been preserved after 1900 in the case of the Baltimore motherhouse, the following account will focus on church debates concerning the conception and reform of parish work.

Parish Nursing in the United States: The Lutheran Deaconess Motherhouse in Baltimore

From the very beginning, when the Baltimore deaconess motherhouse was founded in 1895, it was decided that the primary focus would be on parish nursing and not on hospital care. From the turn of the century onward, further fields of activity were added, mostly in the areas of education and foreign mission. Accordingly, the Baltimore motherhouse—unlike the Henriettenstiftung—did not run its own hospital. Deaconess candidates were trained at the nearby motherhouse in Philadelphia, where they acquired the necessary skills of hospital and at-home nursing, followed by further instruction that included parish nursing at the Baltimore motherhouse. In 1901, the Baltimore motherhouse opened its own school, but its focus was on religion and Christian education to, among other reasons, prepare for the foreign mission.[34] Thus, the training of the Baltimore motherhouse was specialized in caring for the soul. The parish nurse's job description, however, was oriented on the German model and included domestic nursing care, social work, and care of the soul.[35]

Recruitment of deaconesses was slow from the outset. By 1926 only seventy-nine deaconesses had been consecrated in Baltimore.[36] Confronted with a stagnating membership, the future of parish nursing became a regular item on the United Lutheran Church in America agenda in the late 1920s. This occurred at a time when professionalization of church work and reform of confessional training as a whole were up for debate. In the late 1920s and early 1930s, a committee was established to carry out surveys in the parishes to gauge the need for deaconesses and other workers and to get a sense of desired training standards.[37] From the perspective of the motherhouse deaconry, the results were shattering. It turned out that the majority of pastors were not interested in working with deaconesses, preferring laypersons instead. There was one simple reason for this: In the case of secular personnel, the pastor acted as employer. When someone ill-suited to the work had been hired, it was up to the pastor to dismiss the person.[38] A deaconess, however, was deployed by the motherhouse and worked under the directing sister and the directing pastor; the local parish pastor could request the relocation of the deaconess, but he did not have decision-making power. Granted, this was also a problem for pastors in Germany—as well as, incidentally, for German doctors.[39] Particularly when a deaconess lived at the parsonage, she could come into intense conflict with the pastor and his wife. But as long as nursing in Germany was predominantly church-organized and the pastors had a social responsibility to their parishioners who received nursing care, they had to accept these conditions. In the United States, due to the less-established tradition of sisterhoods, the market rule of "hire and fire" took hold much sooner.

The survey results also proved that the American pastors' understanding of parish work was fundamentally different from that of German pastors. Not a single American pastor wished to have a nurse work in the community. In fact, they frequently brought up the many Visiting Nurse Associations (VNAs), suggesting that these associations could look after the physical welfare of community members.[40] To most pastors, a well-trained parish secretary who would take on administrative work was more desirable.[41] Sporadically, the opinion was voiced that deaconesses ought to have a better theological education to master the requirements of the children's service, Sunday school, and similar work.[42]

If we follow the responses of the pastors, there is no room for deaconesses in community work for two reasons. First, with the VNAs, a local nursing infrastructure already existed, one that had become established in the United States as early as the nineteenth century. In addition, following the example of the British district nurses, women from the upper classes in America had also founded charity associations and hired nurses to care for the impoverished sick.[43] Hence the deaconess institutions were in no way founded on barren ground, and it seems plausible that the VNAs perceived them as unwanted competition rather than welcome support. And this may indeed be one explanation for the failure of the German concept of the parish deaconess in the United States.[44]

This response from the pastors suggests that the Lutheran church in America contributed considerably to the secularization of nursing. By delegating physical nursing care to nonchurch organizations, representatives of the church withdrew from the responsibility of providing nursing care to their parishioners and accelerated the rupture of the unity of nursing body and soul. By and large, the female managers of VNAs in the nineteenth century indeed had a Christian motivation, and the associations were partly church-funded. But with the secularization and professionalization of home-based care since the turn of the century, this Christian basis quickly lost significance.[45] What remained in the hands of the church was nonsomatic pastoral care, which was later professionalized in the form of theological education.

Second, there was no room in the community for the real work of a deaconess because the volume of administrative tasks in community work became so great at some point. Why would a young woman choose the life of a deaconess only to end up as the pastor's secretary? Accordingly, the investigation committee in its 1929 interim report asked about "how far the Church is justified in allowing the deaconess to be diverted from her original work of mercy and nursing to that of the pastor's and congregation's office secretary."[46] It was indeed hardly possible to transform the idea of "labor of love"—service to one's fellow man—into administrative service to the pastor. Under these circumstances, the recruitment of female "laborers of love" could only fail.

The Baltimore motherhouse tried to counter this dilemma by dividing its training program into two parts: in the mid-1940s, a one-year course for parish secretaries was set up to invite lay personnel. The deaconess training program was made more academic through its focus on Christian education and, from 1946 onward, was carried out in cooperation with a college.[47] In this way, deaconesses did not disappear from community work altogether, but the understanding of parish nursing had changed fundamentally, and physical nursing care was no longer part of it.

That this process of academization and secularization did not constitute genuine historical progress has become apparent by the reinvention of parish nursing in the context of the present-day parish nurse movement, which was started successfully by Granger Westberg in 1984 and has led to the establishment of a new field of specialization in nursing. Westberg opposed the dominant division of medicine and church, of physical and spiritual care, and demanded that the two areas be united in parish nursing to better meet the needs of the sick. This idea met with enormous response and was taken up in numerous parish nurse programs. Calling Westberg a pioneer of parish nursing, however, is misleading and neglects the older tradition of Christian parish nursing. It would be more appropriate to speak of a revival of parish nursing bearing a definitively modern stamp. Some modern attributes are the decidedly interconfessional orientation of the parish nurse movement, the interest in standardizing parish nursing education (1986), the accreditation of parish nursing as a nursing specialty (1997), and the publication of standards for practice by the American Nurses Association in 1998.[48]

Conclusion

Deaconess motherhouses originated in the context of nineteenth-century German society and remained influential in West Germany until the 1960s because of the attractive opportunities they offered women. They opened highly respected working and living prospects outside of marriage. And as the social practice of parish nursing shows, the range of activities the work entailed was itself very appealing.

In West German parish nursing, an important factor in the nurses' great professional satisfaction was, first, that the tasks and duties of parish nurses were only loosely defined. This gave the sisters ample room to decide how to spend their time and organize their work. This considerable autonomy and the feeling that they were actually able to respond to needs as they arose formed an important prerequisite for the great professional satisfaction experienced by the parish nurses. Second, the directors of a motherhouse had an obligation to provide for the welfare of the sisters and indeed took this obligation seriously: A deaconess was not a worker to whom the "hire and fire" principle would be applied. As a daughter of the motherhouse, she was part of a religious community committed to living and working together. It was well understood that it was in the community's interest to look after its members once they had been socialized into the community. It can be demonstrated that the directing sister and the directing pastor took the welfare of their sisters into account when making decisions. The programmatic ideal of service, strongly emphasizing self-sacrifice, can thus not be equated with the deaconesses' everyday experience.

The concept of parish nursing, attractive as it was in the German context, could not be transferred to American society. Although the Baltimore motherhouse initially adopted the German model of the parish deaconess, it soon became clear that not only was it extremely difficult for the motherhouse to recruit women, there was also hardly any demand for deaconesses in the communities. For one thing, a local infrastructure of ambulant care for the impoverished and sick had already been established by VNAs. For another, Lutheran pastors from, at the latest, the 1920s and 1930s onward, were in favor of a divided nursing concept, whereby the church would focus solely on care for the soul. Under the circumstances, there was no room for the German conception of parish nursing with its unity of physical and spiritual care.

The reinvention of parish nursing in the United States of the 1980s, however, shows that the Christian understanding of illness and nursing did not sink into oblivion. The history of the parish nursing movement shows once again that the history of nursing cannot be written as a story of progress with a linear progression. It is much more the case that, following a cyclical progression, concepts and practices were and are often rediscovered and invented without knowledge of historical predecessors. A simple duplication of old concepts in a new context is certainly inadvisable, however, because their usefulness was rooted in specific historical conditions. More generally speaking, for the purpose of tempering a perhaps overzealous pioneer spirit, it does no harm to remember that old ideas and practices are often rediscovered or reinvented to consider why this is the case and to look into the conditions under which they disappeared in the first place.

Susanne Kreutzer, PhD
Department for Humanities/Nursing Science
University of Osnabrück
Solmsstr 12 10961 Berlin
Germany

Acknowledgments

Research for this article was supported by VolkswagenStiftung, Robert Bosch Foundation, and by a Lillian Sholtis Brunner Fellowship at the Barbara Bates Center for the Study of the History of Nursing, University of Pennsylvania. I also wish to thank Karen Nolte and Lisa Zerull for their comments on this article.

Notes

1. See Norbert Friedrich, "Überforderte Engel? Diakonissen als Gemeindeschwestern im 19. und 20. Jahrhundert," in *Pflege, Räume, Macht und Alltag: Beiträge zur Geschichte der Pflege*, ed. Sabine Braunschweig (Zurich: Chronos, 2006), 85–94. As opposed to hospital nursing, there is little research on parish nursing. One of the few exceptions is a study by Karen Buhler-Wilkerson on ambulant care in the United States in the nineteenth and twentieth centuries: *No Place Like Home: A History of Nursing and Home Care in the United States* (Baltimore: Johns Hopkins University Press, 2001). On the history of parish nursing in West Germany, see Susanne Kreutzer, "Fürsorglich-Sein: Zur Praxis evangelischer Krankenpflege nach 1945," *L'Homme: Europäische Zeitschrift für feministische Geschichtswissenschaft* 19, no. 1 (2008): 61–79; idem, "Freude und Last zugleich: Zur Arbeits- und Lebenswelt evangelischer Gemeindeschwestern in Westdeutschland," in *Alltag in der Krankenpflege: Geschichte und Gegenwart/Everyday Nursing Life: Past and Present*, ed. Sylvelyn Hähner-Rombach (Stuttgart: Franz Steiner, 2009).

2. See Karen Nolte, "Pflege von Leib und Seele: Krankenpflege in Armutsvierteln des 19. Jahrhunderts," in Hähner-Rombach, *Alltag in der Krankenpflege/Everyday Nursing Life*.

3. On the history of the motherhouse deaconry, see Jutta Schmidt, *Beruf Schwester: Mutterhausdiakonie im 19. Jahrhundert* (Frankfurt am Main: Campus Verlag, 1998). Specifically on the Kaiserswerth deaconess motherhouse, see Silke Köser, *Denn eine Diakonisse darf kein Alltagsmensch sein: Kollektive Identitäten Kaiserswerther Diakonissen, 1836–1914* (Leipzig: Evangelische Verlagsanstalt, 2006), and Ute Gause and Cordula Lissner, eds., *Kosmos Diakonissenmutterhaus: Geschichte und Gedächtnis einer Protestantischen Frauengemeinschaft* (Leipzig: Evangelische Verlagsanstalt, 2005).

4. On the reform of the occupational image since the late 1950s, see Susanne Kreutzer, "'Before, We Were Always There—Now, Everything Is Separate': On Nursing

Reforms in Western Germany," *Nursing History Review* 16 (2008): 180–200; and Marianne Schmidbaur, *Vom Lazaruskreuz zur Pflege aktuell: Professionalisierungsdiskurse in der deutschen Krankenpflege 1903–2000* (Königstein/Taunus: Ulrike Helmer, 2002), 147–75.

 5. See Susan M. Reverby, *Ordered to Care: The Dilemma of American Nursing, 1850–1945* (Cambridge: Cambridge University Press, 2004); and Sioban Nelson, *Say Little, Do Much: Nursing, Nuns, and Hospitals in the Nineteenth Century* (Philadelphia: University of Pennsylvania Press, 2001), 134–50.

 6. Nolte, "Pflege von Leib und Seele"; Karen Nolte, "Telling the Painful Truth: Nurses and Physicians in the Nineteenth Century," *Nursing History Review* 16 (2008): 115–34.

 7. See Köser, *Diakonisse*, 83–86.

 8. See Schmidt, *Beruf Schwester*, 207–14.

 9. See Nolte, "Pflege von Leib und Seele."

 10. See Schmidt, *Beruf Schwester*, 110–13.

 11. On the first "free" sisterhood (Berufsorganisation der Krankenpflegerinnen Deutschlands) see Schmidbaur, *Lazaruskreuz*.

 12. See Susanne Kreutzer, *Vom "Liebesdienst" zum modernen Frauenberuf: Die Reform der Krankenpflege nach 1945* (Frankfurt am Main: Campus Verlag, 2005), 33.

 13. All names of sisters except the matron have been anonymized.

 14. Sister Ella Hartung, interview by Susanne Kreutzer, January 28, 2005.

 15. Directing sister Florschütz to Sister Helene Otte, January 15, 1947, S-1–0004, Archive of the Henriettenstiftung.

 16. Note on file by directing Sister Florschütz concerning a visit at the parish nurse station Hameln, May 8, 1962, 1–09–100, Archive of the Henriettenstiftung.

 17. Sister Erika Schröder to directing Sister Florschütz, March 14, 1951, 1–09–181, Archive of the Henriettenstiftung, emphasis original.

 18. See Susanne Kreutzer, "Hierarchien in der Pflege: Zum Verhältnis von Eigenständigkeit und Unterordnung im westdeutschen Pflegealltag," in *Braunschweig, Pflege, Räume, Macht und Alltag*, 203–11.

 19. Marianne Albrecht, interview by Susanne Kreutzer, March 19, 2004.

 20. See Christel Kumbruck and Eva Senghaas-Knobloch, *Das Ethos fürsorglicher Praxis im Wandel: Befunde einer empirischen Studie*, Artec-paper 137 (2006): 30.

 21. Obituary for Sister Emma Weyers, May 14, 1970, S-1–0093, Archive of the Henriettenstiftung.

 22. Sister Helene Otte to directing Sister Florschütz, January 9, 1963, S-1–0004, Archive of the Henriettenstiftung.

 23. Sister Josephine Brandt to Pastor Otto Meyer, March 3, 1944, 1–09–229, Archive of the Henriettenstiftung.

 24. See Ute Gause, *Frömmigkeit und Glaubenspraxis*, in Gause and Lissner, *Kosmos*, 145–73.

 25. See Friedrich, "Überforderte Engel," 92; and Gerta Scharffenorth et al., *Schwestern: Leben und Arbeit Evangelischer Schwesternschaften. Absage an Vorurteile* (Offenbach: Burckhardthaus-Laetare, 1984), 235–51.

 26. See Kreutzer, "Before, We Were Always There," 187–93.

 27. Superintendent Bruns to Pastor Karl Friedrich Weber, April 18, 1959, 1–09–187, Archive of the Henriettenstiftung.

 28. See Nelson, *Say Little, Do Much*, 134–42.

29. See Köser, *Diakonisse*, 118; Ann Doyle, "Nursing by Religious Orders in the United States. Part IV—Lutheran Deaconesses, 1849–1928," *American Journal of Nursing* 29, no. 10 (1929): 1197–207.

30. The individual deaconess motherhouses were in Philadelphia, Brooklyn, Omaha, Minneapolis, Milwaukee, Baltimore, Chicago, St. Paul, Brush (Colorado), and Axtell; see Frederick S. Weiser, "Serving Love: An Early History of the Diaconate in American Lutheranism" (Paper for B.D. degree, Lutheran Theological Seminary, Gettysburg, Pennsylvania, 1960), 168.

31. The largest deaconess motherhouse, with 109 sisters, was in Philadelphia, followed by that in Omaha with 77 sisters. The total number of deaconesses in the United States was 450. See Minutes of the Fifteenth Biennial Convention of the United Lutheran Church in America, Cleveland, October 5–12, 1946, Philadelphia, 545, Evangelical Lutheran Church in America (ELCA) Archives, United Lutheran Church in America (ULCA), 2/1, Box 5. The Henriettenstiftung counted 650 sisters in 1949. Review of the year 1949, Archive of the Henriettenstiftung, S-8–8.

32. See Nelson, *Say Little, Do Much*, 142; Weiser, *Serving Love*, 158.

33. See Barbra Mann Wall, *Unlikely Entrepreneurs: Catholic Sisters and the Hospital Marketplace, 1865–1925* (Columbus: Ohio State University Press, 2005).

34. Training School Affiliated with Susquehanna University, in *Motherhouse Tidings*, Lutheran Deaconess Motherhouse, Baltimore, Md., January–March 1946, ELCA Archives, ULCA 61/8/2.

35. See Frederick S. Weiser, *To Serve the Lord and His People, 1884–1984: Celebrating the Heritage of a Century of Lutheran Deaconesses in America* (Gladwyne, Pa.: Deaconess Community of the Lutheran Church in America, 1984), 14.

36. Committee on Survey to the Board of Deaconess Work of the United Lutheran Church in America, April 24, 1930, ELCA Archives, ULCA 22/7, Box 1.

37. Questionnaire, undated, ca. 1928, and Report of Committee on Survey of the Field, undated, ca. 1929, ELCA Archives, ULCA 22/7, Box 1.

38. Committee on Survey to the Board of Deaconess Work.

39. See Friedrich, "Überforderte Engel," 90.

40. Rev. Frederick B. Clausen, St. John's Evangelical Lutheran Church, to Rev. Foster U. Gift, Lutheran Deaconess Motherhouse, February 26, 1930, ELCA Archives, ULCA 61/6/1, Box 1.

41. Committee on Survey to the Board of Deaconess Work.

42. P.F.W. Teichmann, Christ Evangelical Lutheran Church, to Rev. Dr. Simon, Hagerstown, July 23, 1935, ELCA Archives, ULCA 61/6/1, Box 1.

43. See Buhler-Wilkerson, *No Place like Home*, 17–29.

44. In nineteenth-century Germany as well, women founded associations comparable to the VNAs. As opposed to the motherhouses, however, they did not successfully take hold. See Catherine M. Prelinger, *Charity, Challenge, and Change: Religious Dimensions of the Mid-Ninetheenth-Century Women's Movement in Germany* (New York: Greenwood Press, 1987).

45. See Buhler-Wilkerson, *No Place like Home*, 26.

46. Report of Committee on Survey of the Field, undated, ca. 1929, ELCA Archives, ULCA 22/7, Box 1.

47. Training school affiliated with Susquehanna University.

48. See Lisa Zerull, "One Foot in the Sciences and One Foot in the Humanities: A History of Parish Nursing in the United States 1984–1998" (manuscript).

Finance and Faith at the Catholic Maternity Institute, Santa Fe, New Mexico, 1944–1969

Anne Z. Cockerham
Shenandoah University Division of Nursing
Arlene W. Keeling
University of Virginia School of Nursing

Abstract. In 1944, the Medical Mission Sisters opened the Catholic Maternity Institute in Santa Fe, New Mexico, primarily to serve patients of Spanish American descent. The Maternity Institute offered nurse-midwifery care and functioned as a school to train nurse-midwifery students. Originally planned as a home birth service, the Catholic Maternity Institute soon evolved into a service in which patients chose whether to deliver in their own homes or in a small freestanding building called La Casita. In fact, despite their idealism about home birth and strong feelings that home birth was best, the sisters experienced significant ambivalence concerning La Casita. Births there met many of the institute's pragmatic needs for a larger number of student experiences, quick and safe transfers to a nearby hospital, and more efficient use of the midwives' time. Importantly, as the sisters realized that many of their patients preferred to deliver at La Casita, they came to see that this option permitted these impoverished patients an opportunity to exercise some choice. However, the choice of many patients to deliver at La Casita—which was significantly more expensive for the Maternity Institute than home birth—eventually led to the demise of the Maternity Institute.

In 1944, the Medical Mission Sisters opened the Catholic Maternity Institute in Santa Fe, New Mexico, primarily to serve patients of Spanish American descent.[1] Several factors influenced the sisters to do so, including the Progressive Era's increased interest in maternal-infant health; the success of the first American nurse-midwifery services, the Frontier Nursing Service and Maternity Center Association, in providing nurse-midwifery care to underserved populations; and the dire public health challenges in New Mexico. Another important factor was the availability and interest of the Medical Mission

Sisters, who wanted to provide mission-type medical and nursing care within the United States while World War II limited their international work. The Maternity Institute offered nurse-midwifery care during pregnancy and birth, as well as postpartum and newborn care. It also functioned as a school to train nurse-midwifery students, both lay women and Catholic sisters from the Medical Mission Sisters and other orders who served in maternity-oriented missions around the world. Throughout the twenty-five years the Maternity Institute served the Santa Fe area, the nurse-midwives attended to their patients' physical health and spiritual lives.

Originally planned as a home birth service, the Catholic Maternity Institute soon evolved into a service in which patients chose whether to deliver in their own homes or in a small freestanding building operated by the sisters. They referred to this facility as a maternity home or La Casita, reflecting their Spanish American patients' term for "the little house." In this article we explore the tensions surrounding the location of the Maternity Institute's patients' births. We argue that the sister-nurse-midwives encouraged home births and even romanticized them, but that over time more women began delivering at La Casita. The sisters experienced significant ambivalence concerning La Casita because births there met many of the institute's pragmatic needs for student experiences. Moreover, La Casita births enhanced the sisters' ability to transfer patients to a nearby hospital safely and quickly if needed and allowed them to avoid traveling long distances to patients' homes. Furthermore, as the sisters realized that many of their patients preferred to deliver at La Casita, they came to see that this option permitted these impoverished patients an opportunity to exercise some choice, certainly more than the Spanish American women of Santa Fe would have otherwise had. However, the choice of many patients to deliver at La Casita—which was significantly more expensive for the Maternity Institute than home birth—eventually led to the demise of the Maternity Institute.

The Development of the Maternity Institute

The Maternity Institute leaders and staff were members of the Society of Catholic Medical Missionaries, a community of Catholic sisters better known as Medical Mission Sisters. Building on the work of a Scottish lay woman, Agnes McLaren, who practiced medicine as a Catholic medical missionary in India between 1909 and 1912, the Medical Mission Sisters were founded in 1925 by an Austrian lay woman and physician, Anna Dengel.[2] The Medical Mission Sisters began as a pious society, an organization approved by the church in which the members lived in community like other religious orders but did not take public vows. This was a deliberate decision by Dengel because, at that time, sisters who took public vows were not permitted to practice medicine, surgery, or obstetrics. The purpose of their society was to provide medical and nursing care where needed. Beginning with their founding in 1925, Dengel and the small group of society members, including one other physician and two registered nurses, spent their first year in religious instruction before departing for their mission assignments, primarily in India. Most Medical Mission Sisters entered the community having trained in professional roles as nurses or physicians, or in other disciplines.[3] Dengel and the other Medical Mission Sisters experienced expanded options when in 1936 the Vatican published the encyclical *Constans et Sedula*, which lifted the prohibition against sisters practicing medicine, surgery, or obstetrics. The Medical Mission Sisters were then able to take public vows as an official religious congregation.[4]

Since their founding, the Medical Mission Sisters have been an internationally focused medical missionary order, primarily working in countries, such as India, that had overwhelming needs for professional medical and nursing care. However, in addition to the curtailment of international travel because of World War II, several factors motivated the Medical Mission Sisters to accept a call to Santa Fe, New Mexico, to open the Catholic Maternity Institute in 1944. Most important were the devastatingly high maternal and infant death rates for babies of all ethnic groups in New Mexico in the late 1930s and early 1940s. Additionally, the use of nurse-midwives to provide professional maternity care in areas with few physicians, similar to care provided by nonreligious nurse-midwives at the Frontier Nursing Service in the Appalachian Mountains of Kentucky, provided a model for this type of care in the first half of the twentieth century.[5]

Relationships were key in the inception of the Maternity Institute. Dengel was particularly savvy at developing relationships, especially with people who held goals in common with hers. She enjoyed a collegial and friendly relationship with the archbishop of Santa Fe, Rudolph Gerken, who invited the Medical Mission Sisters to come to Santa Fe in 1942.[6] The presence of a pro–birth control clinic in Santa Fe motivated the archbishop to invite the sisters to counterbalance those influences on his parishioners. The idea of a mission in Santa Fe was appealing to Dengel, because the sisters needed a field to continue to gain experience and serve the ideals of the order while being unable to work overseas during World War II. They carefully considered the archbishop's invitation and, determining that the proposed service met the order's needs, accepted his offer. With the arrival of the trained sister-nurse-midwives in Santa Fe and the opening of the Catholic Maternity Institute in 1944, many Spanish American women had professional maternity care for the first time.[7]

The Maternity Institute opened with a staff of two registered sister-nurse-midwives. The first director was Sister Theophane Shoemaker, born Agnes Shoemaker in 1913 to a large, close-knit Kentucky Catholic family. After graduating from nursing school in Washington, D.C., she joined the Medical Mission Sisters and continued her education with a Bachelor of Science in Nursing Education from the Catholic University of America. Her partner in the Santa Fe mission assignment was Sister Helen Herb, born in Green Bay, Wisconsin, in 1897. She graduated from the nurses' training program at Deaconess Hospital in Buffalo and worked as a private duty nurse there for eight years. In 1928, she entered the Medical Mission Sisters and traveled to England for midwifery training.[8] For nine years during the 1930s, Sister Helen worked in a variety of nursing and midwifery roles in Dacca, India. When Anna Dengel determined that the proposed Santa Fe mission site should be led by Sisters Theophane and Helen, she ordered them to undergo American midwifery training. The two sisters took nurse-midwifery training at the Lobenstine School in New York City and graduated in June 1943.[9]

Location for Maternity Institute Births

Consistent with their goals, between 1944 and 1949 the nurse-midwives attended nearly all births in their patients' homes.[10] However, the sisters began to realize that a few patients needed a place other than home in which to deliver their babies. Some patients simply lived too far away for the midwives to travel to their homes. Others needed a safe place to deliver because they lived in homes the sisters considered unsuitable for births.[11]

Beginning in October 1946, a small number of patients began delivering at a tiny, two-room adobe structure, separate from the Maternity Institute and owned by the archdiocese of Santa Fe. The midwives called this building La Casita, "the little house."[12] It was located about a mile from the Maternity Institute, adjacent to the home of another religious community in Santa Fe, the Order of Our Lady of Mount Carmel. In contrast to the Medical Mission Sisters, the Carmelites were a cloistered religious order.

The proximity to another group of women religious—particularly the Carmelites, whose specific spiritual focus was contemplative prayer—was a benefit, according to a former Maternity Institute nurse-midwife, who recalled later: "We always felt that the Carmelites knew when the lights were on we were having a delivery. And so we felt that we were really prayed for all the time we were taking care of these mothers."[13] Birth setting was important to the sisters; it had to be a place where they could properly carry out their goal to keep birth a spiritual affair. Over the years, this would influence their judgments about the best place for their patients to deliver.

Although La Casita was originally intended only for rare exceptions to home births, the number of patients delivering in the little house grew quickly. Between 1948 and 1950, approximately 8 percent of the Maternity Institute's 300 annual deliveries took place at La Casita. By 1951, however, La Casita births had nearly tripled, to about 20 percent of the deliveries.[14] This increased demand required a new, larger facility than the building they had been using near the Carmelite sisters' residence. In 1951, the Medical Mission Sisters opened a new facility across the small parking lot from the Maternity Institute's main building—a permanent and larger La Casita.

Challenges of Maintaining the Maternity Institute's Financial Health

The Maternity Institute's finances as a charity-focused, nonprofit service were a constant concern for the sisters.[15] Some of the funding came from patient revenues, as the Maternity Institute staff expected patients, regardless of their income, to pay a modest fee to help cover expenses. But charity service and the economic health of the institution were sometimes at odds. As time went by, difficulties in fee collection surfaced, and the Maternity Institute felt financial stress. Some of the difficulties stemmed from the cash-poor economy in which many of their patients lived. One institute director later recalled that, in deference to patients' inability to pay cash, the staff sometimes accepted payment in kind:

> The other principle we had was the families would make some kind of contribution toward their care. Money was not easily available for our patients, but we had a section, along side of our building, and we had a low fence around our property and, in the front, we discovered that people—in the evenings—would sit on that low fence and it would get a little noisy. Our sleep was precious . . . we decided to build a higher fence around and, in that area, you build with adobe. We arranged for, anyone in the family—men—to come and make adobe bricks.[16]

By 1948, a few members of the Maternity Institute staff expressed dissatisfaction with a charity-based approach to the amount and collection of patient fees. They thought that patients could pay more, and that some patients' families were taking advantage of the charity provided by the Maternity Institute. According to the January 1949 Staff Meeting Minutes:

> At the beginning of last year it was decided that many of the patients could well afford to pay more than $10.00 for their care. They were to be told that the actual cost to the service was much more than this and they were to be asked to give more in the form of donations if they felt that they could afford it. This system has been unsuccessful. Many who could well afford to pay the actual cost of their care have given nothing beyond the minimal fee.[17]

Why the Maternity Institute Sisters Preferred Home Birth

From the Maternity Institute's inception, home birth was spiritually and economically consistent with the way the sisters thought birth should be. The sisters romanticized home birth, perhaps because it was congruent with many of their previous experiences. For example, some of the sisters had attended births in areas of the world where women had no access to hospital care and thus delivered in their own homes. Sister Helen, one of the original sisters of the Maternity Institute, had practiced midwifery in India. She and Sister Theophane incorporated many facets of the Lobenstine School program of care into their own work.

For the Maternity Institute nurse-midwives, a woman delivering her baby in her own familiar adobe home, surrounded by her family's presence and prayers, was birth the way God intended it. Even as more patients delivered at La Casita, Maternity Institute nurse-midwives continued to describe home birth as the Christian ideal by teaching women during mothers' classes, "Home delivery is good and proper thing (besides being cheaper). Not only the Birthday but birthplace is important. Bethlehem's stable honored world over."[18] The sisters also preferred home birth because it was more economical for their impoverished patients than either La Casita or hospital birth.

In 1988, Sister Catherine Shean, a nurse-midwife who served as director for many years, recounted her experiences at the Maternity Institute and highlighted the spiritual importance of home birth:

> I think one of the most beautiful [aspects] for me was when you were in the home and the baby was born and . . . the mother had been cleaned up and she was ready to receive the baby . . . many times the other younger children were invited in to meet the baby. . . . We had the tradition in our midwifery service that when we

finished with the mother . . . we would gather together the family and the husband and we would pray with them before we left, thanking God for this new life and for all the help that He had given to us.[19]

Sister Catherine's recollections vividly demonstrate the Maternity Institute nurse-midwives' dual focus on physical and spiritual care of their patients. To them, these all-important elements were best found in the home.

During the 1950s, the Maternity Institute staff indicated their disquiet with increasing patient preference for La Casita over home deliveries. In January 1951, staff minutes noted that "There was discussion on who should be admitted to La Casita. Those who reasonably can be delivered at home should be encouraged to deliver there."[20] A Catholic journal described the Maternity Institute's work: "Deliveries take place at the maternity center or in the patient's home. The nurse-midwives prefer the latter since it is more conducive to the normal pattern of family life."[21] The faculty at the nurse-midwifery school also inculcated in their students the belief that home was the optimal location for birth. A 1950s-era alumna reflected: "The mother remaining in a familiar home environment contributed also towards having a good experience during labor and delivery."[22]

La Casita's Financial Challenges

Another reason the sisters continued to prefer home births was that they were more economical, not only for their patients but for themselves as well. As more and more patients came to La Casita, there were growing concerns related to its operation and the Maternity Institute's financial viability. Although births at La Casita were far less costly to patients than births at the hospital, they cost the Maternity Institute significantly more than did home births. Because of the fee structure set by Maternity Institute leaders, many of these costs were absorbed by the institute. Thus, though patients were drawn to delivery at La Casita, it operated at a deficit.

Discussions at staff meetings reflected the staff's attempts at optimal financial stewardship of La Casita, including minimizing waste, maximizing efficiency, and enhancing fee collection. According to staff meeting minutes:

> Sister Theophane stated that all items in the closets, rooms and on the shelves were enumerated on a label nearby. These are to be used for checking the supplies before the patient is dismissed. The aquastat is to be kept at 160° and the thermostat at 60°. . . . It was agreed upon that since the actual cost for the upkeep of La Casita was $3.00 per diem, [Maternity Institute] patients . . . would be charged the $3.00 fee.[23]

The sisters also economized by reusing linen. Staff minutes noted that "each patient is to have her Turkish towel and wash cloth washed out each day after use and hung outside to dry and brought back in for reuse.... The drape sheet used for delivery is to be used again for the first day demonstration care in the making of the bed."[24]

By the mid-1950s, the financial challenges the sisters faced regarding La Casita provided a renewed push for home delivery. According to the minutes of another staff meeting, Maternity Institute leaders advised their staff:

> Next was discussed the advisability of persuading more patients to deliver at home rather than at La Casita. Sister Theophane said that in doing the distribution analysis on the annual financial report, Anne Fox [a nurse-midwife employed by the New Mexico State Department of Health who provided consultation services to CMI] determined that 1,000.00 dollars had been lost through La Casita [this year].[25]

By the mid-1960s, the Maternity Institute's financial problems had reached an alarming level. One major reason was that many patients did not pay their bills, for either home services or those at La Casita. This was not a new problem; the sisters had discussed it intermittently for many years. However, in early 1965, they attempted to gather information about exactly *why* their patients had difficulty paying their fees. On January 1, 1965, the sisters initiated a four-month study to elicit employment histories and other data from both husbands and mothers. According to one document,

> The purpose of such a study is to determine some of the cogent economic problems and their causes among the people in the community of Santa Fe and the outlying communities from which we draw our patients for maternity care.... Despite the fact that our fee is kept as low as possible we find that many of the people have difficulty in meeting this obligation. Since January, 1965, we have started a graded scale of payment in hopes that this will alleviate the economic burden of the families. At the same time we feel that it is equally important to probe into the causes that beset the families so.[26]

The sisters believed that if they could understand the specific reasons for their clients' dire economic circumstances, then they could work with other professional agencies to help the families reach healthy and more satisfying goals.[27] The results of the study, if they were in fact recorded or published, have not been found.

The Maternity Institute's leaders, after more than two decades of lamenting that their patients were unable to pay their bills, determined again that they should delve into the underlying economic causes of their problems. This likely reflected Catholics' growing concern for social justice that the Second Vatican Council, which met from 1962 to 1965, had implemented. However, in addition to the patients' true financial hardships, there was a sense, at least according to a member of the Maternity Institute's administrative staff, that some patients were able but unwilling to pay their bills:

> What happened at CMI [was] the fact that they had people coming who wouldn't pay. We had one little old man who would come in every month and give us $1 on his daughter's account. He only had a dollar. He came in every month until he had it paid off. He said, "I just don't understand these young people. They have TVs and everything else and they don't pay their bills to the nuns."[28]

Thus, there was a significant difference between the amount the Maternity Institute staff charged patients for services and the amount they collected. A 1966 midwifery service financial report corroborates this former staff member's recollections. Of $41,434 owed for services rendered, the Maternity Institute collected only $26,321, leaving a deficit of $15,113 between billed and collected fees.[29]

Contributions from other sources such as the United Fund, student tuition, local and out-of-state donations, and proceeds from events such as a rummage sale helped the Maternity Institute remain viable.[30] However, by far the largest contributor was the Medical Mission Sisters congregation, with a $29,435 contribution in 1966 that enabled the Santa Fe operation to continue. These annual contributions from Medical Mission Sisters were tenuous and subject to being revoked at any time. Indeed, the sisters somewhat reluctantly supported the Maternity Institute, in part because it was a mission within the United States rather than part of their preferred overseas missions.[31] Still, the support of the Medical Mission Sisters was truly the economic lifeblood of the Maternity Institute. If the sisters withdrew their support, it could not remain in operation.

La Casita's Appeal to Patients

Despite the overriding philosophy of the Maternity Institute staff that home birth was superior, many births moved into La Casita, for several reasons. La Casita provided an option for women to choose where they wanted to deliver, and patients increasingly demonstrated a preference for birth at La Casita. An important practical advantage to patients was that delivery somewhere other than their homes resulted in several days free from household responsibilities. One sister noted that patients reported they were able to rest more adequately after their births at La Casita than if they had delivered at home.[32] Additionally, the maternity home, with its comfortable surroundings, could be a luxury to patients unaccustomed to electricity or running water. In fact, the Maternity Institute staff had to assist these patients in navigating the different world of La Casita. Meeting minutes recorded: "Since these patients and their helpers may not be familiar with the proper use of the telephone, running water, gas stove, etc., careful instructions should be left with them when they are admitted."[33]

The sisters also believed that patients enjoyed a certain prestige in delivering at a medical facility rather than in the home, although no patient records are available to verify this assumption. A Maternity Institute nurse-midwife stated: "It was a staff opinion that a status-seeking factor was . . . in operation."[34] These sisters were from middle-class backgrounds and were products of mid-twentieth-century college educations. They likely were aware of white middle-class women's growing preferences for hospital births and their denigration of home births as only for poor women.[35] According to the sisters' perceptions, some patients declined to return to the Maternity Institute, exercising one of the few choices they had, if they perceived that they would be forced to deliver at home rather than at La Casita. The staff discussed this at a meeting:

> The drop in the caseload was next discussed, and factors which might possibly be influencing it. It was the opinion of all present that a number of patients who had been delivered by CMI and did not return for future care, might have returned . . . if they were given an option, either to have their delivery at home or in the maternity home.[36]

Because data about patients' perceptions are unavailable, it is debatable whether the increase in La Casita births was related to patients' demands to deliver there to enjoy the relatively luxurious surroundings and restful atmosphere away from the responsibilities of home or if the sisters projected their middle-class educations of what they thought women might want. Nevertheless, La Casita gave Maternity Institute patients *choices*.

Maternity Institute Sisters Also Drawn to La Casita Births

In spite of the sisters' philosophical preferences for home birth, there were also advantages to the nurse-midwives themselves when their patients delivered at

La Casita. Located just steps away from their main building, La Casita allowed the midwives to avoid travel that sometimes entailed a long, cold drive over dark and poorly marked roads to attend women who lived miles from Santa Fe. Indeed, La Casita deliveries allowed Maternity Institute nurse-midwives to avoid startling experiences like the following home birth described by a school alumna.

> We were called to Pecos [25 miles from Santa Fe through extremely mountainous terrain] one Sunday evening. We were making the turn off to Pecos, when BAM! We hit something, or something hit us! It was a horse and the windshield was shattered (but still holding together) . . . the horse ran off—at least he was nowhere to be seen. . . . We then went on to the patient and it was early morning when we again set out for Santa Fe. It was a spooky ride with my head out the side window most of the way.[37]

A significant factor in the sisters' decision making about Maternity Institute policies was the presence of student nurse-midwives at the school. The Maternity Institute's school of nurse-midwifery educated students in two educational tracks: It awarded certificates to students who did not desire a master's degree and served as the clinical site for nurse-midwifery students in the Catholic University of America Master of Nursing program. The school averaged four graduates each year, approximately half women religious and half lay women. Many of the religious graduates used their education to serve in a medical missionary role abroad.[38] The proximity of La Casita to the Maternity Institute's main building and clinic enhanced the clinical opportunities for these nurse-midwifery students. They could gain more clinical hours than if they had to travel great distances to observe births. Sister Theophane was well aware of this advantage. She instructed staff members to call her if someone in labor came to La Casita so that more students could observe deliveries.[39]

Additionally, La Casita's proximity to Santa Fe's only hospital, St. Vincent's—two blocks from the Maternity Institute—facilitated rapid transfer of mothers or babies who experienced complications. A former Maternity Institute director recalled that La Casita deliveries were useful for "mothers that we wanted to watch more closely."[40] Typical of these were women with Rh negative blood, who were at increased risk of delivering an isoimmunized—and potentially very ill—baby. Leaders advised their staff: "Mothers with Rh negative blood will be encouraged to come to La Casita for delivery if they have been sensitized as shown by previous difficulties."[41] Thus, staff used La Casita as a way to decrease the rate of complications associated with home delivery in patients with high risk factors.

The increasing number of births at La Casita, with its convenient location, represented a conflict for the Medical Mission Sisters. Their spiritual ideals of service encouraged home births to keep the birth with the family. But these conflicted with their teaching priorities to enhance the number of opportunities for their students to be involved with births, as well as their clinical priorities to keep patients safe by facilitating appropriate hospital transfers.

Conclusion

From the end of the 1940s to the 1960s, the number of Maternity Institute patients delivering at La Casita increased, while home births decreased commensurately. At the same time, the number of hospital deliveries held constant at approximately 5 to 10 percent of all Maternity Institute births.[42] Whereas a nurse-midwife who attended a birth in the first few years of the Maternity Institute would likely travel down a dark, rural road to find a woman laboring in her own home, in the late 1960s she was more likely to welcome a woman into La Casita.

Because of the conflicting interests of idealized home births and the realities of increasing La Casita births, the sisters worked toward reconciling the two seemingly disparate approaches. One way was to keep La Casita births as similar to home births as possible. Sister Rosemary Smyth, a Medical Mission sister who completed nurse-midwifery education at the Maternity Institute, argues that the sisters emphasized the importance of keeping La Casita as similar as possible to the homes of their patients, instead of like a hospital.[43] Advertisements highlighted that births at La Casita were "set up as nearly like a home as possible."[44] One nurse-midwifery school alumna remembered La Casita as being "very homey; it wasn't a hospital atmosphere at all."[45] Another alumna of the same era similarly recalled:

> The concept and actual functioning of La Casita was very unique, providing such a wonderful homelike atmosphere for the patient. It was a big factor in helping all of us, including the mother and husband, realize how normal and natural the experience of giving birth is meant to be.[46]

Thus many of La Casita's characteristics, including its modest furnishings, contributed to its similarity with the homes of Maternity Institute patients.

Financial problems associated with an increasing number of La Casita births were important to the sisters, and their fear of debt was realistic. However, beyond finances, the sisters also believed that the home was the *correct* place for birth. This resulted in a disconnect between what they envisioned as the best care and what they did to respond to the realities of their patients' lives. Indeed, this shift from home to La Casita births represented a response to practical realities such as a need for efficient use of Maternity Institute personnel, enhanced experience for student nurse-midwives, and quick and safe transfer for hospital care in the event of emergencies. Moreover, La Casita allowed impoverished patients to experience an environment that was different from their rural homes; indeed, it was a place where they could enjoy rest after delivery. In so doing, they added to the national trend of delivering somewhere other than the home.

Maternity Institute care—with the midwives' original plan for home births—had emerged as a new solution to maternity care problems in New Mexico in 1944. But after the sisters began attending births at La Casita and the numbers of births at La Casita grew, care grew increasingly expensive. Although the sisters preferred home care, they still provided their patients a choice to deliver at La Casita. This ultimately led to the demise of the mission, however, as the facility grew too expensive to maintain. After twenty-five years of providing nurse-midwifery care to a predominantly Spanish American patient population, the Catholic Maternity Institute closed in July 1969.

ANNE Z. COCKERHAM, PHD., CNM, WHNP-BC
Course Coordinator
Frontier School of Midwifery & Family Nursing
195 School Street
Hayden, KY 41749

ARLENE W. KEELING, PHD, RN
The Centennial Distinguished Professor of Nursing
Director, Center for Nursing Historical Inquiry
University of Virginia School of Nursing
P.O. Box 800782
Charlottesville, VA 22908–0782

Acknowledgments

The authors gratefully acknowledge Barbra Mann Wall, Ph.D., for her skillful and patient editing during the publication process. This work was supported by the Shean Family Foundation, 2006–2008; the American Association for the History of Nursing Student Research Award, 2007; and the Barbara Brodie Doctoral Scholars Endowment Award, 2007–2008.

Notes

1. There is little scholarly consensus about the appropriate manner in which to refer to persons of Mexican origin in the American Southwest, particularly with the terms *Spanish American, Mexican,* or *Mexican American.* These terms have multiple meanings and may be considered politicized, value laden, or pejorative. Additionally, terms vary in the context of different states in the Southwest and at different times. In this article, we use the term Spanish American because the Catholic Maternity Institute staff referred to their patients as Spanish American and the patients self-identified as Spanish American in that time and place. Moreover, the majority of the Latino population in Santa Fe at that time did not consist of recent Mexican immigrants; instead they had roots in Santa Fe dating to the nineteenth century.

2. Katherine Burton, *According to the Pattern: The Story of Dr. Agnes McLaren and the Society of Catholic Medical Missionaries* (New York: Longmans, Green, 1946). For more about the founding and subsequent service of the Medical Mission Sisters, see Sister M. Bonaventure Beck, "The Society of Catholic Medical Missionaries: Organization and Development" (master's thesis, Catholic University of America, 1955); Anna Dengel, *Mission for Samaritans: A Survey of Achievements and Opportunities in the Field of Catholic Medical Missions* (Milwaukee: Bruce Publishing, 1945); Anna Dengel, "The Society of Catholic Medical Missionaries," in *The Mission Apostolate,* ed. National Office of the Society for the Propagation of the Faith in the United States (New York: Paulist Press, 1942); Angelyn Dries, *The Missionary Movement in American Catholic History* (Maryknoll, N.Y.: Orbis, 1998); Medical Mission Sisters, *History of the Society of Catholic Medical Missionaries: Pre-Foundation to 1968* (London: MMS, 1991).

3. It is unclear how it was determined which Medical Mission Sisters would train in which discipline after joining the community.

4. Dengel, *The Mission Apostolate,* 182–83; Burton, *According to the Pattern,* 215.

5. The Frontier Nursing Service has been well documented by many historians. See, for example, Melanie Beals Goan, *Mary Breckinridge: The Frontier Nursing Service and Rural Health in Appalachia* (Chapel Hill: University of North Carolina Press, 2008); Laura E. Ettinger, *Nurse-Midwifery: The Birth of a New American Profession* (Columbus: Ohio State University Press, 2006); Katy Dawley, "Origins of Nurse-Midwifery in the United States and Its Expansion in the 1940s," *Journal of Midwifery & Women's Health* 48 (2003): 86–95.

6. Archbishop Rudolph A. Gerken, letter to Mother Anna Dengel, September 8, 1942, Record Group (hereafter RG) 15-6-1, Folder 129, Ecclesiastical Correspondence, Medical Mission Sisters Archives, Fox Chase, Pa. (hereafter MMSA).

7. *Santa Fe New Mexican,* "Institute to Open Aug. 15," August 9, 1944.

8. Sister Helen Herb's personal information card, MMSA. Sister Helen remained at the Catholic Maternity Institute until 1947, when she returned for service at the order's motherhouse in Philadelphia. She died in 1968.

9. Sally Austen Tom, "Agnes Shoemaker Reinders: A Biographical Tribute," *Journal of Nurse-Midwifery* 25 (1980): 10. After she left the Medical Mission Sisters and married, Sister Theophane Shoemaker was known as Agnes Shoemaker Reinders.

10. Sister Rosemary Smyth, "History of the Catholic Maternity Institute from 1943 to 1958" (master's thesis, Catholic University of America, 1960), 27. Sister Rosemary was a nurse-midwife at the Catholic Maternity Institute.

11. Ibid., 28.

12. Ibid.

13. Oral history of Sister Catherine Shean, July 18, 1988, p. 10, Manuscript Collection (hereafter MSC) 330a, box 13, folder 24, American College of Nurse-Midwives Collection (hereafter ACNMC), National Library of Medicine (hereafter NLM).

14. Data from Smyth, "History of the Catholic Maternity Institute," 27.

15. By-Laws of Catholic Maternity Institute, RG 15–6-1, Folder 3, MMSA.

16. Oral history of Sister Catherine Shean; interview with author, November 17, 2006, p. 6 of transcript.

17. Catholic Maternity Institute Staff Meeting Minutes, January 4, 1949, RG 15–6-1, folder 186, MMSA.

18. Class Outline, undated (likely ca. 1950s), RG 15–6-1, folder 55, MMSA.

19. Oral history of Sister Catherine Shean, July 18, 1988, MSC 330a, box 13, folder 24, ACNMC, NLM.

20. Catholic Maternity Institute Staff Meeting Minutes, January 26, 1951, RG 15–6-1, folder 186, MMSA.

21. Jacques Lowe and Jillen Lowe, "Nurse-Midwives of Santa Fe," *The Sign* (April 1955): 50, MSC 330a, box 12, ACNMC, NLM.

22. Submission by Sister Rosemary Leier, in *CMI Graduates and Faculty Remember Nurse-Midwifery in Santa Fe, New Mexico*, eds. Rita Kroska and Catherine Shean (Tucson: Medical Mission Sisters/Catholic Maternity Institute Historical Project, 1996), 31.

23. Catholic Maternity Institute Staff Meeting Minutes, January 22, 1950, RG 15–6-1, folder 186, MMSA.

24. Catholic Maternity Institute Staff Meeting Minutes, July 10, 1950, RG 15–6-1, folder 186, MMSA.

25. Catholic Maternity Institute Staff Meeting Minutes, January 24, 1956, RG 15–6-1, folder 186, MMSA.

26. Employment history and other important data regarding husbands and mothers in maternity service, January 1–April 30, 1965, RG 15–6, folder unknown, MMSA.

27. Ibid.

28. Oral history of Barbara Rochford, interview with author June 27, 2007, p. 1 of transcript.

29. Data from Catholic Maternity Institute Financial Report—1966, Midwifery Services, dated January 30, 1967, RG 15–6; Education Staff Minutes 1966–1967, folder 182, MMSA.

30. According to a 1964 newspaper article, "The Medical Mission Sisters bear most of the cost of operating the Catholic Maternity Institute. The United Fund makes up the difference in the bill of those families who can't afford to pay all of the cost of their maternal and baby care. *New Mexico Register*, "United Fund Helps . . . Catholic Maternity Institute Provides Vital Services," January 31, 1964, RG 15–06, Folder 209, MMSA.

31. As far back as 1947, discussion within the MMS demonstrated that at least some members did not support funding home missions (missions within the United States). During the 1947 Fourth General Chapter, "Home missions were discussed. Some felt home missions seemed to obscure or even contradict the special object of the Society. It was strongly recommended to have no more home missions." Medical Mission Sisters, *History of the Society of Catholic Medical Missionaries*, 61.

32. Smyth, "History of the Catholic Maternity Institute," 29.

33. Catholic Maternity Institute Staff Meeting Minutes, January 22, 1950, RG 15–6-1, folder 186, MMSA.

34. Smyth, "History of the Catholic Maternity Institute," 29.

35. About the societal change from home to hospital births, see Ettinger, *Nurse-Midwifery*, 108–15; Judith Walzer Leavitt, *Brought to Bed: Childbearing in America, 1750–1950* (New York: Oxford University Press, 1986).

36. Catholic Maternity Institute Staff Meeting Minutes, January 22, 1952, RG 15–6-1, folder 186, MMSA.

37. Submission by Sister Rosemary Smyth, in Kroska and Shean, eds., *CMI Graduates and Faculty*, 53.

38. Smyth, "History of the Catholic Maternity Institute," 48.

39. Catholic Maternity Institute Staff Meeting Minutes, October 15, 1954, RG 15–6-1, folder 187, MMSA.

40. Oral history of Sister Catherine Shean, July 18, 1988, p. 10, MSC 330a, box 13, folder 24, ACNMC, NLM.

41. Catholic Maternity Institute Staff Notes, November 29, 1956, RG 15–6-1, folder 187, MMSA.

42. Data from Smyth, "History of the Catholic Maternity Institute," 27; and Peggy Elrington, 1966 Report, Catholic University of America School of Nursing, General Administration Files, Box 4, Santa Fe, N.M., Nurse-Midwifery Program file.

43. Smyth, "History of the Catholic Maternity Institute," 28.

44. Description of Catholic Maternity Institute School of Nurse-Midwifery in "Education for Nurse-Midwifery," American College of Nurse-Midwifery, RG 15–6-1, folder 214, MMSA.

45. Oral history of Sister Joan Marie Doud, interview with author, February 21, 2008, p. 3 of transcript.

46. Submission by Sister M. Paula D'Errico in Kroska and Shean, eds., *CMI Graduates and Faculty*, 38.

METHODOLOGY

Looking Closely: Material and Visual Approaches to the Nurse's Uniform

CHRISTINA BATES
Canadian Museum of Civilization

I start by looking at a rare and remarkably complete uniform that belonged to Edna Muir while she was a student at Montreal's Western Hospital School for Nurses in 1917 (Figures 1 and 2). Her ankle-length dress buttons up center-front, with long sleeves and V-neck. The fabric is blue cotton, soft from repeated washing, and printed with the entwined initials of the hospital—WHM.

Let us follow Miss Muir as she dons her uniform. First she inserts the heavily starched collar carefully into the neckline of the dress. She reaches behind her neck to attach the collar to the back of the dress with a stud. She also studs the tabs together at the front of the collar, but this is not sufficient to keep the collar in place, so she draws long tapes attached to the collar tabs over her bosom and ties them at the back of her waist. No matter how carefully it is placed, the starched collar is going to chafe her neck.

Next she puts on her cumbersome bib, with shoulder straps that cross over the back, secured with pins to a separate waistband underneath her apron. The center front of the bib is pleated at the top and held in place with a pin. Her dress is worn thin around the shoulders from the rubbing of the starched bib. Miss Muir will now have to stand erect lest she crease the bib! Next, she puts on her apron, attached with a stud at the back, then her starched cuffs, closed with studs, and finally, her cap, the crown of which she has carefully folded into box pleats and sewn into place. The brim at the back is worn, patched, and full of pin marks where she has inserted hat pins to keep her cap on her head.

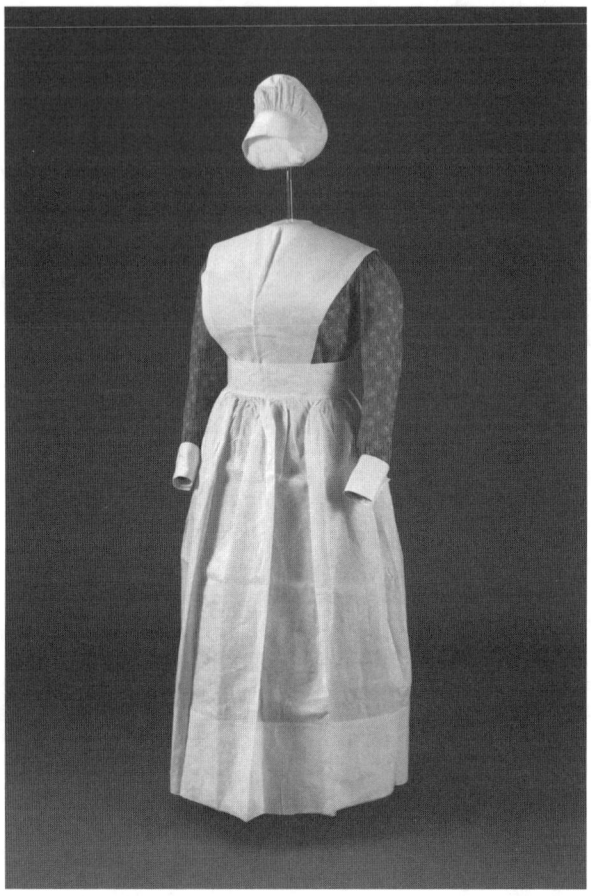

Figure 1. Uniform of Edna Muir, student at Western Hospital, Montreal, 1916–1920. Canadian Museum of Civilization, 2000.111.421, Canadian Nurses Association Collection. Photo by Harry Foster.

Now let us look at the photographic portrait of Miss Muir. Her hair is neatly parted in the middle and pulled over her ears into a bun at the back. Her spectacles and expression give her a serious and demure demeanor. Her uniform is immaculate and precisely arranged. Her stiff bib stands out from her upper body and her rounded cap sticks up above her head.

Taken together, this object and image form a discourse about nursing in the early twentieth century. Nursing uniforms were practical, symbolic, and active in creating patterns of behavior, attitudes, and values that defined generations of nurses for just over one hundred years. The uniform was a major

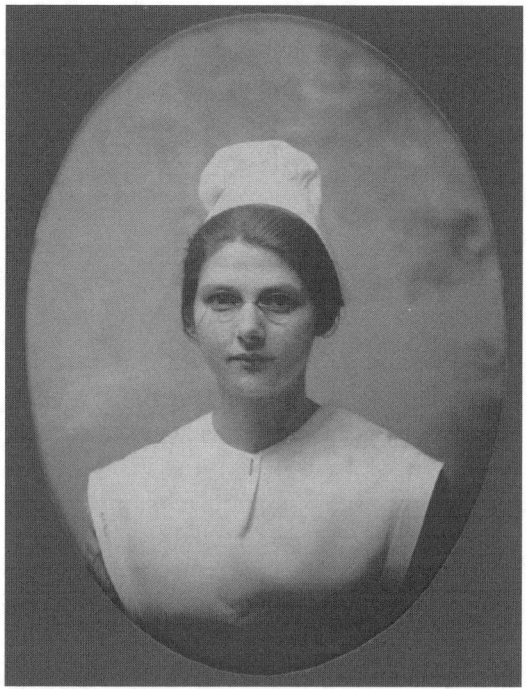

Figure 2. Portrait of Edna Muir, student at Western Hospital, Montreal, 1916–1920. Canadian Museum of Civilization, 2000.111.421, Canadian Nurses Association Collection. Photo by Harry Foster.

strategy in introducing nursing reform and also in creating a strong sense of identity for hundreds of thousands of women.

I am fascinated with this remarkable outfit. For those of us born before nurses began to don scrubs, this was just how they looked; the look was naturalized, not questioned. Yet the combination of soft dress, cardboard-stiff overgarments, and pop-up cap is perplexing: How did it come to be? My study of this integral aspect of nursing combines contextual information on the history of nursing with my long interest in dress to write a cultural history of the nurse's uniform. The purpose of this article, however, is not primarily to present the results of my research but rather to explore the methodology I have found useful, with emphasis on rich visual and material evidence for our understanding of labor, social, and women's history, in particular that of a significant female occupational group. This article presents my interpretation of the uniform using an analogy to the photographic process. When you take a photograph, you frame your subject (the nurse's uniform); you focus the lens (your questions); you decide on depth of field (moving back and forth from the artifact to the historical context); you search for the best exposure (uncovering meanings); and finally, you develop the film (the whole picture).

Very little was written explicitly about the nurse's uniform during its formative period. Therefore, photographs and artifacts are the salient sources. They are powerful conduits to assumptions and beliefs that are so taken-for-granted that they are not expressed in words. Images of graduating nurses are compelling; they bring us face to face with the experience of nurse training. The students' expressions, the way they wear their uniforms, their gestures, and their props enact a performance about nursing culture. Equally evocative are the uniforms themselves: their colors, textures, construction, fit, and condition. The photographs put the static uniforms into action, and the uniforms detail what cannot be seen in the photographs. The two together show the connections and contradictions between the social and private body and between the ideological presentation of nursing and the real experience of work on the wards. For example, we can see in Edna Muir's uniform and portrait the contrast between the polished finished image and the bodily effort it took to pull it all together.

Though my interpretation of these sources has been informed by cultural theory, I do not follow formal quantitative methods. I am interested in the significance of the uniform, but I have also tried to stay close to the material sources themselves, avoiding the temptation to "ignore the artifact in favour of social meaning."[1] I view the uniform as significant, both as symbol and as artifact. Theoretical overviews of the visual and material, such as Peter Burke's *Eyewitnessing*, Gillian Rose's *Visual Methodologies*, and Grant McCracken's *Culture and Consumption* have provided inspiration on a variety of interpretive models.[2] What the methods have in common, as summarized by Rose in her chapter on discourse analysis, is the imperative to look closely and critically at the sources with fresh eyes, to focus on details, to pay attention to complexity and contradictions, to look for the invisible as well as the visible, and to examine how the sources influence the viewer.

The history of the nurse's uniform has been the topic of a limited number of publications by nurses, social historians, and dress historians. In the 1920s and '30s, nurses began to reflect on the uniform through nostalgic articles such as "The Picturesque Past of the Nurse's Uniform," which contain valuable archival pictures and information about the history of the uniform and its differences among schools of nursing.[3] In the 1970s, English historians of occupational dress such as Elizabeth Ewing included in their books detailed histories of the nurse's uniform, from the Middle Ages through Florence Nightingale and into the twentieth century.[4] Despite the uniform's similarity to the apparel of other occupations, they viewed it as distinct, championing the arrival of women in a professional role in the workplace. With the rapid changes in health care in the

1970s and '80s, a flood of articles by nurses, such as "The Tyranny of Uniforms" by Shermalayne Southard Szasz, disparaged the history of nurses' uniforms in the context of the profession's changing image and feminist outlook.[5]

More recently, balanced articles have looked critically at the uniform in its historical context. Notably, Lynn Houweling traced the U.S. uniform as a source of controversy and pride, a site of conflict between individual expression and group identity. Jane Brooks and Anne Marie Rafferty explored the uniform in England as a metaphor for the class divisions and fractures within the profession. Kathryn McPherson examined how the uniform and disciplined behavior mediated femininity, sexuality, and nursing. Though these insightful studies position nursing uniforms in terms of nursing reform, training, and gender identities, they do not really look at the uniform itself in a concerted way. Mary Juszynski Curran's thesis took a step in this direction, studying in detail photographs and a limited number of actual uniforms from some of the first American schools of nursing.[6]

Artists Mark Dion and J. Morgan Puett looked closely at the visual and material properties of uniforms in their 2003 exhibition, *RN: The Past, Present and Future of the Nurses' Uniform*, at the Fabric Workshop and Museum in Philadelphia.[7] Dion and Puett used uniforms, other artifacts, and photographs to explore identity, hierarchy, and labor in the history of nursing through a unique artistic approach that dared the viewer to look at uniforms in a new way. Uniforms from a former nursing uniform company hung like ghosts from the ceiling; intricately folded caps were displayed like origami; and starched bibs were stacked like paper in a display case. Part of the project was to design a contemporary nurse's uniform based on feedback from a focus group of nurses. The artists also imagined the future by designing and displaying uniforms based on science fiction and new material technologies, such as the Bioterrorism Nurse and the Post-Apocalyptic Nurse. The artists challenged conventional wisdom about what a nurse's uniform should look like. By presenting the uniform in unconventional and artistic settings, they asked viewers to see it for what it is: an artificial construction that played a part in the creation of nursing as a profession.

Frame: Choosing Your Subject

Why study the nurse's uniform? As is often the case in the study of objects, a well-developed collection can spark interrogation. The Canadian Museum of Civilization has a large holding of uniforms from across the country in its

Canadian Nursing History Collection.[8] This collection, as well as those preserved by nursing alumnae associations,[9] allowed my material approach to the nurse's uniform.

The collection at the Museum of Civilization includes sixty complete uniforms from twenty schools, more than 300 caps, and 200 school graduation pins from approximately 250 schools of nursing across Canada, dating from 1890 to 1985. This is the largest collection of its kind, and it is representative in several ways. Because all students from a school wore the same uniform, there is no bias in what was kept or discarded. The collection represents major institutions in big cities and tiny rural outposts. It includes a good sample of the uniform changes that occurred as students moved through the academic stages of probationary, junior, and graduate.[10]

Another reason for studying uniforms is that they are clothing—the category of material culture that arguably has the greatest potential for exploring personal and social identity and values. Whether by choice or convention, what we wear is intimately connected with who we are. Dress is both personal and social, private and public, modest and daring, barrier and bait. This ambiguity is described by fashion historian Elizabeth Wilson: "A part of this strangeness in dress is that it links the biological body to the social being, and public to private. This makes it uneasy territory, since it forces us to recognize that the human body is more than a biological entity. It is an organism in culture, a cultural artifact."[11] This very unease makes dress a potent means to illuminate how culture works.

Dress and adornment, because they are internally coded rather than explicit like written evidence, can reveal nuances and complexities that escape historical methods that rely on traditional sources. Clothing, as suggested by Grant McCracken, is an unwritten code that speaks "sotto voce," whose messages are "less overt and their interpretation less conscious than those of language . . . allowing culture to insinuate its beliefs and assumptions into the very fabric of daily life."[12] Studying the way people look through their clothes and portraits can deepen our understanding of a particular issue and even challenge conventional knowledge from textual sources.

Uniforms are the most public clothing type. They immediately identify the social role of the wearer, conveying authority, virtue, expertise, obedience, or responsibility. Uniforms are the public face of an institution, designed to communicate the functions and values of that institution. They also function within the organization to create group identity and loyalty. They are mandated for institutional workers by those in power who carefully monitor the wearing of the uniform and severely reprimand transgressions. The uniform is often used as a reward (such as capping the probationary nurse) or punishment (such as removing the cap).

Yet as much as uniforms appear to be carefully controlled, they also have a life of their own. The nurse's uniform was more than the outward representation of received behaviors and values of the school and hospital on its students. It literally disciplined the student's body to create those behaviors and values. As we have seen with Edna Muir, each day student nurses pinned, pulled, buttoned, fastened, and put together their complex outfit. Their starched collars chafed their necks, and their heads were held high to support their precarious caps. Every day they were physically reminded of the discipline of their occupation. Like all clothing, the uniform is not just a symbol but an active participant in the formation of personal or social mentalités.

A third reason for studying the nurse's uniform is its power to inform women's history. Nursing uniforms were designed for, and worn by, women. As stated by Barbara Burman and Carole Turbin in *Material Strategies: Dress and Gender in Historical Perspective*, "clothing is one of the most consistently gendered aspects of material and visual culture.... Because clothing is highly gendered it is often emotionally charged, and always with us, literally carried on our backs."[13] Clothing is a potent entrée to our understanding of how gender is manifested and how it works. Nurses' uniforms are particularly suited to revealing the construction of a unique ideal of femininity within the masculine structure of the hospital.

Focus: Asking Questions, Seeing Patterns

The first task in this study was to establish a genealogy of the uniform by comparing images of nurses in various countries to those of other female workers, members of religious congregations, and women of fashion. Where did the design ideas come from? How closely did the uniform follow or divert from conventional dress? What were the differences among British, U.S., and Canadian uniforms, if any? What were the elements of the uniform (bib, cap, cuffs), when did they appear, and how did they change? Despite the wealth of visual evidence, the development of the nurse's uniform has not been clear cut, and some mysteries remain. I have yet to figure out the true origin of the nursing cap's black band.

Where to begin? I decided to concentrate on the Montreal, Toronto, and Winnipeg hospitals schools of nursing collections because they all had examples of uniforms representing their entire history, as well as almost complete sets of graduation photographs. I also looked at about twenty other Canadian school uniforms in the nursing history collection at the Museum of Civilization.

Without attempting any particular methodology or theory, I began to examine the uniforms, noting their visual and tactile qualities. I got a sense of the changes in the uniform over time and the differences in uniforms from various schools. I was struck with the worn, faded, and patched condition of uniforms lovingly preserved. For comparison purposes, I also examined a few rare extant nineteenth-century uniforms of domestic servants and factory workers.

At the same time, I searched published Canadian nursing school histories for information on their uniforms and images of graduation, individuals, and nurses at work. I was impressed with how the image of nurses changed over time from feminine poise to professional precision. To determine the relationship between the Canadian uniforms and those from other countries, I assembled about a hundred pictures of nurses from the United States, England, Scotland, Ireland, Australia, and other countries. I photocopied, cut out, arranged by place, date, and design, and taped these pictures all over my dining room walls

How to make sense of this barrage of images? I could see what they had in common and how they differed, but what was the significance of these

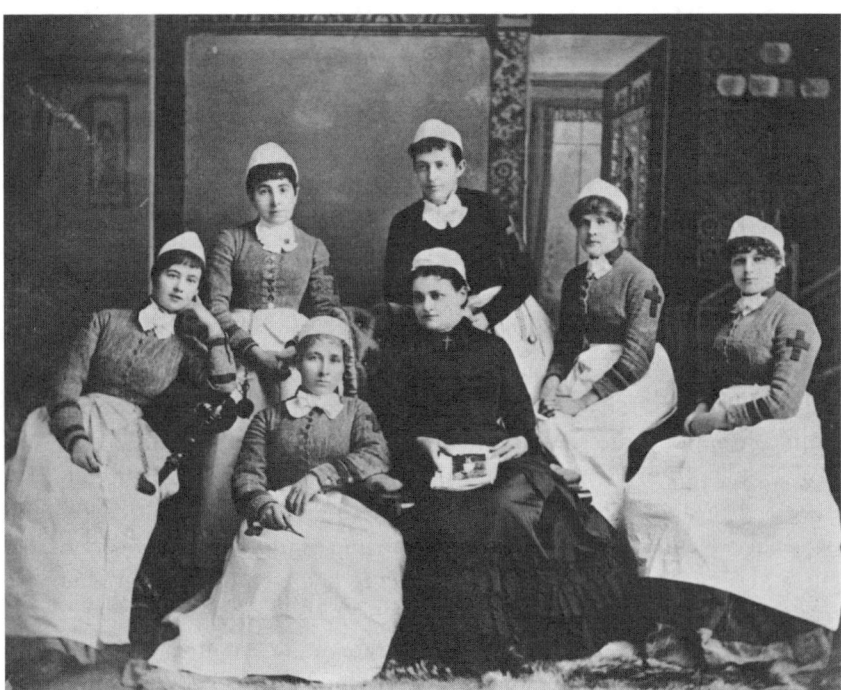

Figure 3. Graduate nurses and probationers, Mack Training School for Nurses, St. Catharine's, Ontario, ca. 1875. Canadian Museum of Civilization, 2001-H0006.4, Canadian Nurses Association Collection.

observations? The approach that made the most sense to me is suggested by sociologist Nathan Joseph in *Uniforms and Nonuniforms*. To analyze uniforms we can use the rhetorical device of metaphor by asking "Who [or what] is adopted as the model for the metaphor; who uses the metaphor; to what extent is the model adopted?"[14]

I tested several models. First, I examined how the uniform related to contemporary women's fashion by comparing the silhouettes, individual garments, and materials of uniforms with those in fashion plates in women's journals, mail-order catalogues, and contemporary female portraits, as well as actual garments. It became clear that the first uniforms, introduced in the 1870s and '80s, used the vocabulary of women's conventional dress, but in a comparatively simple and unadorned manner. For example, in the photograph of the staff of the first nursing school in Canada, called the Mack, each nurse wears a similar white fichu around her neck, which is ruffled but much simpler than those made of lace or whitework worn by fashionable women (compare Figures 3 and 4).

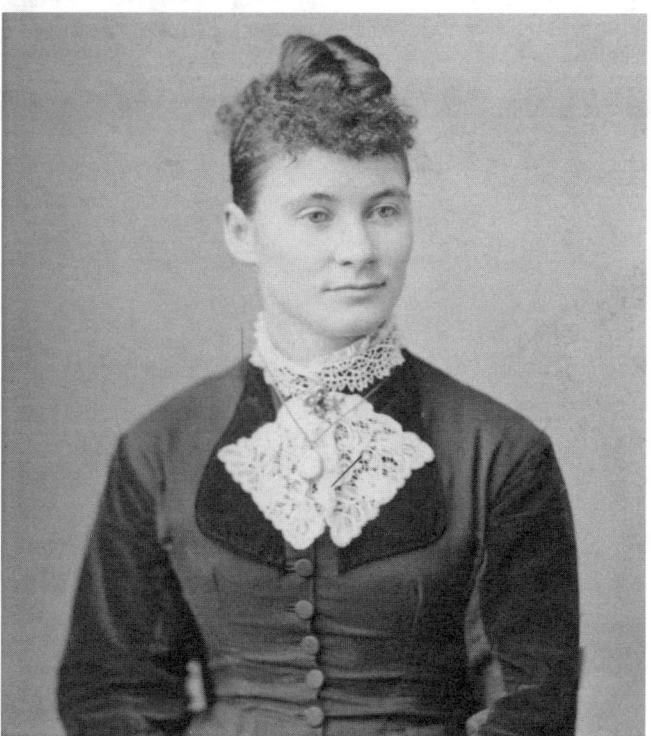

Figure 4. Mrs. Cook. Alexandra Photography Studio, Toronto, ca. 1880, Library and Archives Canada, RD 000702.

I also compared the uniform with clothing worn by other working women. I collected pictures of women in trained occupations such as clerical workers, teachers, and dressmakers, as well as students in other kinds of training schools. By the late nineteenth century, and increasingly into the twentieth, more and more women were entering the business and professional workplace and favored an outfit consisting of a white tailored shirtwaist and plain dark skirt (Figure 5). This ubiquitous "white-collar" working woman

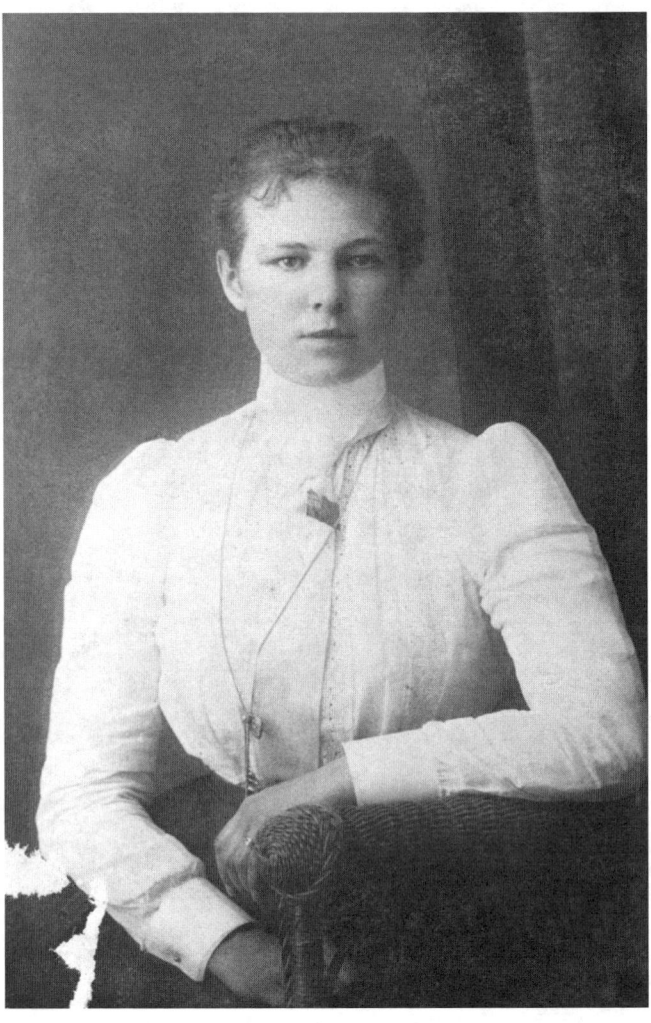

Figure 5. Miss Emily Muriel Mason, schoolteacher, Airdrie, Alberta, 1899. Glenbow Museum, NA-598–4.

look was not adopted for nursing uniforms. Hospital authorities favored more conservatively fitted "wash" dresses, with accessories such as aprons that signaled the manual nature of the work. We can see these fitted dresses in the photographs, but even more clearly in the construction and fit of the dresses themselves (Figure 6).

The apparent similarity between nursing uniforms and clothing worn by household servants led me to concentrate on this model. However, I was careful not to make assumptions before intense examination. Are the garments for the two occupational groups an exact match, or are there small but significant differences? For example, both groups wore caps and

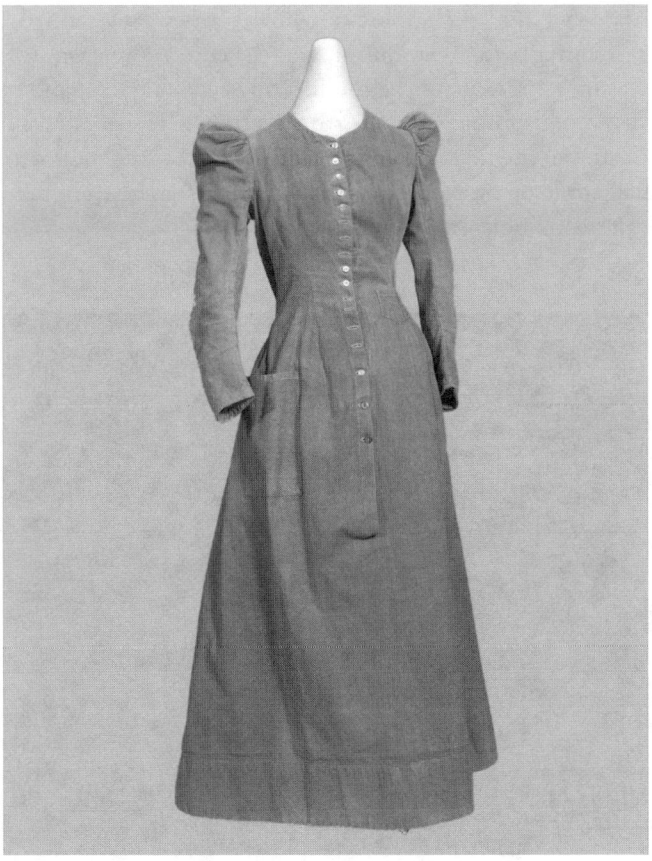

Figure 6. Uniform of Margaret Elizabeth Lamb, Saskatchewan, ca. 1892. Photo © Canadian Museum of Civilization, artifact 982.8.1, image 2008–0594.

aprons, but servants wore fancy garments and nurses wore plain. Household servants wore rough brown aprons for morning cleaning and changed into decorative white aprons in the afternoon to receive and wait on family and guests. Nurses wore white aprons consistently. So, the plain white nurse's apron was a conflation of two messages: the plainness referring to their domestic labor, but the white the higher status color of social contact (compare Figures 7 and 8).

Another crossover between servant and nursing dress was the practice of changing from washable cotton dresses for morning work to dark woolen dresses for formal afternoon duties (Figure 8). The binary dress code of morning/afternoon, cotton/wool, light/dark was adopted for the first nursing apparel in England and was transplanted to North America. For example, the nurses of the Mack training school in 1875 wore dark woolen uniforms (see Figure 3). The practice, however, was abandoned in North America soon after being introduced, and the cotton dress was worn exclusively. It was more suitable to the English nurse training system, where class distinctions were prominent. In North America there were no doubt social differences among the first nursing recruits, but they were not institutionalized, and all students performed the same tasks (for their level of training) and wore the same uniform.

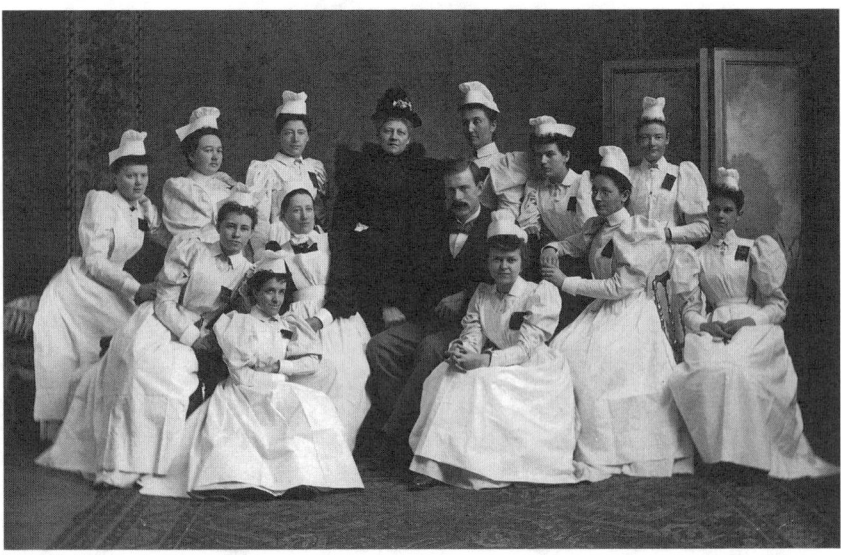

Figure 7. Nurses of Montreal General Hospital, 1894. Wm. Notman & Son, 1894. © McCord Museum, II-105877.

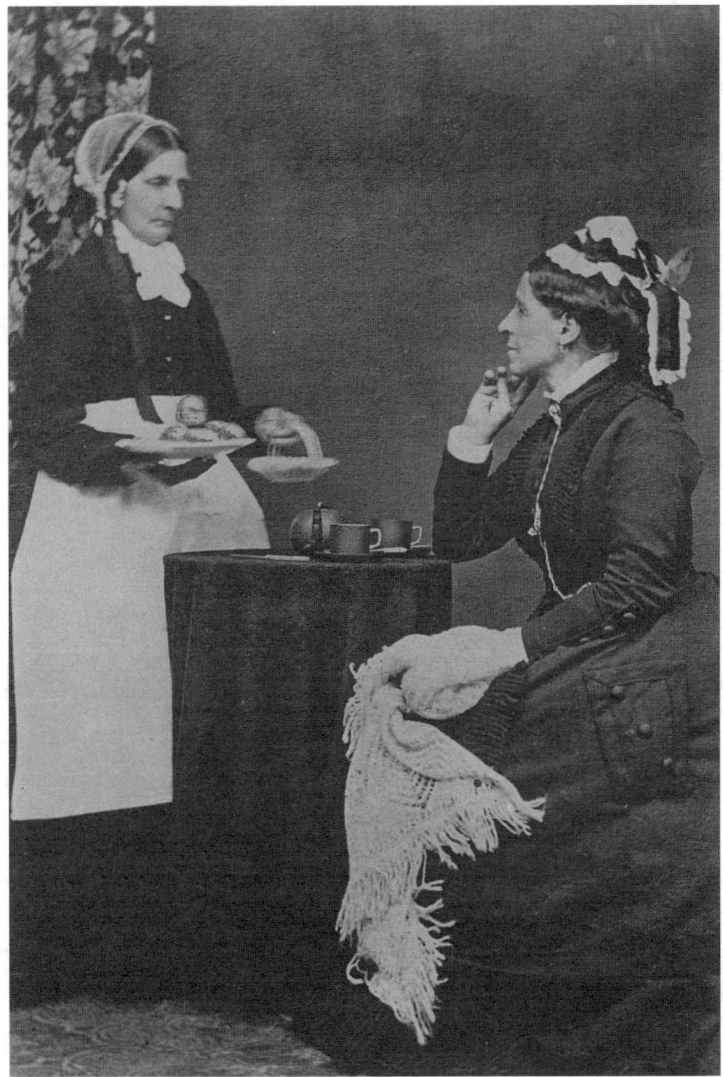

Figure 8. Serving tea, copied 1888. © McCord Museum, II-88120.0.

By the early twentieth century, starched and streamlined uniforms like Edna Muir's suggest another model related to medical science. As the rise of bacteriology and microbiology led to an understanding of the risks of contagion, nurses became the experts in contamination prevention. Immaculate uniforms were equated with the new science of hygiene. But it was a particular, feminized version of medical wear. The metaphor of medical science was limited as it applied to nursing. Of course nursing was in no position to usurp symbols of the medical profession like lab coats. The white severity of the nurses' uniform made nursing a serious and respected occupation related to medicine, at the same time that it assured nursing's inferior status.

Conventional women's wear, domestic servants' uniforms, and medical science are three of several models that can be discerned in the uniform. In the end, the nurse's dress was a mixed metaphor. It was a restrained garment elevating nurses as a disciplined and respectable occupational group, but its humble origins are clear in its reference to the dress of household servants doing manual labor. The hygienic starched surface layered on top of essentially conservative female garments revealed the contradictions of modern nursing, treading a fine line between women's work (domestic, inferior, social) and professional work (empirical, expert, objective).

Depth of Field: The Object and Its Historical Context

A material culture researcher first comes face to face with the object. An informed but intuitive grasp of its design and the messages the design appears to deliver is the starting point, but it is also imperative to take a broader view of the historical and cultural context in which the object was made or used. Most artifact analysis methodologies begin with an analysis of observable or intrinsic details. The materials, design, construction, marks, and condition of the object are studied, and its characteristics are compared with those of similar objects. These data are expanded by other sources of information such as provenance, historical environment, and cultural affiliations, leading to an interpretation of the object to determine its significance or meaning.[15]

But first is the sensory encounter with the object, without assumptions, and with as little theorizing or contextualizing as possible. What are we really seeing? Not, what do we want to see? Historian Richard Grassby warns that "theory has too often obscured the proper analysis of visual images and artifacts . . . cultural historians often describe what the world would be like if their theories were correct."[16] The close observation of an object can confirm, inform, or contradict its historical context. Going back and forth between the object and its context is a powerful heuristic method that brings out new questions and understandings.

The uniform developed along with modern nursing, which in North America began in the 1870s and had solidified institutionally by the early twentieth century. This period is accepted by historians as a transitional time in which urbanization and industrialization changed society to create social instabilities leading to reform movements. Massive reform in health care transformed hospitals from charitable hospices for the poor to socially respectable therapeutic institutions, a change that depended on a formally trained and disciplined nursing corps. One by one, hospitals opened nurse training schools. Nursing care was transferred from the hands of older working-class women to young trainees. Every school, of which there were hundreds in Canada, immediately instituted a proprietary uniform.[17]

The uniform, then, was a major strategy for the acceptance of nursing reform. According to nursing historians, hospital authorities imposed rules and regulations on their young students, including a uniform, yet the images of the first generation of these nurses, and the uniforms themselves, indicate that the introduction of the uniform was anything but monolithic. In the 1891 graduation portrait of the Toronto General Hospital School of Nursing (TGH) (Figure 9), the nurses wear similar but not identical uniforms. They sport personal brooches, handkerchiefs, and other accessories. Examining the uniforms themselves reveals differences in cut and construction. Over time, TGH caps puffed up and down; dress bodices went from plain to covered in scarves, bibbed aprons, or starched bibs; fabric changed from brown check (shown here) to blue stripe. This experimentation underlines the shaky ground in which nursing reform was attempting to establish itself.

By the early twentieth century, a look was solidified for nursing. If we return to Edna Muir's uniform and portrait, we might notice the severity of the outfit and the predominance of starched white garments, and we might be tempted to compare her uniform with that of the nun, making assumptions about the uniform as sexual boundary. But her actual dress is medium blue and closely fitted, with the fabric quite fine and soft (partly through countless washings). If we were to animate Miss Muir in her uniform, we would catch tantalizing glimpses of the soft inner body underneath the crisp carapace. Though some historians maintain that prescribed uniforms and behavior conveyed nurses' asexual status, a closer look at the uniform presents a different story. The visual and tactile dissonance between the "don't touch" starched bib and apron and the feminized dress underneath can help reevaluate the sexual role of these young women. When Miss Muir entered nursing, all the student nurses on the ward were young and female. They were of marriageable age, and it was expected, in the ideology of late Victorian heterosexual gender roles, that they would make themselves available and desirable for the sake of

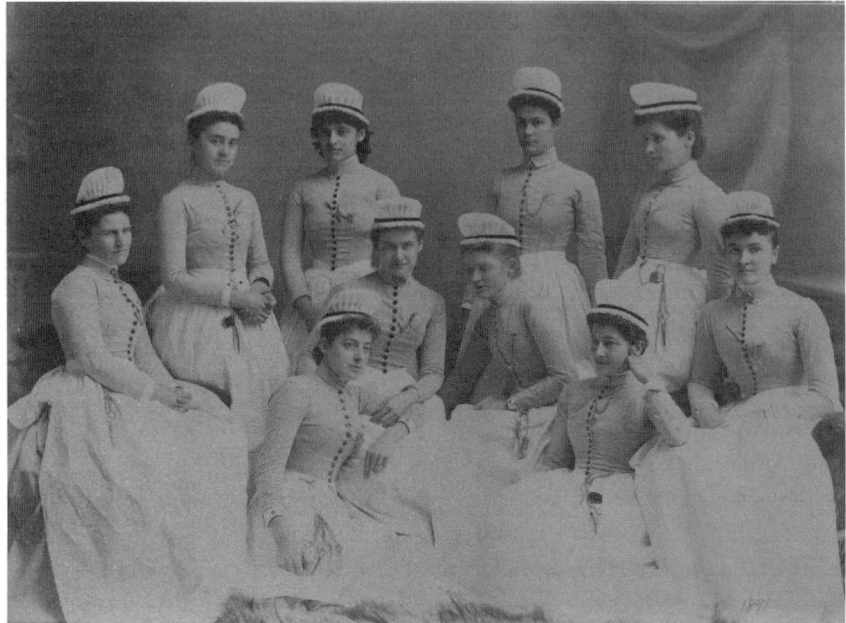

Figure 9. Graduating class, School of Nursing, Toronto General Hospital, 1891. Canadian Museum of Civilization, 2004-H0037.8. Alumnae Association of the School of Nursing Toronto General Hospital Collection.

future marriage and motherhood. In that context, the uniform conveys both the acceptance of, and the anxiety about, that role.

Contextualization can inform and correct spontaneous impressions of the object. For example, the most prevalent colors for nursing uniforms in Canada were blue and pink. We might ascribe symbolic meanings to these colors, but there were important practical and technological reasons for their use in uniforms. Blue from indigo and red from madder were the two dyes most resistant to fading in the late nineteenth century, and they could take the constant laundering required of nursing apparel. We might assume gender connotations in the choice of pink (feminine) and blue (masculine), but this assumption has to be tested. Dress historian Jo B. Paoletti has found through an analysis of magazine articles, department store surveys, and mail-order catalogues that gender color coding in the late nineteenth century was the opposite of that of today: Pink was appropriate for boys' clothing, being considered a strong color, and blue for girls because it was more delicate.[18]

Through contextualization, it is also possible and important to note what is *not* in the picture. During the period of this study all the faces in the photographs are Caucasian. Unlike in the United States, women of color were not accepted into nursing schools in Canada until well into the twentieth century, nor were there separate Black nursing schools.[19] It will be important to examine the uniform around the 1930s, when people of color began to be allowed into nursing programs, and after the 1950s, when immigrant Black and Asian nurses, as well as men and married women, were actively recruited in Canada. How did they experience wearing the white uniform?

Exposure: Uncovering Issues

Once the models have been established and contextual information has been checked, what can these observations contribute to our understanding of the significance of the uniform to nursing history? Pervading all the models are two issues. One is how the uniform constructed an image of femininity for an all-female occupation. The other is how the uniform created a middle-class identity.

Consider an 1895 portrait of two Brantford, Ontario, nursing students (Figure 10). They sit close to each other, gently touching, their expressions soft and dreamy. They wear soft collars with large bows at the neck, gathered bibs, and diminutive caps. One nurse has a floral bouquet on her white aproned lap. The photograph would have been read at the time as a portrait of femininity: gentle, passive, delicate. Based on this and other images, I would suggest that nurses' uniforms were an integral part of the creation of a feminized look in the hospital, described in diminutive and condescending terms such as "neat," "pretty," "becoming," "pleasing." The uniforms both sexualized and infantilized their wearers.

The gentle expressions and ladylike gestures of the Brantford nurses can also be interpreted as a performance to persuade the viewer that these student nurses are enacting middle-class ladylike refinement. At the outset, the aim of nursing schools was to attract what they called a "better class of women." The need to define nursing as a respectable White middle-class occupation was heightened when hospitals established private wards to attract paying patients. In her history of nursing, Kathryn McPherson maintains that "respectability was constructed in a racial and national context," as virtually all students were Canadian born and English or French speaking.[20] According to hospital administrators and nursing leaders, women of non-European background (women of color) were believed to lack the moral and social

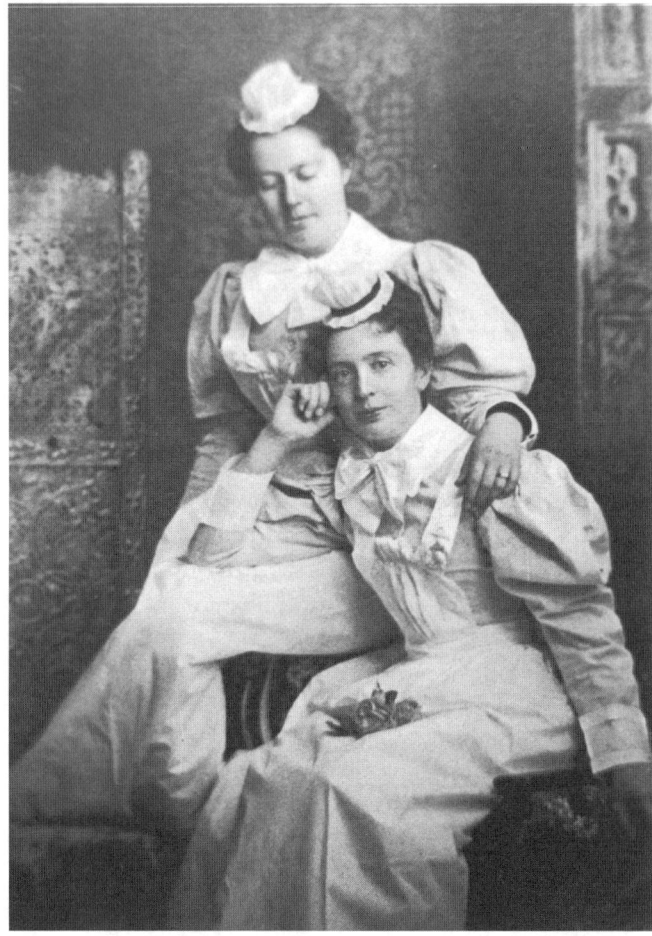

Figure 10. Student nurses at the John H. Stratford Hospital Training School for Nurses, Brantford, Ontario, 1897. Library and Archives Canada, e002414893.

superiority to care for either their inferiors (poor patients) or their superiors (elite private patients). The uniforms with their white aprons and white bibs always appeared on white bodies.

Underneath the veneer of classed and raced gentility are the worn and patched uniforms that have survived. Figure 11 shows a rare 1894 Montreal General Hospital uniform preserved by the school's alumnae association. Students were responsible for making their own uniforms at this time. The bodice is quite roughly machine sewn, with crude handmade buttonholes.

Material and Visual Approaches to the Nurse's Uniform 185

The fabric is very soft and thin from repeated washing, still retaining its pink color, although much faded. There are many tears, especially around the collar and underarms, which are roughly darned.

This bodice—wash-worn, threadbare, unlined, ripped, and worn until it almost fell apart—is material evidence of the other side of nurses in "pretty pink dresses." It alludes to the need for extreme economy on the part of some of the young students whose families could barely afford to

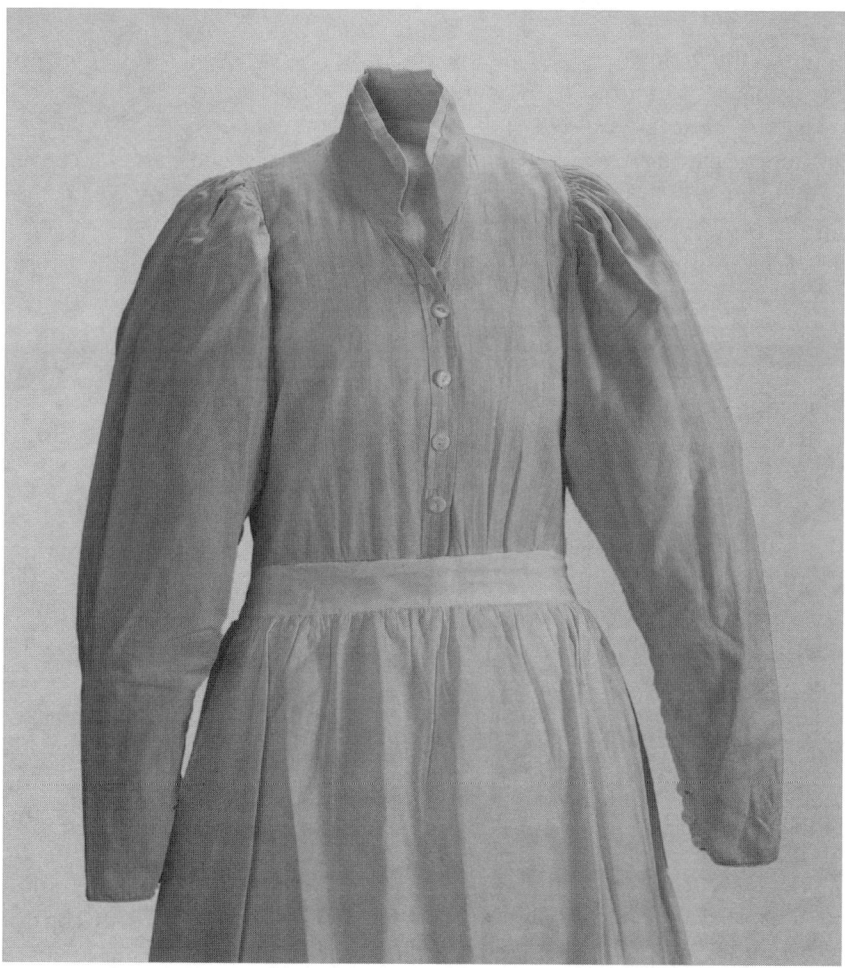

Figure 11. Student uniform, Montreal General Hospital, 1891. Alumnae Association of the Montreal General Hospital School of Nursing. Photo by Steven Darby, Canadian Museum of Civilization.

send their daughters to school rather than straight into paying jobs. Most evocative, it bears witness to the reality of nurses' work—lifting, cleaning, and restraining patients, disposing of blood and guts, staunching bleeding wounds, scrubbing bedpans—work deliberately not even hinted at in graduation photographs.

Develop: The Whole Picture

After focusing closely on the silhouette, materials, vocabulary, and design of the nurse's uniform to determine the models it emulates; after comparing the images to the artifacts and placing them within the context of nursing reform; and after exploring the underlying messages about gender and class they convey (among other things), is it possible to develop an all-encompassing explanation for the creation of this curious outfit?

Like so much of material culture, especially dress, the nurse's uniform defies simple interpretation. Perhaps anthropologist Claude Lévi-Strauss's notion of *bricolage* can explain how the uniform incorporated all sorts of metaphors from different sources to create something new.[21] There was no blueprint or overarching plan. Rather, the uniform evolved by trying out different garments and forms that came to hand. In examining the uniforms themselves, and the images of nurses wearing the uniform, it is possible to discern several different elements—often conflicting ones. The uniform was built from bits and pieces of fashionable, occupational, academic, ecclesiastical, military, and scientific wear. It managed quietly to mediate some of the challenges faced by nursing reformers at the same time as it held its own contradictions. It was part of reformers' strategy to professionalize nursing, but it clung stubbornly to its subservient roots.

Looking closely at uniforms and images of nurses in uniform is useful in two ways. It can shed light on this remarkable chapter in purpose-made dress, the most prevalent and, arguably, most significant women's working apparel. Second, it can contribute to our understanding of nursing reform and the introduction of formal nursing schools. No one can deny the role of the nurse's uniform in forming the nursing identity. The temptation is to view it as an *illustration* of nursing reform values, such as control and conservatism, rather than as an active player in creating that identity. The uniform was a significant part of the culture of the hospital ward and nurses' residence where young women like Miss Muir each day donned their occupational identity.

CHRISTINA BATES
Curator for Ontario History and the Canadian Nursing History Collection
Canadian Museum of Civilization
100 Laurier Street
Gatineau, Quebec K1A 0M8
Canada

Notes

1. Christopher Breward, "Cultures, Identities, Histories: Fashioning a Cultural Approach to Dress," *Fashion Theory* 2, no. 4 (December 1998): 301–13.
2. Peter Burke, *Eyewitnessing: The Uses of Images as Historical Evidence* (Ithaca, N.Y.: Cornell University Press, 2001); Gillian Rose, *Visual Methodologies: An Introduction to the Interpretation of Visual Materials* (London: Sage, 2001); Grant McCracken, *Culture and Consumption: New Approaches to the Symbolic Character of Consumer Goods and Activities* (Bloomington: Indiana University Press, 1990).
3. Lillian Sabine, "The Picturesque Past of the Nurse's Uniform," *Trained Nurse and Hospital Review* (*Nursing World*) 82 (February 1929): 197–203 (Part I); 331–36 (Part II).
4. Elizabeth Ewing, *Women in Uniform Through the Centuries* (Totowa, N.J.: Rowman and Littlefield, 1975).
5. Shermalayne Southard Szasz, "The Tyranny of Uniforms," in *Socialization, Sexism and Stereotyping: Women's Issues in Nursing*, ed. Janet Muff (St. Louis: C.V. Mosby, 1982), 197–220.
6. Lynn Houweling, "Image, Function, and Style: A History of the Nursing Uniform," *American Journal of Nursing* 104, no. 4 (April 2004): 40–48; Jane Brooks and Anne Marie Rafferty, "Dress and Distinction in Nursing, 1860–1939: 'A corporate (as well as corporeal) armour of probity and purity,'" *Women's History Review* 16, no. 1 (February 2007): 41–57; Kathryn McPherson, "'The Case of the Kissing Nurse': Femininity, Sexuality, and Canadian Nursing, 1900–1970," in *Gendered Pasts: Historical Essays in Femininity and Masculinity in Canada*, ed. Kathryn McPherson, Cecilia Morgan, and Nancy M. Forestell (Oxford: Oxford University Press, 2003), 179–98; Mary Juszynski Curran, "Women in White: The Development of the American Nurses' Uniform, 1860–1915," (master's thesis, Department of Consumer Studies, University of Massachusetts, 1994). On early Canadian uniforms, see Sheila J. Rankin, Glennis Zilm, and Valerie Grant, "Nursing Uniforms—Early 1800s," in *Labour of Love: A Memoir of Gertrude Richards Ladner, 1879 to 1976* (Delta, B.C.: ZGZ Publications, 2006), 89–96.
7. Mark Dion and J. Morgan Puett, *RN: The Past, Present, and Future of the Nurses' Uniform* (Philadelphia: Center for the Study of the History of Nursing, University of Pennsylvania School of Nursing and Fabric Workshop and Museum, 2003), http://www.fabricworkshop.org/exhibitions/uniforms.php
8. For a discussion of the development of this collection, see Christina Bates, "The Material of Practice: The Canadian Nursing History Collection," *Canadian Bulletin of*

Medical History 21, no. 2 (2004): 377–85; an online database to the collection is located at http://www.civilization.ca/tresors/nursing/ncint01e.html

9. From the beginning, nursing school alumnae associations had a strong sense of their own identity and preserved many documents, photographs, and artifacts. Most prevalent among their collections are uniforms, evidence of the importance of the uniform to nursing identity. Sometimes these collections are in peril: The holdings of the alumnae association of the Toronto General Hospital were dispersed when the association lost its archival space in the hospital. A selection of the objects was donated to the Canadian Museum of Civilization, including twenty-two uniforms. Happily, some alumnae associations retain archival facilities, including those of the Montreal General Hospital and the Winnipeg General Hospital schools of nursing.

10. Many museum collections of dress privilege highbrow fashion or special occasion clothing over everyday wear. Museums of decorative arts purposely acquire and study elite fashionable and designer wear. Even history museums are biased toward the finest clothing, as that is often what is saved and donated, along with garments associated with transcendent moments (such as christening and wedding gowns), rather than quotidian or work wear. In contrast, the uniforms in the Canadian Nursing History Collection form an extraordinarily thorough and unbiased study group.

11. Elizabeth Wilson, *Adorned in Dreams: Fashion and Modernity* (New Brunswick, N.J.: Rutgers University Press, 2003), 2.

12. McCracken, *Culture and Consumption*, 68–69.

13. Barbara Burman and Carole Turbin, eds., *Material Strategies: Dress and Gender in Historical Perspective* (London: Blackwell, 2003), 1.

14. Nathan Joseph, *Uniforms and Nonuniforms: Communication Through Clothing* (New York: Greenwood, 1986), 14.

15. [Darrel Butler], "Towards a Material History Methodology," *Material History Bulletin* 22 (Fall 1985): 31–40; E. Fleming McClung, "Artifact Study: A Proposed Model," in *Material Culture Studies in America*, ed. Thomas J. Schlereth (Walnut Creek, Calif.: Altamira Press, 1999), 162–73; Susan M. Pearce, "Thinking About Things," in *Interpreting Objects and Collections*, ed. Susan M. Pearce (London: Routledge, 1994), 125–32; Jules David Prown, "Mind in Matter: An Introduction to Material Culture Theory and Method," *Winterthur Portfolio* 17, no. 1 (Spring 1982): 1–19.

16. Richard Grassby, "Material Culture and Cultural History," *Journal of Interdisciplinary History* 35, no. 4 (Spring 2005): 591–603.

17. In the last fifteen years a wealth of material dealing with the history of nursing in Canada has been published. The most thorough work on nursing since the establishment of training schools is Kathryn McPherson, *Bedside Matters: The Transformation of Canadian Nursing, 1900–1990* (Toronto: Oxford University Press, 1996).

18. Jo B. Paoletti, "The Gendering of Infant's and Toddler's Clothing in America," in *The Material Culture of Gender, the Gender of Material Culture*, ed. Katharine Martinez and Kenneth L. Ames (Winterthur, Del.: Henry Francis du Pont Winterthur Museum, 1997), 27–35.

19. Agnes Calliste, "Antiracism Organizing and Resistance in Nursing: African Canadian Women," *Canadian Review of Sociology and Anthropology* 33, no. 3 (August 1996): 361–90; McPherson, *Bedside Matters*, 118–20.

20. McPherson, *Bedside Matters*, 17.

21. Claude Lévi-Strauss, *The Savage Mind* (Chicago: University of Chicago Press, 1974), 16–33.

NOTES AND DOCUMENTS

Nurse Irene Shea Studies the "Kenny Method" of Treatment of Infantile Paralysis, 1942–1943

Janet Golden
Rutgers University

Naomi Rogers
Yale University History of Medicine

> **Abstract.** In the 1940s nurses in the United States set out to learn the Kenny method of treating polio patients, which relied on hot packs and muscle strengthening exercises instead of the standard system of prolonged immobilization. Named for Sister Elizabeth Kenny, an Australian nurse who based herself in Minnesota during the 1940s and early 1950s, and viewed with suspicion by many physicians, nurses, and physical therapists, the treatment nonetheless proved effective. It changed the practice of polio nursing and the experiences of patients in the years before vaccine prevention largely eliminated paralytic polio.

The documents discussed here show how one nurse, Irene Shea, sought to learn the Kenny method and how she viewed both Kenny and her treatment protocol. The documents provide a window into an important aspect of nursing history, elucidating the ways nurses in the past sought to learn new clinical techniques and how their efforts to do so required an understanding of the local medical and political environment. They also suggest how issues of hospital authority, disease philanthropy, health care financing, and relations between nurses and physicians shaped the scope of nursing practice and thus nurses' options for advanced continuing education.

In June 1942, Irene F. Shea, R.N., superintendent of nurses at Baltimore's Sydenham Hospital, the city's infectious disease hospital, wrote to Dr. Huntington Williams, head of the city's health department (see Document 1).[2] She sought funding for one or two staff nurses to attend a one-week course in the Kenny method for the treatment of infantile paralysis (polio).[1] Shea had recently returned from the annual meeting of the American Medical Association (AMA) in Atlantic City, New Jersey, which she attended with support from both the health department and the Maryland chapter of the National Foundation for Infantile Paralysis (NFIP), popularly known as the March of Dimes. While there she had the opportunity to see a special exhibit organized by the NFIP and to attend lectures by three physicians who spoke to packed audiences about the Kenny method. Two of Kenny's Australian assistants demonstrated elements of her work to the audience. Kenny herself, who was living in Minneapolis and teaching local professionals with support from the March of Dimes, had not been invited. The March of Dimes wanted medical skeptics to judge the work and not the woman.

Polio patients received care in hospitals with contagious disease facilities. In Baltimore, Sydenham, the city's infectious disease hospital, housed these patients. After speaking with one of the Kenny technicians at the AMA meeting, Shea concluded that, despite the new method's unusual concepts and new terminology like spasm, in-coordination, and mental alienation, "it seems to be a rather simple nursing procedure." She believed it could easily be learned at a one-week course offered at the University of Minnesota under Kenny herself, or at Warm Springs, Georgia, the polio rehabilitative center established in the 1920s by Franklin Roosevelt.

In the 1930s and 1940s polio epidemics in the United States became increasingly common and more serious. Most frequently polio struck down young children, but teenagers and adults were also vulnerable. No one knew how the disease spread—although water, flies, and contaminated food were blamed—or how the virus entered and left the body, or how to prevent paralysis. An effort to develop a vaccine in the mid-1930s ended in disaster, and a trial of a nasal spray a few years later also proved disappointing.

Pain, muscle sensitivity, and paralysis characterized the early or acute stages of polio, and the particular manifestations of these symptoms could neither be predicted nor halted. During the 1910s physician Robert Lovett and his physical therapist Janet Merrill developed a system of rest and splinting based on the fear that inappropriately stretched muscles would become weak and further deform a patient struggling to regain muscle function. Health care professionals came to view splinting with plaster casts and sometimes steel frames as necessary to prevent children from moving their limbs in ways that could result in further deformity.³ Nurses and physical therapists traveled to Boston to learn Lovett and Merrill's polio therapy.⁴ The children they returned home to treat frequently cried in pain and struggled to free themselves. For nurses, work with polio patients proved tremendously hard.⁵

Polio patients endured other treatments as well. Based on the belief that after two years little improvement was likely, orthopedists developed a variety of surgical techniques for muscle transplantation and stabilization. In addition, public interest in Warm Springs, thanks to its association with President Roosevelt, led some clinicians to urge that muscle education underwater be added to the standard conservative therapeutic regimen in the hopes of regaining some muscle power—a hope Roosevelt shared.⁶ Many parents, however, unable to pay for long-term rehabilitative care and unwilling to allow their children to undergo orthopedic operations, simply took their children out of the hospital as soon as they were deemed noncontagious and treated them at home. Kenny's techniques thus addressed a widespread dissatisfaction with polio therapy, and her dramatic results with patients who had been paralyzed for many years as well as with acute patients impressed everyone. She proved able to ameliorate their pain with heated blankets or "hot packs," and she introduced early muscle training, closely supervised by her technicians, enabling patients to develop muscle strength, flexibility, and improved function.⁷

Elizabeth Kenny, a tall, fierce woman, showed no deference to physicians; she told them that their ideas about polio were "wrong" and that only by their adopting both her methods and her concepts would their patients improve. Gritty determination marked her life as a nurse and educator. Born in rural Australia, Kenny spent the 1930s struggling to have Australian physicians take her work seriously. She came to the United States in 1940, convinced that it offered a more open medical culture. She gained the support of Minneapolis physicians, including orthopedist John Pohl, who began to teach with her and in 1943 coauthored with her the defining text of her work and ideas.⁸ Kenny was sure of the truth and logic of her own ideas and wanted to convince and convert skeptics, but she was not interested in a middle ground. She refused to see her ideas as derivative or even based on established concepts. When visitors remarked that certain ideas or techniques seemed familiar, she dismissed them, saying she was presenting a different disease, one they had never encountered before, and that all efforts to make it familiar represented a refusal to listen. She declined to alter her terms or make analogies to familiar ideas. Kenny understood herself as a character, larger than life, overwhelming men and women unused to being overwhelmed. She hoped doctors and nurses would come to Minneapolis to learn her theory of the disease, but, as Shea's letter shows, many proved more interested in the one-week hot-packing course that taught the method's practical techniques than in Kenny's theories of polio.

The March of Dimes was America's largest disease philanthropy in the 1940s. Directed by Franklin Roosevelt's former law partner, Basil O'Connor, and headquartered in New York City, the organization had chapters across the country raising money to fund care for polio patients, training for doctors and nurses in the latest polio methods, and scientific research. The March of Dimes paid for the work of virologists Jonas Salk and Albert Sabin, who produced polio vaccines in the 1950s that led to the widespread eradication of the disease.[9]

With the support of Baltimore's health commissioner, the Maryland state chapter of the NFIP agreed to pay $150 for Shea to attend a six-day hot-packing course in Minnesota, urging that the money be used carefully. It was to Catherine C. Gaule, assistant secretary-treasurer of that chapter, that Shea directed her subsequent report (see Document 2).[10] In Minneapolis Shea learned Kenny's technique for muscle training and the use of hot packs. Nurses, her notes detailed, were taught how to relieve pain and spasm, how to keep muscles receptive and relaxed, and how to improve circulation and metabolism.[11]

With a growing reputation in America, Kenny found many health professionals like Shea eager to travel to Minnesota to meet with her and study her methods. By 1942 Kenny received clinical privileges at both the university hospital and the city's general hospital. Wards at both were available for clinical visitors like Shea to see patients treated by Kenny methods and to learn how to use hot packs. As Shea noted in her letter, while taking the course she saw acute cases being treated in the hospital and discharged patients who returned for checkups and muscle tests. Her fellow students consisted of nurses from various parts of the United States.

Most Americans learned about Kenny's work from the popular media; nurses and physicians encountered her work in the professional literature as well. Feature articles about Kenny appeared in *Reader's Digest*, the Hearst Sunday supplement *American Weekly*, and *Life* magazine among others.[12] In the early 1940s Kenny published two textbooks with a Minneapolis press: *Treatment of Infantile Paralysis in the Acute Stage* and *The Kenny Concept of Infantile Paralysis and Its Treatment*. After the March of Dimes urged all chapters to pay for doctors and nurses to learn her method, many professionals began to look at her work seriously. She received favorable although cautious reviews in the *Journal of the American Medical Association* and the *New England Journal of Medicine*. In the *American Journal of Nursing*, a Denver orthopedic nurse commented that Kenny's methods were detailed and "extremely valuable," but warned that "the experienced orthopedic nurse" would be "reluctant" to accept "her theories *en bloc*" until there was "more solid, scientific proof of the permanent efficacy of this method."[13] Although professionals proved cautious, public presentations of her work were nearly all laudatory. In 1946 American moviegoers enjoyed a heavily fictionalized account of her life in the RKO biopic *Sister Kenny*, starring Rosalind Russell as Kenny—a role for which Russell received an Oscar nomination.[14]

Kenny's techniques demanded that patients themselves, even toddlers, be active and knowledgeable participants in muscle exercises.[15] Making a patient "muscle conscious" was contrary to standard rehabilitative work with children, who, professionals feared, would become uncooperative and later too self-conscious. But with the Kenny method even two- and three-year-olds were taught the Latin terms for their muscles. A *Reader's Digest* article featured "Suzy," an African American child who, when asked if she could move one muscle replied, "you mean my *gluteus maximus* Sister?"[16] A New York physician mocked the idea that paralysis could be improved "by hot packs and finger manipulation, or by educating 4 or 5 yr old children by talking." In particular, the idea of telling "'Sissy' the little colored girl to flex her Gluteus Maximus & she did" was "absurd."[17]

In reply, pediatrician Philip Stimson protested that he had verified this element of Kenny's work from his personal observation and his own clinical experience. "As for teaching little children to know the names of muscles, I myself have heard the four year old colored girl name and flex 8 or 10 of her muscles."[18] That Kenny's methods gave even young patients the psychological confidence to talk back to medical skeptics was a delightful example of Kenny's lack of deference to medical authority; that the girl in question was identified as "colored" made it for contemporaries even more shocking. Shea met the girl, whose real name was Dolores, and saw for herself her ability to name all the muscles and heard her say she "was going to be a 'Kenny Hot Packer'" when she grew up. Not all patients proved to be as inspired. A number of polio survivors who experienced the Kenny hot pack treatments recalled the unpleasant smell of the hot wool and described the treatment as torturous.[19]

Shea's notes provide a detailed description of the ways hot packs were to be used in the Kenny method. She also learned a little about Kenny's new terms, her refusal to conduct muscle tests, and her efforts to have health professionals see her work as a scientific contribution that had to be performed by professionals, not by parents doing a few techniques at home. Shea's letter quoted from Kenny's 1941 text, *Treatment of Infantile Paralysis in the Acute Stage*, which Kenny had written to ensure the permanency of her work.[20] Kenny clearly recognized that "it must be understood by all that it is impossible to teach without a book of reference."[21] Nurses in particular, she believed, were "impressed by the authority associated . . . with the printed word" and preferred a "text book" so it could be used "for intensive study."[22]

What Shea's notes and letter also make clear is the disorganization pervading much of this early teaching. Assigned to a patient "without preliminary introduction or orientation," Shea succeeded in applying hot packs only because her patient was not a toddler but an articulate young man who could give her cooperation and aid. It was difficult and complicated work, but she was determined to master it. Frustratingly, Vivian Hannon, one of the Kenny technicians, abruptly removed all the packs applied by Shea and the rest of her class, saying "it was wrong" but giving no further explanation. During informal rounds, any effort by the nurses in Shea's class to compare the new method with older techniques was "tactfully avoided" by Kenny and by the medical school's physical medicine specialist Miland Knapp. There were in fact many significant practical and theoretical differences, as Kenny's early textbook pointed out, but this technical short course was not the place to explicate them. Kenny was more forthcoming in the one week physicians' courses she and her medical allies taught during this period, and by the time the Elizabeth Kenny Institute was established in December 1942, she had come to argue that only a full six- or nine-month course would adequately prepare a nurse or physical therapist to comprehend her method and earn the right to call him or herself a "Kenny technician."

After returning to Baltimore, Shea submitted copies of her detailed notes and a letter describing her experiences to Catherine Gaule. Her letter provides a vivid firsthand account of Kenny and this distinctive moment in continuing nursing education. In it she notes Kenny's size—"a rather large woman"—and indeed Kenny frequently used her height (five feet ten inches) as a way to dominate medical audiences. In an era in which physicians expected nurses to defer to their authority and when women rarely taught medical or science subjects to men, it must have been a shock to see and hear Kenny. Shea described meeting Kenny at the university hospital, calling her "somewhat abrupt in manner but courteous," and noting- "she possesses an extreme belief in her work." The letter also describes several patients in the hospital and those who came back for checkups after their discharge. Her observations led her to conclude cautiously that the Kenny method "seems effective" and that patients did well with the treatment.

Shea's hesitancy to embrace the Kenny system may have reflected a reticence to pass medical judgment or an awareness that, despite its growing practice, the Kenny method along with Sister Kenny did not meet with universal acceptance from the medical profession. Local medical politics may have played a role in this hesitation. Baltimore contained a cadre of professionals at the Children's Hospital School who came to define themselves as proponents of anti-Kenny polio techniques. They included orthopedists George Bennett and Raymond Lenhard and physical therapists Florence and Henry Kendall, a husband and wife team who had written an important guide to polio rehabilitative care published and distributed by the U.S. Public Health Service.[23] A hint of this anti-Kenny method appears in a letter from Huntington Williams to Catherine Gaule. He thanked Gaule for the support given to Shea, enclosed a check for $2.12 (the balance of unspent funds), and included a copy of Shea's report, which he marked "Confidential." He explained that "The City Health Department does not want to get into any controversial difficulties regarding the matters that might jeopardize our relationship that are traditionally excellent with the physicians in the city in which we must work."[24]

Shortly after completing this course, Shea left Sydenham Hospital for wartime service in the Army Nurse Corps. Mrs. Gwendolyn Betz, Shea's successor as superintendent of nurses at Sydenham Hospital, followed in her footsteps, enrolling in a one-week Kenny method course at the Jersey City Medical Center with support from the Baltimore chapter of the NFIP.

Studying Polio Nursing History

The desire of senior nurses at Sydenham Hospital to learn the somewhat controversial Kenny method suggests both the commitment of nurses to seeking the most up-to-date care for their patients and the power of one nurse, Sister Elizabeth Kenny, to transform that care. The letters from Shea also reveal the challenge presented by the polio epidemics of the 1940s. Further study in each of these areas—the history of continuing education in nursing, polio nursing, and the work and influence of Kenny—promises to yield important insights into the ways nurses confronted epidemics and expanded their professional reach while negotiating an increasingly complex health care system. In pursuing these topics students can turn to the Kenny papers housed at the Minnesota Historical Society in St. Paul, Minnesota, and the March of Dimes archives in White Plains, New York. The Syndenham Hospital records—including records of polio patients and the nursing care they received—are located at the National Library of Medicine in Bethesda, Maryland. Archival records of nursing schools, nurses, and voluntary nursing associations can be found at the Barbara Bates Center for the Study of the History of Nursing at the University of Pennsylvania in Philadelphia, which also holds nursing textbooks published over the course of the twentieth century. An online exhibit from the National Museum of American History entitled "What Ever Happened to Polio" includes a useful bibliography and historical summary for those interested in beginning research on this topic; see http://americanhistory.si.edu/polio/ In addition, a number of important and useful primary and secondary sources are cited in the notes to the present article.

JANET GOLDEN, PhD
Rutgers University
c/o 19 W. Levering Mill Rd.
Bala Cynwyd, PA 19004

NAOMI ROGERS, PhD
Yale University History of Medicine
333 Cedar Street
Sterling Hall of Medicine, L132
New Haven, CT 06520

Baltimore City Health Department
Memorandum

June 16, 1942

To: Dr. Huntington Williams
From: Miss Irene F. Shea
Subject: Report of the Observation of the Kenny Method of Treatment of Infantile Paralysis at the A.M.A. Convention

At the annual meeting of the A.M.A. held in Atlantic City, it was my privilege, through the courtesy of the National Foundation for Infantile Paralysis, to observe for two days the Kenny technique used for the treatment of infantile paralysis and the opinions of Drs. Cole, Knapp, and Pohl of Minneapolis, Minnesota, and Dr. Phillip Stimson of New York as derived from their recent experiences with this treatment.

Four lectures and demonstrations were given each day which were followed with open discussions by members of the groups attending . . .

My general observations and opinions of these demonstrations are as follows:

1. That the Kenny method of treatment is intended primarily for the acute stage of poliomyelitis.

2. Personal training is necessary to carry out this method, especially after the acute stage when the period of muscle reorganization begins. This part of the treatment is done by technicians or physiotherapists, who must have had at least six months training in muscle theory.

3. The method is instituted after observation of the patient by the physician. No muscle testing or massage is done until after the acute stage.

4. Observations of Miss Kenny of this disease indicate that (1) "Spasm" is present in the muscle, (2) "Incoordination" results due to a change in the pattern of muscles, and (3) that there is "Mental Alienation" or a pseudo-paralysis in unaffected muscles.

5. Treatment should begin as soon as diagnosis is made.

6. Hot fomentations are then started and applied either to the entire body or only the affected part as prescribed by the physician. For the ordinary case these packs are applied every two hours from 8 a.m. to 8 p.m. each day for a period of days, until the spasm is relaxed. For the more acute cases they may be applied every 15 minutes to 1/2 hour for several hours and then every two hours thereafter . . . The hot fomentations are made preferably from old woolen blankets, cut to the size to fit the various parts of the

patient's body, boiled in hot water, taken in a tub to the patient's bedside and placed through a wringer twice before being applied. No lubrication has been applied to the skin and no burns have resulted from their experiences. Packs are usually removed at night and the patient rests without sedation. A bed board is placed on the bed to give a sense of firmness. A foot board is placed at the bottom of the bed and after the acute stage, the patient's feet are placed against this to stimulate a normal standing reflex.

7. Respirators are not used with this type of treatment because they feel that respiratory difficulty in poliomyelitis is not due to actual paralysis, but spasm of the muscles of respiration and therefore can be relieved by hot fomentations. With the spinal type of paralysis, the respirator, they feel, oxygenates the individual and tends to make them live longer but they cannot do without the respirator thereafter.

8. There are three factors in regard to muscle reeducation and training which is instituted by the physiotherapist after the acute stage. (1) "Awareness," making the patient aware or the muscle that is to be reeducated, (2) "Passive Motion" in which the technician or physiotherapist does the exercise twice for the patient, and (3) "Active Motion" in which the patient does the exercise once by himself. This type of exercise is usually done twice a day.

Conclusion: My general opinion from observation of this treatment is that in the acute stages of poliomyelitis there apparently is given to the individual a great deal of relief without undue harmful aftereffects. As to the actual application of the fomentations, it seems to be a rather simple nursing procedure which could be carried out effectively without too great an increase in the nursing personnel. If this treatment were to be instituted here, I feel that it would be beneficial for one or two nurses at Sydenham Staff to take the one-week course either at Minneapolis or Warm Springs, Georgia . . .

Very sincerely yours,
Irene F. Shea, R. N.
Superintendent of Nurses
ifs/mlg
cc: Miss Catherine C. Gaule
cc: Dr. Tull
Sydenham Hospital
Baltimore, Maryland

October 12, 1942

Miss Catherine C. Gaule
National Foundation for Infantile Paralysis
Baltimore, Maryland

Dear Miss Gaule:

... The course of one week which I pursued is offered to nurses in executive capacities and public health nursing and pertains merely to the application of the hot foments in the acute stage of the disease. It does not include the muscle reeducation program which follows the acute stage or hot packing period and for which a six months course is offered to nurses and physiotherapists, to enable them to complete by Kenny method this realm of treatment.

On Monday, at 8:00 a.m. our first day, we were inducted to the ward on Station 43 of University Hospital by Miss Davies, our teacher during the course. Here we were shown how the hot packs were applied to the various parts of the body and were about to proceed with the actual application when we were interrupted by the presence on the floor of Sister Kenny herself. Here I might say a word about Sister Kenny. She is a rather large woman, somewhat abrupt in manner but courteous. She possesses an extreme belief in her work, thereby trying to impart her knowledge in all sincerity to others ...

At the General Hospital Sister Kenny with Dr. John Pohl, who is in charge of this work there, showed us several muscle tests on old patients. Among these patients was the young five year colored child Dolores, whose statements appear in a recent issue of Reader's Digest. She performed beautifully for the group, naming all the muscles and assuring us that when she grew up she was going to be a "Kenny Hot Packer" and that she would put them on "hot." The cases there were all old cases, numbering around 12, and most of which were continuing to receive the hot foments, at least in part. One case presented was a boy of 17 years who had come to them completely paralyzed several weeks after the onset of the disease and had received the orthodox treatment. When we saw him he was able to sit up by himself, use his respiratory muscles properly, had complete control of both arms, but could not walk without the use of the "sticks." He had been there then several months and according to Sister Kenny was progressing rapidly with their treatment, and would soon be able to walk correctly.

That afternoon we returned to University Hospital where we were assigned to patients' care without preliminary introduction or orientation, to the ward and the content of its equipment. After some confusion, I discovered that there were two electric washing machines and a hand wringer and large sterilizer full of boiling 100% cool packs of various sizes. With the cooperation and aid of my assigned patient, who fortunately was a young adult man of 25 years, I proceeded to apply the packs. My first application was a rather clumsy procedure and although I have applied numerous hot packs in my work in previous days,

I soon learned that this technique is really an art. However, I was determined to master it and at the end of the week, after numerous applications, I was able to completely pack an entire patient in 10 minutes...

... Thirteen cases are being treated at the University Hospital, the majority of which were from two to eight months old. In each case they had either been hot-packed at home prior to admission or were admitted directly and hot packing begun at onset of disease. All of these patients were still receiving hot foments, at least in part, but in the majority of cases had regained a large part of the functioning of the muscles of their extremities. There were also two acute cases, both adult males, one of which was still on isolation. In both cases they were said to have both been on admission completely paralyzed and were therefore started on a complete set of hot packs. Although there was partial movement of the upper extremities they continued to receive the complete packs and we were told would continue to do so until all evidence of spasm was removed, spasm, according to their theory, being the cause of the paralysis.

Several patients who had been discharged came back to the hospital during the course of the week for checkups and muscle tests. One, which we observed, was a man who on admission was completely paralyzed and had received the Kenny treatment. At the time I saw him he was able to walk and use all muscles correctly. This was 3 months after treatment had been started. Another patient was a young female of 4 years of age, who although not completely recovered, was walking well with the aid of the sticks.

... From my own observations and experience with poliomyelitis, which no doubt is limited in comparison with others, I would say after having this course, that the Kenny treatment in the acute stage seems effective. Patients on the whole appear and act more comfortable and apparently regain muscle functioning as rapidly, if not more rapidly with this treatment. Whether or not the muscle reeducation program, which follows and is the work of physiotherapists is as effective, I am not able to state...

Very sincerely yours,
Irene F. Shea, RN
Superintendent of Nurses

Notes

1. On the history of Sydenham Hospital, see "Baltimore's Sydenham Service for Hospital Case of Communicable Diseases 1909–1924–1949," *Baltimore Health News* (July 1949): 147–57. Sydenham Hospital, a 110-bed communicable disease hospital run by the Baltimore City Health Department, cared for almost all the acute polio cases in the city.

2. Letter from Irene F. Shea to Dr. Huntington Williams, June 16, 1942, Sydenham Hospital Records, Box 82, National Library of Medicine, Bethesda, Md. (hereafter NLM).

3. On the early history of polio in the United States, see Naomi Rogers, *Dirt and Disease: Polio Before FDR* (New Brunswick, N.J.: Rutgers University Press, 1992); on polio nursing, see Lynne M. Dunphy, "'The Steel Cocoon': Tales of the Nurses and Patients of the Iron Lung, 1929–1955," *Nursing History Review* 9 (2001): 3–34. On polio care and polio patient experiences, see Daniel J. Wilson, *Living with Polio: The Epidemic and Its Survivors* (Chicago: University of Chicago Press, 2005); Marc Shell, *Polio and Its Aftermath: The Paralysis of Culture* (Cambridge, Mass.: Harvard University Press, 2005); Edmund J. Sass with George Gottfried and Anthony Sorem, eds., *Polio's Legacy: An Oral History* (Lanham, Md.: University Press of America, 1996); Amy L. Fairchild, "The Polio Narratives: Dialogues with FDR," *Bulletin of the History of Medicine* 75 (2001): 488–534. See Hugh C. Gallagher, *Black Bird Fly Away: Disabled in an Able-Bodied World* (Arlington, Va.: Vandamere Press, 1998); Leonard Kriegel, *Flying Solo: Reimagining Manhood, Courage, and Loss* (Boston: Beacon Press, 1998); Regina Woods, *Tales from Inside the Iron Lung (and How I Got Out of It)* (Philadelphia: University of Pennsylvania Press, 1994).

4. On the significance of polio in the shaping of the American physical therapy profession, see Marilyn Moffat, "The History of Physical Therapy Practice in the United States," *Journal of Physical Therapy Education* 17 (2003): 15–25; Wendy Murphy, *Healing the Generations: A History of Physical Therapy and the American Physical Therapy Association* (Alexandria, Va.: American Physical Therapy Association, 1995); Beth Linker, "The Business of Ethics: Gender, Medicine, and the Professional Codification of the American Physiotherapy Association, 1918–1935," *Journal of the History of Medicine and Allied Sciences* 60 (2005): 320–54; Beth Linker, "Strength and Science: Gender, Physiotherapy, and Medicine in Early Twentieth Century America," *Journal of Women's History* 17 (2005): 106–32.

5. Carmelita Calderwood, "Nursing Care in Poliomyelitis," *American Journal of Nursing* 40 (1940): 624–30. In the acute stage nurses, supervised by orthopedists, were the only ones who worked with patients, and the difficult job of caring for frightened, crying children lying in casts had to be justified by a sense that these were the proper medical procedures. "The entire success of the treatment depends upon the loyalty of the nurse in maintaining the position effected by splinting," warned Evelyn C. Pearce, *A Textbook of Orthopaedic Nursing* (New York: C. P. Putnam's Sons, 1930), 40–41.

6. Hugh Gregory Gallagher, *FDR's Splendid Deception* (New York: Dodd, Mead, 1985); Davis W. Houck and Amos Kiewe, *FDR's Body Politics: The Rhetoric of Disability* (College Station: Texas A&M University Press, 2003).

7. On Kenny, see Victor Cohn, *Sister Kenny: The Woman Who Challenged the Doctors* (Minneapolis: University of Minnesota Press, 1975); John R. Wilson, *Through Kenny's*

Eyes: An Exploration of Sister Elizabeth Kenny's Views About Nursing (Townsville: Royal College of Nursing Australia, 1995); Wade Alexander, *Sister Elizabeth Kenny: Maverick Heroine of the Polio Treatment Controversy* (Rockhampton: Central Queensland University Press, 2002); Naomi Rogers, "Silence Has Its Own Stories: Elizabeth Kenny, Polio and the Culture of Medicine," *Social History of Medicine* 21 (2008): 145–161; Naomi Rogers, "Sister Kenny Goes to Washington: Polio, Populism and Medical Politics in Postwar America," in *The Politics of Healing: Histories of Alternative Medicine in Twentieth-Century North America*, ed. Robert D. Johnston (New York: Routledge, 2004), 97–116; and Naomi Rogers, *The Polio Wars: Sister Kenny and the Golden Age of American Medicine* (New York: Oxford University Press, forthcoming).

      8. John F. Pohl and Elizabeth Kenny, *The Kenny Concept of Infantile Paralysis and Its Treatment* (Minneapolis, Minn.: Bruce Publishing, 1943).

      9. There is no complete history of the National Foundation. See John R. Paul, *A History of Poliomyelitis* (New Haven, Conn.: Yale University Press, 1971), 357–94; Tony Gould, *A Summer Plague: Polio and Its Survivors* (New Haven, Conn.: Yale University Press, 1995), 41–126; Richard Carter, *The Gentle Legions: National Voluntary Health Organizations in America* (New Brunswick, N.J.: Transaction Publishers, 1961, 1992); Jane S. Smith, *Patenting the Sun: Polio and the Salk Vaccine* (New York: William Morrow, 1990), 64–87; David M. Oshinsky, *Polio: An American Story* (New York: Oxford University Press, 2005); Angela N. H. Creager, *The Life of a Virus: Tobacco Mosaic Virus as an Experimental Model, 1930–1965* (Chicago: University of Chicago Press, 2001); Sydney A. Halpern, *Lesser Harms: The Morality of Risk in Medical Research* (Chicago: University of Chicago Press, 2004); and David W. Rose, *March of Dimes* (Charleston, S.C.: Arcadia, 2003).

      10. Letter from Irene F. Shea to Catherine C. Gaule, October 12, 1942, Sydenham Hospital Records, Box 82, NLM.

      11. Irene F. Shea, "Notes on Kenny Method of Hot Foments Taken at the University of Minnesota, September 28 to October 4, 1942," Sydenham Hospital Collection, MS C 243, Box 82, History of Medicine Division, National Library of Medicine (hereafter NLM). For a finding aid see http://www.nlm.nih.gov/hmd/manuscripts/ead/sydenham.html

      12. Elizabeth Kenny, *The Treatment of Infantile Paralysis in the Acute Stage* (Minneapolis, Minn.: Bruce Publishing, 1941); Robert D. Potter, "Sister Kenny's Treatment for Infantile Paralysis," *American Weekly* (August 17, 1941): 4–13; Robert M. Yoder, "Healer from the Outback," *Saturday Evening Post* 214 (January 17, 1942): 18–19, 68, 70; "Sister Kenny: Australian Nurse Demonstrates Her Treatment for Infantile Paralysis," *Life* 13 (September 28, 1942): 73–75, 77; Lois Maddox Miller, "Sister Kenny vs. Infantile Paralysis," *Reader's Digest* 39 (1941): 1–6; and "Paralysis Treatment Boosted," *Newsweek* 18 (September 8, 1941): 62.

      13. "Kenny Paralysis Treatment Approved by U.S. Medicine," *New York Times*, December 5, 1941; "Sister Kenny's Triumph," *Newsweek* 8 (December 15, 1941): 77; Editorial, "The Kenny Method of Treatment in the Acute Peripheral Manifestations of Infantile Paralysis," *Journal of the American Medical Association* 117 (December 20, 1941): 2171–72; "The Kenny Method of Treatment of Infantile Paralysis," *New England Journal of Medicine* 226 (April 23, 1942): 700–2; F. H. Krusen, "Observations on the Kenny Treatment of Poliomyelitis," *Proceedings of the Staff Meetings of the Mayo Clinic* 17 (August 12, 1942): 449–60; Wallace H. Cole and Miland E. Knapp, "The Kenny Treatment of Infantile Paralysis: A Preliminary Report," *Journal of the American Medical Association* 116 (June 7, 1941): 2577–80;

Carmelita Calderwood, Review of Elizabeth Kenny, *The Treatment of Infantile Paralysis in the Acute Stage*, *American Journal of Nursing* 42 (January 1942): 121.

14. Naomi Rogers, "American Medicine and the Politics of Filmmaking: *Sister Kenny* (RKO, 1946)," in *Medicine's Moving Pictures: Medicine, Health, and Bodies in American Film and Television*, ed. Leslie J. Reagan, Nancy Tomes, and Paula A. Treichler (Rochester, N.Y.: University of Rochester Press, 2007), 199–238.

15. Pohl and Kenny, *The Kenny Concept of Infantile Paralysis*, 152.

16. Lois Maddox Miller, "Sister Kenny Wins Her Fight," *Reader's Digest* 41 (1942): 28.

17. Charles C. Zacharie to My Dear Dr. Stimson, January 11, 1943, Stimson Papers, Box 2, folder 4, Correspondence re: Medical Talks, Medical Center Archives, New York-Presbyterian/Weill, Cornell, New York City (hereafter NYPWC).

18. Philip Stimson to Dear Dr. Zacharie, January 12, 1943, Stimson Papers, Box 2, folder 4, Correspondence re: Medical Talks, Medical Center Archives, NYPWC.

19. Oshinsky, *Polio*, 73

20. Kenny to Dear Sir [O'Connor], December 4, 1940, Public Relations, Kenny Files, Box 6, March of Dimes Archives, White Plains, N.Y.

21. Kenny to Dear Mr. Connor, September 30, 1941, Basil O'Connor 1940–1942, Elizabeth Kenny Collection, Minnesota Historical Society, St. Paul.

22. Quoting Kenny's remarks, R. W. Cilento, "Report on the Muscle Re-Education Clinic, Townsville (Sister E. Kenny), and Its Work," [August 9, 1934], Box 13, McCracken Collection, Fryer Library and Special Collections, University of Queensland, St. Lucia, 4.

23. See, for example, Raymond E. Lenhard, "The Results of Poliomyelitis in Baltimore," *Journal of Bone and Joint Surgery* 25 (1943): 132–41; Florence P. Kendall, "Sister Elizabeth Kenny Revisited," *Archives of Physical Medicine and Rehabilitation* 79 (April 1998): 361–65; Henry Otis Kendall and Florence P. Kendall, *Care During the Recovery Period in Paralytic Poliomyelitis*, Public Health Service Bulletin 242 (Washington, D.C.: Government Printing Office, 1938, rev. 1939); Lucie P. Lawrence, "Florence Kendall: What a Wonderful Journey," *PT Magazine of Physical Therapy* 8 (May 2000): 36–45.

24. Williams to Miss Catherine Gaule, October 19, 1942, Sydenham Hospital Collection, MS C 243, Box 82, NLM.

MEDIA REVIEWS

History of Nursing: Early Years. 2008. Insight Media. Producer: Jessica Tannenbaum, Director: Ken Lam. Insight Media. 2162 Broadway, New York, N.Y. 10024. DVD, 35 minutes. ($199.00) www.insight-media.com

History of Nursing: The Development of a Profession. 2008. Insight Media. Producer: Jessica Tannenbaum, Director: Ken Lam. Insight Media. 2162 Broadway, New York, N.Y. 10024. DVD, 36 minutes. ($199.00) www.insight-media.com

After a flurry of black and white films on the history of nursing appeared in the 1970s and 1980s, the use of this powerful medium to illustrate nursing's role in history ceased. It is therefore with pleasure that one welcomes the arrival of this attractive well-illustrated film production of the history of nursing. Developed by *Insight Media* and packaged as two DVDs, *History of Nursing* is an ambitious project that covers the history of the profession from antiquity to the present. Although primarily designed as an educational film for nursing students and those interested in health history, the DVDs will also appeal to audiences who simply want to learn the story of how nurses have cared for the sick over time.

The first segment, *The History of Nursing: Early Years*, explores the original appearance of nurses and nursing in society. Using a variety of colored images from ancient paintings, sculptures, maps, and more contemporary black and white photographs, the story opens in ancient Mesopotamia around the fifth century B.C. Drawing from evidence extracted from artifacts and writings from ancient civilizations, the struggle of mankind is revealed as men try to understand why humans suffer and die and how certain people in every society became healers, sometimes as priests, physicians, medicine men, and nurses. The two videos wisely use two expert nurse historians, Jean Whelan and Barbra Mann Wall, to clarify facts and add a sense of vitality to the presentation. Their comments aid viewers in recognizing the contributions to medical knowledge and the development of Western medicine made by the ancient medical traditions of the Egyptian, Indian, and Islamic cultures. I was pleased to see highlighted the role Islamic medicine took in shaping Western medicine as other nursing histories too often slight Islamic contributions.

Nursing History Review 18 (2010): 204–216. A Publication of the American Association for the History of Nursing. Copyright © 2010 Springer Publishing Company.
DOI: 10.1891/1062-8061.18.204

After discussing the origins of nursing, an important dimension of the story of the profession, the film considers the creation of religious and then secular nurses and explores the powerful function gender exerted in fashioning the roles and interactions of physicians and nurses.

Moving quickly in time the video captures the dramatic development of biological sciences that occurred in the nineteenth century and how information gained from these sciences spurred the rise of Western medicine. Armed with new knowledge about the human body and diseases, physicians were able to heal many of the sick, helping to transform hospitals into therapeutic healing institutions. Equally important to the scientific advancement of medicine was the appearance of knowledgeable and skilled trained nurses to care for the sick and work alongside physicians.

A discussion of the pre- and post-Nightingale periods introduces the emergence of formal nursing education. The early training programs, most notably the one at London's St. Thomas Hospital Training School, established by Florence Nightingale in 1860, laid the foundation for today's professional nurses' education. Both hospitals and physicians realized that an inexpensive work force of intelligent, hard-working student nurses radically improved patient care services and the efficiency of hospitals leading to the rapid expansion and spread of Nightingale-modeled nursing schools in countries around the world, assuring the development of professional nursing.

As an educational guide, the film identifies various salient themes that shaped the nursing profession, which helps the audience focus on major changes and issues important in the profession's evolution. This is an essential tool because the film quickly covers many centuries and multiple historical dimensions pertinent to illness, society, and the rise of modern medicine, nursing, and hospitals. However, this teaching aid cannot meet all student needs. A faculty member versed in the history of nursing and medicine needs to be present to answer viewers' questions and lead class discussions that stimulate students to critically view the past and explore ways it may affect their own clinical practice and the profession. Finally, because today's nursing students are, to a large degree, lacking in historical knowledge about the past and the nursing profession, the lack of suggested historical readings and a reference list diminishes the power of the film to intellectually engage students to understand the power of the past in shaping today's world.

The second part of the production, *History of Nursing: The Development of the Profession*, picks up the story of nursing's development in the early twentieth century. From the appearance of its opening credits this film quickly captures the attention and interest of its audience as it, through its well-crafted narrative and use of hundreds of archival images and films, follows the struggles of nurses as they undergo transformation from kindly but untrained caregivers to college-educated highly competent professional nurses.

This transformation begins when nurse leaders move to gain control of nursing education and the clinical practice of professional nurses. The creation of professional nursing organizations, around the turn of the twentieth century, aided nurses in establishing educational standards for nursing programs and in securing state nurse licensure laws that protected the public from incompetent untrained women who claimed to be nurses.

Leaders of the profession, who created new roles for professional nurses such as public health and military nursing or established innovative advanced practice nursing programs, are identified. The film illustrates the positive role nurses played in the country's many armed conflicts of the twentieth century and the discrimination faced by African American and male nurses as they sought to claim their rightful place as professional nurses within the profession, the military, and in society. The powerful role the federal government wielded, beginning in 1943 with the creation of the U.S. Cadet Nurse Corps, in meeting the needs of the country for well-educated professional nurses is also well documented.

Advances in nursing education in the late twentieth century and the creation of new programs such as undergraduate associate degree programs, master-level clinical specialty programs, nurse practitioner programs, and doctoral programs are depicted. Each new program reflected the increasing complexities of modern nursing and the expanding abilities of nurses to provide patients expert care.

The last portion of the film clearly clarifies that nursing's history is still being forged in today's world. One of the more important issues facing the profession today is how to recruit more males and individuals from minority and ethnic groups into the profession. Both nurse consultants, Drs. Whelan and Wall, discuss why this issue must be resolved if the profession is to continue to meet its social responsibility to provide competent, skillful, and compassionate care to patients.

The History of Nursing: The Development of a Profession, the stronger of the two films, possesses a kinetic and intellectual energy that propels the story of nursing's development into an essential component of the health care system, and does so with a verve and style that will appeal to students. The story is grounded in the events of America's past, but instead of being weighed down by historical facts the film captures nursing's ability to meet the needs of the country, whether it is at peace or engaged in war.

Although this video also lacks a suggested reading list of nursing history articles and books, there is a wealth of such literature available, and today's computer savvy students can easily access it. Faculty can use this historical literature in tandem with the films to engage students in exploring not only the history of their own specific clinical areas of interest but also in identifying the basic values of the profession throughout history.

BARBARA BRODIE, PHD, RN, FAAN
Madge M. Jones Professor of Nursing Emerita
Associate Director, Center for Nursing Historical Inquiry
University of Virginia School of Nursing
Charlottesville, VA 22908

Contagion: Historical Views of Diseases and Epidemics. Harvard University Library, Open Collections Program, Cambridge, Mass 2008. Web site design: Robert Levers/Levers Advertising and Design. Funding by the William and Flora Hewlett Foundation, Arcadia, and Prince Alwaleed Bin Talal Bin Abdulaziz Alsaud. http://ocp.hul.harvard.edu/contagion/

Open access to Harvard University's digital library is of incalculable value to historians in need of access to sources concerning diseases and epidemics. On the opening page of *Contagion: Historical Views of Diseases and Epidemics,* the authors propose that the Web site ". . . contributes to the understanding of the global, social-history, and public-policy implications of diseases and offers important historical perspectives on the science and the public policy of epidemiology, today."[1] This ambitious goal is reached on this extensive Web site, which provides a timeline, discussion of disease entities, and historical summaries of some of the major events surrounding contagious diseases that traveled around the world.

The disease synopses cover a multitude of ailments that have long plagued humans including cholera, plague, smallpox, syphilis, Spanish influenza, tuberculosis, yellow fever, and tropical diseases. Eight health and science leaders and their work are also presented with links to their digitalized materials. The time frame of the Web site spans 500 years with well-documented narrative and direct links to online sources located at Harvard University Library. A quick click on the red-lettered titles in the reference list under each summary directly opens a separate window with the complete referenced work. Additional outside sources, though footnoted in the summaries, are unfortunately not linked to a direct Web site. The Web site supplies summations of general topics and concepts connected to the public health domain providing context for the disease development and policy responses.

Contagion: Historical Views of Diseases and Epidemics presents an array of information on designated topics and provides digitized copies of books, journals, and other documents offered in English, Spanish, French, German, and Chinese. The volumes and documents included on the Web site date from the late fifteenth century to more recent twentieth-century materials. A search of several of the catalog titles showed a variety of works related to the diseases and epidemics featured, allowing a researcher to read about the pathophysiology of the disease as well as the social, economic, and political influences surrounding the malady. This Web site provides sources to build understanding of the context surrounding epidemic diseases and the philosophy behind attempts to control illnesses that destroyed large segments of populations.

There is an eclectic mix of papers, journals, manuscripts, and presentations for which one can search on this Web site, adding to its significance. As it is often difficult to find the original documents from conferences and symposiums on public health, the ability to locate and view so many on one site represents an important contribution to historical knowledge and a critical source of material for historians. Committee reports are available as well as a selection of papers on topics such as vaccines, tuberculosis, and many other public health issues. In addition, one can view the original handwritten script on the Blackwell family documents as well as other famous physicians and scientists. This site is important for the variety it offers and the ease with which the sources are accessed. It adds background and richness to many research reports that might otherwise remain hidden or at the very least require travel to Harvard University's library for accessing.

One of the greatest features of this Web site is the ease in which users can move around the site and view journals, books, and documents related to major public health scourges that occurred around the world. After choosing a source, a new viewing window opens, allowing the user to either examine the document or return easily to the original search spot. The Web site provides four different image sizes and a zoom feature so that users can view charts, pictures, and words from a close perspective. In the item window, one can easily search for specific words within the document, allowing a quick assessment of the content. Documents can be downloaded entirely for later reading or printed by page or by the entire document. Permission and copyright information, easily identified with its own tab, specifies the conditions under which Web site visitors can use the materials.

Harvard University Library offers a unique digital collection of global works about attempts to control the morbidity and mortality of diseases. And it is all available with the click of a mouse! Nurses, physicians, public health personnel, historians, and researchers all over the world can access the books, papers, and journals documenting the international endeavors and programs to institute measures to prolong life and minimize the suffering that trails epidemics and diseases. But beware, you will find yourself spending much more time at this site than you can ever anticipate.

JEANNINE URIBE, PhD, RN
Drexel University
College of Nursing and Health Professionals
1505 Race Street
Mail Stop 501
Philadelphia, PA 19102–1192

Note

1. *Contagion: Historical Views of Diseases and Epidemics.* http://ocp.hul.harvard.edu/contagion/

Making Visible Embryos. 2008. Tatjana Buklijas and Nick Hopwood. An online exhibition developed by the University of Cambridge with support from the Wellcome Trust http://www.hps.cam.ac.uk/visibleembryos/index.html

Tatjana Buklijas and Nick Hopwood's Web site *Making Visible Embryos* traces the evolution of the embryo as a cultural concept, as an object for scientific exploration, and the interplay between these two. For most of the 700 years covered by this Web site, the scientific specifics of the human embryonic phase of development, which begins with implantation and ends with the eighth week of gestation, the beginning of the fetal phase, were unknown, and popular concepts of the embryo were nonexistent. Today images of embryos are ubiquitous as shorthand for political, religious, and pop culture messages. An Internet search for embryos nets information for expectant parents, craft instructions including those for a fetus coin purse, and propaganda from pro- and antiabortion proponents. In the fourteenth century images of human gestation were far less common and more fantastic. *Making Visible Embryos* exposes the conceptual and imagined evolution of the embryo from the 1300s to present day.

Buklijas and Hopwood use images from collections throughout Europe and the United States to follow the changing notions of the embryo over time. Although the Web site authors primarily focus on human embryos they also include fetal and nonhuman images within the collection. In the fourteenth century, the embryo was not known or considered independent of pregnancy. With the rise of anatomic studies and more powerful microscopy in the eighteenth century the study of embryos became more precise. By the end of the nineteenth century, scientific images of embryos were much more accurate, and publishing methods made the images available to a wider audience than ever before. In the twentieth century, popular and scientific images of embryos coalesced. The popular media reported on test tube babies and published photos of life in the womb while proud parents displayed ultrasound images as their first baby photos. Rather than simply chronicling the development of the science of embryology, Buklijas and Hopwood have interspersed their account with interesting details such as a discussion of "ensoulment" (when the soul first entered the body), explanations of how medieval laws regarding abortion and infanticide were linked to an understanding of gestational development, and how the first human egg and the earliest embryos were obtained at a Boston women's clinic. Throughout the years covered by this site, scientists' depictions of embryos and fetuses reflect the political, religious, and scientific debates of their day, and this is where Buklijas and Hopwood are most successful. *Making Visible Embryos* is one of many sites detailing the development of human embryos. What sets this site apart is that it provides a useful contextual reference to the social, scientific, and political background for all embryonic images.

Making Visible Embryos, a very large Web site, is structured chronologically with eight different distinct phases in addition to an introduction and conclusion page. Each phase has four to five subpages with two images that supplement the text and another box with an image and a related question. The three images per subpage are linked to enlarged versions with further explanation of the source and photo credits. The authors have included a link to the "resources" page with the bibliographic information on each page of the site, as well as a user's guide. The site is easy to use and very thorough. One critique is that the periodization is not instinctive and the names of the phases do not reflect their era, for example 1300–1700 is "Unborn." The phase names are explained in the user's guide, but it is easy to get lost in time within the structure of the site, especially once scientific developments start coming closer chronologically together. The bibliography is comprehensive and includes other sites dedicated to embryology and its history.

Though the history of embryology is laid out in an interesting and accessible way, this site also serves as a history of the modeling and printing of anatomical images. For scholars of print culture this provides a useful example of the various ways the images of embryos were produced and consumed by scientists and the public. For students of women's history the site provides an analysis of how the image of the embryo (and fetus) fueled women's rights campaigns as well as antiabortion movements. Finally, clinicians and students of obstetrics and women's health will find the phases and development of the field of embryology as fascinating as embryonic development itself.

WINIFRED C. CONNERTON, CNM, MS
Doctoral Candidate
Barbara Bates Center for the Study of the History of Nursing
Claire M. Fagin Hall
University of Pennsylvania School of Nursing
Philadelphia, PA 19104

MCH Timeline: History, Legacy and Resources for Education and Practice. Maternal and Child Health Bureau, Health Resources and Services Administration, United States Department of Health and Human Services, Rockville, Md. Contributors: Greg Alexander, Alice R. Richman, Sun Hee Rim, Bonnie Means Lane, Colleen E. Huebner, Holly Grason, Maribeth Badura, Laura Kavanagh. Web design: Jack Neuner. http://mchb.hrsa.gov/timeline/

This Web site, established by the Maternal and Child Health Bureau (MCHB) of the Health Resources and Services Administration, describes the history of maternal, infant, and child care in the United States beginning in 1798 and concluding in 2006. An introduction states that the bureau's hope is for the site to ". . . be used as an orientation tool for those new to maternal-child health (MCH) professions, for grantees of the [MCHB] and MCH students. [They] also hope that those with experience in the field will find it a rich resource and a source of inspiration."[1] The MCH timeline is focused on the highlights of the United States Public Health Services record in providing resources and direct services to childbearing women and children. It provides the material using an interactive timeline that takes the user from general information to more specific facts with a few clicks of the mouse.

Information contained on the main timeline includes major events in the care of women and children, including health care as well as social and cultural events that impacted the provision of such care. For example, the establishment of the Marine Health Service (MHS) in 1798 is the first citation. This service focused on the health of merchant marines and other men working at sea. The connection to mothers and children, initially not an obvious one, is the MHS's assistance to authorities on epidemics and quarantine issues. The MHS is also considered the forerunner of the United States Public Health Service (USPHS).

At first glance (or first click!) many entries on the timeline appear to be mere mentions of very important issues. The Sheppard Towner Act is summarized in ninety-six words. However, links to other sites provide the user with digitized copies of the actual act passed in 1921 and a summary of the programs developed with the grant monies, edited by Grace Abbott and published by the Children's Bureau in 1929. The Web site handles other major legislation affecting women and children in a similar manner.

The Web site gives the user options for searching for a particular topic. The user can filter the main timeline topics by public health and medicine or by government and policy. Some topics such as infant mortality, a module entitled MCH Public Health 101, oral histories and genetics, can be isolated on the timeline and explored in much more depth through connecting links. Users can also type terms or topics of interest into a search bar, results indicating, with appropriate links, where to find the information within the timeline. A tab on the main page brings up a listing of timeline resources that enhance the material covered on the timeline. Included here are downloads for a slide show of the timeline, a power point presentation of the slide show, a glossary of MCH terms, a thesaurus, links to federal MCH legislation, Children's Bureau documents, a history of MCH training programs, and the Centers for Disease Control and Prevention Public Health Image Library.

Controversial topics such as abortion, the repeal of the Sheppard Towner Act, and calls for government-based health care for all are covered; however, though facts are presented, no discussion is included. For example, abortion is mentioned in the context of family planning, the only hint of controversy has to do with the ban on federal funding.

The site's content is wide ranging and achieves its stated purpose. The links to other Web sites, both governmental and private, are appropriate, and with very few exceptions, easily accessed. These links include videos, access to primary documents, and digitized books and manuscripts. The site is easy to navigate and information is readily accessible.

A major drawback for nurses is the paucity of information on their role in the care of women and children. Lillian Wald is highlighted along with the Henry Street Settlement, and links to various sites include the Henry Street Web site, the USPHS, and biographies of Ms. Wald. But the vast numbers of nurses working in maternal and child health are largely ignored, referred to only peripherally within other topics. The emergence of pediatric nurse practitioners as primary care providers during the 1960s is not mentioned at all.

Despite this lack of subject matter on nurses and nursing, this Web site can be very useful for historians of maternal, infant, and children's health. It places, in one location, access to both general and specific information related to the topic. Opportunities for further research via links to legislation, government programs, and private organizations are vast. Useful also is situating topics within the context of the times. Economic and social issues influencing the development of programs such as the Social Security Act, Title V, are rightly described. On some issues, such as child abuse, the amount of time between identification of a problem, acknowledgment of the extent of the problem, and legislative reform is put in perspective.

This Web site is an excellent addition to the resources available for the study of MCH in the United States. Further digitalization of documents within the MCHB will only add to the usefulness for researchers, teachers, and the general public. The site asks for feedback, and this reviewer suggests that Nursing History Review readers comment on the lack of information on the vital role nurses play in this area.

ELIZABETH A. REEDY, PHD, RN
306 Burton Road
Oreland, PA 19075

Note

1. *MCH Timeline: History, Legacy and Resources for Education and Practice.* http://mchb.hrsa.gov/timeline/

Army Nurses of World War One: Service Beyond Expectations. 2006. Lorraine Luciano and Casandra Jewell (Eds). Army Heritage Center Foundation, Carlisle, Pennsylvania. Producer and Director: Anthony V. Rotolo. Narrator: Lisa Stofko. (DVD, 52 minutes $24.95), (book, 267 pages, $14.95), (DVD and book set $34.95). www.armyheritage.org

As part of The Army Heritage Foundation's series, *Voices of the Past Speak to the Future*, editors Lorraine Luciano and Casandra Jewell reconstructed the experiences of two nurses deployed as part of the United States Army Nurse Corps during World War I. Luciano and Jewell use two different media to illustrate the stories of these nurses: a book and a film documentary, employing the diaries, letters, photographs, newspaper clippings, and other primary source documents of nurses Elizabeth Lewis and Emma Weaver to create the landscape of experiences that typify World War I military nursing.

Luciano and Jewell's book begins with brief yet thorough prologue and introduction sections. These components provide the reader with the context necessary to understand the role of the featured nurses who served overseas during World War I with the American Expeditionary Force (AEF). Following the initial sections are more than 250 pages of prose and excerpts from primary data, effectively illustrating the compelling stories of Lewis and Weaver. The reader is enticed by the chronicles of these nurses and can easily overlook the way in which the introduction ends abruptly and lacks a segue into the subsequent section that features Lewis's letters.

Elizabeth Lewis, a young nurse from New England serving in the AEF, wrote letters home to her sisters and mother describing her experiences with Base Hospital Unit #9, which arrived in France in August of 1918. Although her wartime nursing experience was short in duration, ending after the 1918 Armistice, Lewis's written correspondence is rich in detail and description offering insight into how a young woman transitioned into a military nurse.

Lewis voices her concerns about breaching censorship regulations and worrying mom, and these themes come to the forefront of nearly all of her letters to her sisters. These letters, often quite graphic in their description of personal safety, speak to how Lewis establishes herself amidst a military routine. In a time of unrestricted submarine warfare, Lewis matter-of-factly describes the identification disc she wears that would identify her if injured. In Lewis's letters to her mother, however, she is instead reassuring minimizing the threats of war. Spelling and grammatical errors found throughout the text, although a likely distraction to the lay reader, for scholars, paradoxically, add to the richness of the data provided and add evidence of the authenticity of the transcription. Photos and scanned images of letters, photographs, and ephemera throughout the entire book are of excellent quality.

Emma Weaver, the second featured nurse, is Lewis's more mature counterpart. Nurse Weaver volunteers for service with the AEF at the age of thirty-nine and has the foresight to record her wartime experiences in a diary. Upon her return to the United States, Weaver turns her journal into a memoir wherein she contemplates the nature of war, provides rich detail of her care of wounded and gassed soldiers, and offers the reader a perspective on morale among service people usually reserved only to those possessing vast life experience. These data possess depth and breadth that few young nurses could offer.

Although the editors profess this to be a project done for a lay audience, they miss the opportunity to provide the reader with an analysis of how

Media Reviews 215

these firsthand accounts reveal prominent issues reflective of the World War I era, such as gender, rank, standards for entry into service that changed with demand for personnel, and race. Some, if not all, of these topics might have been presented in a way as not to be beyond the reach of the audience. In some sections erroneous assumptions and hasty conclusions imply causality between events that may not exist. For example, the audience is left with an oversimplified idea about the recruitment and enlistment of African American nurses and an inaccurate representation of how nurses' aides were employed only when influenza exacerbated the shortage of nurse personnel. The glossary provided is a useful feature, as is the list of resources where readers can find more information on these and other topics.

Between many of the nurses' letters and diary entries are segments that provide general information about various wartime phenomena. Although I appreciate the attempt at supplying a great deal of information in a short amount of space, these segments interrupt the flow of the letters and make the book choppy.

Included with the book is a companion documentary film adding a multimedia sensory accompaniment. The editors use many of the same images featured in the book, posting them beside the film's narrator, who reads passages from either Lewis or Weaver's writings. Footage from battlefields and contemporary recordings of World War I-era songs add a dimension of illustration not possible in book form.

The documentary includes interesting commentary by Michael Knapp, historian and chief of Oral History Branch of the U.S. Army Heritage and Education Center, who offers insight and analysis into topics like the dichotomy of men and women in the war effort and poses questions about the place of women in war. He also concludes that documentation of women's role in war is illustrated in recruitment posters of the era. In these posters, the nurse is depicted as progressing from a role as a passive observer to one of active participation. As noted above, this commentary in the book breaks up the flow, yet in the film it enhances and helps the documentary move along.

One can almost forgive the editors for inaccurately implying causality between the sinking of the Lusitania and America's entry into war, or how the war helped women overcome obstacles posed by gender, leading to the passage of the nineteenth amendment because of the section of the documentary entitled, "Preparation." Nurses are shown on a train to Ellis Island, participating in roll calls and drills, acquiring their equipment and uniforms, and receiving inoculations and vaccinations while the narrator reads passages about the threat of typhoid infection and the amount of red tape involved in deployment. Better still is the section on "The Work," which illustrates nurses in France transforming hotels into hospitals and caring for soldiers. The nursing shortage is well illustrated. Eventually the Armistice celebration arrives, yet for the nurses the work is far from over. Nurses are shown continuing to care for patients and taking inventory of their supplies as they begin to prepare for home. As the war comes to an end, the influenza epidemic hits, posing more of a threat to military nurses than enemy attack. The sound of patients coughing in the background as a photograph is displayed of a tuberculosis and pneumonia ward provides a powerful illustration. Despite the threats of illness, some nurses, including Emma Weaver, volunteered for service with the allied occupation force. One of the most moving scenes of the documentary shows footage of ships coming into port past the Statue of Liberty where soldiers are walking down gangplanks.

The most important contribution of this project is the inclusion of an "Extras" folder on the DVD. Instructions on how to access this file are not provided, making it unnecessarily difficult to navigate. However, once the reader overcomes this challenge and opens the folder, the data are well worth the struggle! This feature includes an image gallery and printable PDF files of the primary source documents of nurses Lewis and Weaver. These images aid in the preservation and wide accessibility of ephemera and help to make the characters in film and book authentic.

Jennifer Casavant Telford, PhD, ACNP-BC
Assistant Professor
University of Connecticut School of Nursing
231 Glenbrook Rd. U-2026
Storrs, CT 06269–2026

BOOK REVIEWS

Intensely Human: The Health of the Black Soldier in the American Civil War
By Margaret Humphreys
(Baltimore: The Johns Hopkins University Press, 2008) (197 pages; $40 cloth)

Military mortality rates during the Civil War led to sweeping changes in military medicine, nursing, and ultimately, civilian medicine. Many publications addressing Civil War soldier health and mortality focus more on the White soldier. However, within all troops existed a subgroup whose health has not had the closer examination of the whole: the Black soldier. The Black soldiers had higher mortality rates than their White counterparts. Margaret Humphreys's *Intensely Human* addresses and explores the reasons behind these higher mortality rates. The book's title derives from the reply of a military physician responding to the reasons for a Black regiment's susceptibility to disease and response to treatment.

Black soldiers were more likely to die than their White comrades as they entered the war with innate disadvantages of poor nutrition and immunologic isolation. Coming proportionally from a more rural environment on the whole from the White soldier, the Black soldier entered camp with an increased susceptibility to disease. Indifference to their deprivations encountered prior to camp and the sometimes calculated decisions made by authorities resulted in a greater death rate for the Black soldier.

Humphreys presents a compelling preface detailing the challenges faced in researching this particular group of soldiers within the larger Civil War archive. Recordkeeping was not exact during this time. Name changes among Black regiments were fluid in a way not seen in White regiments. Consistently short of medical personnel and probably led by less experienced officers, soldiers in Black regiments were an inherently higher risk group for recovery when injured or ill. Regiments led by conscientious commanders fared better. While researching the archives for information on Black soldiers' health, Humphreys found information specific to this group remains somewhat sketchy and anecdotal. Black troops were the frequent recipients of inferior provisions and supplies, which most likely extended to medical care. Not all military physicians were indifferent to the Black soldier's health, and within the text are several accounts of excellent care extended to these men—not so much because of race, but more to the underlying humanity and compassion of the caregiver. Still, evidence remained to the inborn belief of the inferiority of the Black man among many military physicians and commanders and all too often, translated to Black soldiers receiving inferior, poor, or no care at all when ill, compounded by lack of supplies and even less nutritious food.

An interesting subject Humphreys presents is chapter 5, addressing the influence of region upon disease epidemiology as it affected the Black soldier's health. The coastal regions of the Carolinas accounted for the healthiest of the Black troops, whereas Black soldiers who originated from regions of the Mississippi Valley fared more poorly. Presented statistics of comparative mortality, however, come with caveats as to the incompleteness of records kept for these soldiers. Still, Black soldiers originating in the Atlantic region were healthier, with some having the added advantage of an endemic immunity to malaria not seen by those in more internal areas of the country.

Approximately 180,000 Black men went to war during the Civil War, with 143,000 returning home at its end. *Intensely Human* provides a compelling insight into the overall health of the significant contributions made by Black soldiers in the Civil War. Detailed notes at the book's end from extensive archives provide additional documentation. *Intensely Human* presents a picture of race, epidemiology, and bureaucracy, and its effects on the ability of Black soldiers to make their contribution in the Civil War.

TERESA M. O'NEILL, RNC, PHD
Professor
Our Lady of Holy Cross College
4123 Woodland Drive
New Orleans, LA 70131

This Republic of Suffering: Death and the American Civil War

By Drew Gilpin Faust
(New York: Vintage Civil War Library, 2009) ($15.95; paper)

Modern nurses focus on caring and competence at the bedside, but we need to remember that the presence of death permeated our practice in the nineteenth century. In no other time was that more true than in the Civil War. Drew Gilpin Faust has produced a work that will become a standard reference for all nurse historians with an interest in or focus on Civil War nursing. She puts the massive loss of life into perspective and gives us a detailed analysis of what the deaths of more than 600,000 soldiers and thousands of civilians meant to our society. In her previous research on women during this era the author realized that much of women's perceptions of the war were shaped by the enormous impact of all the deaths (p. 323).

The book opens with a powerful preface where the author introduces the reader to the scope of her topic. It wasn't just the numbers of deaths that were significant but the impact on society. She compares the 2 percent loss of population in the 1860s to what a similar loss would be today of 6 million soldiers (p. xi). Military losses were compounded with the deaths in the civilian population from communicable diseases and deaths from battles fought in communities. Death became a shared experience as losses spread throughout the nation. Frederick Law Olmstead is credited with the expression of a "republic of suffering," as he witnessed hospital ships unloading dead and injured soldiers returning from the conflict (p. xiii). She closes the preface with the thesis of her work: "The work of death was Civil War America's most fundamental and most demanding undertaking" (p. xviii).

In eight topical chapters the author covers every aspect of death in the war era. They share common threads in the study. First, the reader is oriented to the realities of the nineteenth-century culture, mores, and perceptions of the war and its outcome. Contrasts with modern thinking are drawn to keep the reader oriented to the rationale for the behaviors described. Second, the saga of death, its meaning, and management is told through the lives of the people who lived and died in the war. The author's expertise in the period is obvious as one analyzes the scope of references and specific details for each topic examined.

The chapters on "Dying and Killing" profile what caused the deaths and how they happened. The concept of a "good death" and contemporary views of dying are presented (p. 8). Stories of the men and women coping with waves of death from battle and communicable diseases are profiled. The author points out that killing others was a bigger problem than dying because killing violated Christian mores, which were strong in the prewar society. Religious and military leaders on both sides tried to mitigate the values conflict by invoking scripture to exonerate soldiers in battle. The presence of killing in the war-torn areas of the country are described in great detail to reflect the nature of how groups coped with the reality of local war.

The most brutal chapter in the book is on "Burying." The sheer numbers of dead overwhelmed all the systems in place for burial in a proper sense by nineteenth-century standards. The chapter highlights how the burying was done or at times not done because of the pressures of conflict. The loss of mores regarding the care of the dead as the result of wartime realities is described in detail. The grotesque responses of troops to the need for disposing of the dead were painful to read.

The rest of the chapters address the aftermath of the wartime death experience. The chapter on "Naming" focuses on the problem of determining who was in those trenches used as mass graves. Faust traces the patchwork of processes in place for getting word back to families and how many people were never located or named officially. Voluntary organizations, peers, superior officers, nurses, and even profit-oriented agents were involved in the system to name the victims and communicate their deaths. The idea of dying and being unknown compounded the loss for families and communities.

"Realizing," is a chapter subtitled "Civilians and the Work of Mourning" (p. 137). The author describes the specifics of the death experiences of civilians caught in the war. This opening section lays the groundwork for depicting the universal grief experience that enveloped most of society in the North and South. Death was everywhere and was not limited to the battlefield. The realization that the losses were so extensive, impacting soldier and civilian alike, changed the people and society profoundly. How could this loss have meaning? The author addressed this question with the chapter on "Believing and Doubting," as she explored the nineteenth-century struggles with science, innovation, religion, and the realization of the devastation of the war.

The "Accounting and Numbering" chapters describe the search for the dead. The efforts of Clara Barton at Andersonville and others dispersed across the country are described as the postwar society searched for missing graves and unidentified men lost in the war. Proper burials and this search became a focus of the country in the first postwar years. Numbering became important after the war. How many actually died? How many are still missing? The chapter describes the numbering process and closes with the notation that numbering in this period was also about philosophical and transcendent questions about what had happened to the country in the slaughter that had unfolded.

The book ends with an epilogue on "Surviving," where the author returns to some of the people used to depict the story of death in war and their lives after the era closes. The issues of meaning and faith following such a painful encounter with mass death are explored. The author closes with the reflection that this war opened an era of mass destruction and death that we still live in today.

When one finishes this study, there is a sense that one has taken a long journey into the soul of our nation. The text is supported with a massive overview of Civil War documents representative of both sides. Nursing is well represented in the study in relation to our role in the care of the dying and assistance to families. This book has changed this writer's view of what that bare number of over 600,000 dead meant to the people of that time.

LINDA E. SABIN, RNC, PHD
Professor of Nursing
University of Louisiana at Monroe
700 University Avenue
Monroe, LA 71209

Florence Nightingale: The Making of an Icon
By Mark Bostridge
(New York: Farrar, Strauss and Giroux, 2008) (647 pages; $35 cloth)

Like Cleopatra, whose infinite variety time could not make stale, Florence Nightingale continues to fascinate us. Since Sir Edward Cook's 1,000-page, two-volume biography published in 1913 there have been almost fifty further biographies: Mark Bostridge's 647-page work therefore stands in a long line. Cook's magnum opus has stood the test of time, challenged only briefly by Cecil Woodham-Smith's popularly written *Florence Nightingale*, published in 1950. Cook managed to strike a fine balance between sympathetic admiration for his subject and a critical approach, all the more difficult because the Nightingale heirs commissioned his work. Woodham-Smith did not footnote her work, and although she gained access to the Claydon archives, which Nightingale's executors denied Cook, she relied heavily on Cook as have most of Nightingale's biographers. Her *Florence Nightingale* is much more in the tradition of the hagiographies and lacks Cook's judicious critical sense.

So much new information has come forward since Cook published ninety-five years ago that Bostridge's contribution is well justified. For nurses in particular this is especially relevant because Cook either was unaware of the tremendous problems at the Nightingale Training School or, more likely, considered it impolitic and possibly harmful to the struggling new profession to detail them. It took a former union organizer, Monica Baly, to make public the failings of the much respected Nightingale training when she published *Florence Nightingale and the Nursing Legacy* in 1988. Bostridge studies Nightingale, as the subtitle *The Making of an Icon* indicates, with a special interest in how the Nightingale legend and the real multifaceted historical woman interacted with each other. He points out that Nightingale's reputation as the iconic nurse was greatly helped by the secluded life she led after her famous collapse in August 1857. Her disappearance from public life made it possible to sentimentalize her as the saintly and compassionate lady whose shadow the soldiers kissed. At the same time it diminished the brilliance of her personality and intellect and her extensive work in other areas. He tells us that one of his inspirations in writing the biography was Margaret Thatcher, the Iron Lady who also knew how to both deny and exploit her femininity. Her career gave him insight into the political advantages and vicissitudes experienced by a woman operating in a male-dominated world. Thatcher herself admired Nightingale as a great historical figure, a lady who, she said, "had an idea, who knew what she wanted to do, and wasn't going to be put off by anyone" (pp. xxii–xxiii). Thatcher is certainly an apt comparison, but the gendered barriers she faced in the male-dominated world of the late twentieth century, though significant, pale in comparison with the domestic sphere that constrained ladies of Nightingale's generation.

Bostridge's *Florence Nightingale* is an extraordinarily scholarly work providing a wealth of detail, a good deal hitherto unknown, about Nightingale's family and network. His encyclopedic knowledge of her society helps us understand why she acted as she did, and he writes with the same sympathetic yet critical view as Cook, not glossing over her flaws. Both students of nineteenth-century nursing history and the general reader will find the new information enlightening. The book also includes a number of fascinating pictures that I for one have never seen before—for example, Nightingale's father in his forties, her mother in court dress in 1823, a photograph of Lea Hurst taken in the 1860s, Aunt Mai and Uncle Sam Smith and the Bracebridges who chaperoned and helped Nightingale in Scutari, and Mary Stanley and Sister Sarah Anne Terrot, two of the Crimean War nurses. Like Barbara Dossey, Bostridge completely accepts the D.A.B. Young thesis that the "Crimean fever," which almost killed Nightingale in May and June 1855, was what has now been identified as a disease called brucellosis. In fact, Bostridge, quite convincingly, relies heavily on this modern diagnosis to explain the difficult course of Nightingale's long invalidism.

Unfortunately, perhaps because footnotes are so expensive to print or because the book is aimed at the trade rather than students of nineteenth-century history, it is not footnoted. In a sense this is understandable because the sources utilized are massive. For example, one collection alone, the Nightingale papers in the British Library, is the library's second-biggest single collection, second only to the Gladstone papers. Bostridge references every direct quote and makes some comments in a section called "Notes," which is very helpful but, for general information, sources are not given. For example, we learn that Nightingale's ferocious matron, Mrs. Clarke, who was an army in herself at Harley Street and Scutari, was formerly matron of the Sheffield union workhouse. For those of us who are interested in the Crimean War nurses, it is disappointing not to know where this information came from, allowing us to possibly track down more information about Clarke. For students of nursing history (although perhaps not for the general reading public, who will enjoy this book just as much as scholars) this is all the more disappointing because the book is so thoroughly researched, both in the vast primary sources and numerous contextual works.

Readers of *Nursing History Review* will be pleased that Bostridge has carefully read the revisionist nursing history of the past twenty-five years, and indeed *Nursing History Review* itself, citing, for example, Joyce MacQueen's "Florence Nightingale's Nursing Practice." Bostridge spends more time on nursing than may be justified given all the work Nightingale did on army and public health reform both in Britain and in India. Lynn McDonald's *Collected Works of Florence Nightingale*, of which eleven of the sixteen projected volumes are now in print, will devote only two volumes to nursing, which may perhaps be an accurate reflection of Nightingale's interest in and time spent on nursing, especially in her more active years. The need to deal with all the myth grown up around Nightingale and nursing may justify Bostridge's allocation of space.

There is an excellent bibliographical review in the last chapter, beginning with Stanmore's less than flattering portrayal of Nightingale in his 1906 biography of Sidney Herbert. Bostridge includes movies and plays as well as books and ends the chapter with the largest British trade union representing nurses rejecting Nightingale as the founder of modern nursing. One book that he omits and that deserves his well-informed view is Evelyn Bolster's *Sisters of Mercy in the Crimean War*, which treats Nightingale, who is a major figure in her story, in such a way as to make F. B. Smith's *Florence Nightingale: Reputation and Power* look almost mild. The Bolster book is important because a number of recent scholars have accepted as accurate its delineation of the role of Mother Francis Bridgeman and her Sisters in Nightingale's effort to establish a coordinated nursing team in the East. Bostridge describes Smith's work as character assassination masquerading as serious history and finds that he makes many statements that are not supported and sometimes even contradicted by his citations.

There are the inevitable small errors to be expected in a first edition. To name one or two: the six St. John's House nurses who went to Scutari with Nightingale were not St. John's House Sisters but rather paid, working-class nurses; Nightingale's matron Mrs. Clarke did not leave Scutari in 1856 but was dismissed in April 1855 when it was discovered that, as well as being disagreeable, she had a major drinking problem and was leading other nurses astray. There was a Mary Ann Clark, who was one of Miss Skene's Oxford district nurses, who did leave Scutari at the end of the war. (There was even a third Clarke, Elizabeth, who worked at the Renkioi Hospital.) These are minor mistakes and can be easily corrected in the second edition, which I am sure this book will go to.

In summary this is a highly readable, very scholarly, up-to-date, and important contribution to the Nightingale story.

Carol Helmstadter
Adjunct Assistant Professor
University of Toronto
34 Chestnut Park Road
Toronto ON M4W 1W6
Canada

Die Entwicklung der Krankenpflege zur staatlich anerkannten Tätigkeit im 19. und frühen 20. Jahrhundert: Das Zusammenwirken von Modernisierungsbestrebungen, ärztlicher Dominanz, konfessioneller Selbstbehauptung und Vorgaben preußischer Regierungspolitik [The Development of Nursing into a State-Approved Occupation in the Nineteenth and Early Twentieth Century: The Entwined Influences of Modernization, Medical Domination, Assertion of Confessional (Religious) Independence, and Prussian State Politics]
By Christoph Schweikardt
(München: Martin Meidenbauer, 2008) (339 pages)

In a thoroughly researched and well-written account, Christoph Schweikardt analyzes the development of nursing within the Prussian health care system in the nineteenth and early twentieth centuries. Taking Prussia as a case example within the larger context of the German Empire, his particular focus is on the legislatory decision-making process that eventually resulted in an approved state exam for nurses in Prussia in 1907. Schweikardt examines and explains this end result as the outcome of a negotiation process or power struggle shaped by the political structures of the Prussian state administration as well as the various political interests of the main stakeholders, such as physicians, hospital administrators, religious orders and confessional associations, unionized hospital personnel, and, to a minor degree, the women's movement. Given the power constellation in Prussia at the time, the outcome was markedly different from the professionalization process of, for example, their British and North American counterparts.

The analysis provides valuable insight into these differences. Schweikardt argues that a strong influence of a liberal women's movement on nursing did not take hold in Germany during this time period. Although a small group of independently organized, internationally connected female nurses around Agnes Karll and an evangelical deaconal association became politically engaged and supported by the women's movement, their influence remained minor in the face of the large majority of nurses bound by the motherhouses and of untrained attendants who formed the majority of public hospital personnel. The state's interest in not having to commit funds to nursing education aligned well with the motherhouses' interest in keeping control over their own affairs. As a field of work, nursing remained politically divided, medically dominated, and grounded in occupational traditions, with little movement toward the development of nursing as an independent, self-regulated female profession as in the Anglo-American and Scandinavian world, Schweikardt argues. Modernization of health care, development of scientific medicine, and the need for better skilled nurses did have its effect though, and a minimal commitment to nursing education was eventually made.

The book has six chapters. Chapter 1 gives an introduction. Chapter 2 forms the main body of the book. It consists of nine sections presenting the analysis. Section 1 maps out the legal and political framework of medical care since the 1600s. Being part of poor relief, lay attendants of low social status gave nursing care in public hospitals. When these grew in size as of the eighteenth century and scientific medicine emerged, training of personnel became an issue. An early initiative to establish education for ward personnel came from medical official Franz Anton Mai in 1782. In 1832 efforts of physicians at the Charité Hospital in Berlin resulted in the opening of a three-month study program. Both initiatives did not result in legislation but did become signposts in later negotiations over nursing education and enhanced medical control over care. Confessional motherhouses began to fill the gap and became the most important producer of trained nursing personnel. During the Restoration after Napoleon's defeat in 1815, Catholicism grew in influence and Roman Catholic Caritas as well as Protestant Inner Mission evolved in a large network of motherhouses having their own hospitals. The state hardly involved itself in regulation of nursing care.

Section 2 gives a useful review of British developments, using a discussion of Florence Nightingale's influence as a frame for comparison. Essential differences of the British system as compared to Germany were less state control over health care, more liberal self-organization of the professions, and less influence of Catholicism. The 1832 initiative of physician Rudolf Virchow at the urban Charité stood out as a liberal exception in a conservative German state medical bureaucracy. The influence of confessional organizations was so powerful that Red Cross nursing associations, which arose in the wake of the Crimean War, adapted to the traditional motherhouse structure. In section 3, Schweikardt examines how the Prussian state failed to initiate a secular counterpart to the strong religiously dominated structures, despite several public health crises resulting from cholera and other epidemics. Section 4 analyzes available statistics on nursing personnel, confirming how in numbers Catholic and Protestant organizations generated almost two-thirds, if not more, of all nursing personnel—the majority being Catholic nurses—though Catholics formed only one-third of the population. Section 5 describes how the expansion of the health care system and increase in hospital care, with more surgery being performed, eventually formed the push for change, increasing the demand for more and better skilled nursing personnel.

Section 6 analyzes the impact of progressive groups on the establishment of better training, such as Roman Catholic physician-initiated reform within the religious structures as well as the influence of smaller, more progressive groups linked with the women's movement, such as the group of independent nurses led by Agnes Karll, who formed an independent nurses association, and the physician-led Evangelical Deaconal Association. Gradually these groups made inroads on the traditional power structures, although the small progressive organizations' lobby for a three-year nursing education found little political support.

Section 7 examines the role of the medical profession in nursing reform. An interesting initiative was the short-lived movement of scientific nursing, an effort of a small group of physicians to establish nursing as a medical specialty within university medicine. Some medical groups clearly viewed education of nurses and attendants as a threat to medical authority. Physician Martin Mendelson had a central role in the movement, coining the term "hypurgie" for (medical) therapeutic nursing. He published a book *Comfort of the Sick* that showed remarkable resemblance to Nightingale's *Notes on Nursing*, yet without any acknowledgment. More broadly, physicians, relying on their scientific authority, gained control over nursing personnel as they took up positions as medical superintendents of hospitals. Section 8 further analyzes the reform efforts of progressive organizations in the context of early twentieth-century politics. Increased political debate, especially from the socialist side, over poor work conditions of hospital personnel, and public health measures to control infectious disease, further triggered a call for state-approved education of nurses to improve health conditions. How a state approved exam finally became legislated in 1907 is the focus of the final section. As the parliamentary power of the German Empire grew, and political debate over conditions in hospitals increased, the Prussian state government eventually supported the implementation of a state approved nursing exam following one year of training. The exam remained voluntary but eventually did gain commitment from all groups involved, including the powerful motherhouses.

Although the political shift was important, Schweikardt notes that it also was a minimal solution without any regulation of qualifications or work conditions. The final chapters of the book are shorter, summarizing the findings (chapter 3) and implications for later developments (chapter 4) and listing sources as well as areas for further research (chapters 5 and 6). Nursing was the stepchild of the Prussian medical system, Schweikardt concludes. Having its origins in poor relief, and dominated by a charitable motherhouse structure without the political support to regulate basic educational and work conditions, nursing work remained of low social status, constraining the development of nursing as an independent profession for middle-class women. The state nursing exam, established in 1907, was a minimal compromise that reflected the relatively unfavorable German political context for nursing reform at the time. The existing power constellation, however, restricted the social status and political influence nurses were able to gain.

The analysis provides important historical insight in the influences that continued to constrain German nursing as it sought to improve education and work conditions to meet the demands of twentieth-century health care. Schweikardt notes that much more work needs to be done in nursing history as German nurses move toward increased academization and professional independence. This excellent study, however, offers a compelling analysis of the political and legislative process that generated the beginning of state-regulated nursing in Germany. The book will be of interest to academic and professional audiences in nursing, social science, and health care history, providing a valuable contribution to the international nursing history scholarship.

Geertje Boschma, RN, PhD
Associate Professor
School of Nursing, University of British Columbia
T201—2211 Wesbrook Mall
Vancouver, BC V6T 2B5
Canada

Community Nursing and Primary Healthcare in Twentieth-Century Britain
By Helen M. Sweet with Rona Dougall
(New York: Routledge, 2008)
(266 pages; $95.00 cloth)

Organized health services for the sick and vulnerable poor in their own communities have been established for well over a century and a half in Britain, and the district nurse has been to the forefront in planning and providing such services. For much of this period, district nursing services were organized on a voluntary basis through district nursing associations, the most prominent being the Queen's Nursing Institute. Working with communities as diverse as urban poor and remote island dwellers, the district nurse was a key health professional in developing public health services.

In this authoritative account of the history of community nursing and primary health care in Britain in the twentieth century, Helen Sweet and Rona Dougall offer a critical study that examines the development of district nursing and related community health services, including health visiting and general practice. They examine aspects of the content of nursing care as well as the wider context of social change and professional developments within which the district nurse operated in the period under review. The narrative is based on multiple primary sources that include documentary materials from the archives of the Queen's Nursing Institute, official papers, reports, contemporary journals and textbooks, and oral testimonies of district nurses and general practitioners (GPs). The book contains several well-chosen images interspersed throughout the pages, which usefully illustrate the work of the district nurse. The book complements Monica Baly's study of the Queen's Nursing Institute[1] and Mary Stocks's study of district nursing in the period up to 1960.[2] The historiographic framework is an applied prosopographical and institutional interdisciplinary approach, and the authors draw on the paradigm of social, gender, and political history to examine district nursing over a chronological period of more than a century.

The narrative is set out in two major parts. Part I presents a historical analysis of district nursing and primary health care services in four distinct chronological periods from the mid-nineteenth century until the end of the 1970s when primary care became well established. The dominant role of the Queen's Nursing Institute is examined, and the effects of its declining influence toward the end of the period, when responsibility for health care provision came under local authority control, are considered. With the introduction of the National Health Service in Britain soon after WWII, the professional context of district nursing was changing as were the lives of the families served by the district nurse. The authors account for these changes with clarity and insight.

Themes examined in the chronological periods include training and regulation and interprofessional rivalries, what the authors refer to as "contested professional territory." The authors examine the particular relationship between nursing and medicine in a practice context in which there was little day-to-day contact between the doctor and the nurse. In theory, role boundaries existed between the district nurse and other community health professionals, most especially the GP and the health visitor, and these boundaries were often the subject of watchful policing on the part of some GPs and health visitors. Nevertheless, role boundaries were inevitably crossed in the everyday delivery of community health services, because the exigencies of a family's health needs could not be deferentially deferred. The district nurse was a flexible and multi-skilled professional who "was known to everybody and understood every family [and] while washing grandpa . . . could do the health visiting" (p. 41). Evidence from oral testimonies is usefully deployed to give a balanced picture of both good and sometimes fraught interprofessional working relationships. In this way the archetypal doctor-nurse relationship as one of superior-subordinate is rendered less obvious in the reality of public health practice.

Although contested territory could give rise to interprofessional tensions, most district nurses worked harmoniously and in a complementary way with GPs and with other community health professionals. Using some district nurses' personal accounts, the authors explain that, with the introduction of a range of new community health roles and the advent of greater professional accountability, role boundaries became less fluid toward the end of the period under review. The authors also trace transitions in the primary function of the district nurse from that of provider of nursing service to the sick poor in their own homes, to provider of a private nursing service to the middle classes, and later to provider of a state nursing service in a multidisciplinary team context. As the focus of nursing work became subject to social drift, the emphasis on nursing work changed, although many core nursing functions remained.

In part II, the authors examine a number of distinct themes. These include the great variation in a community's needs from one geographical region to the next, the social position of the district nurse in the community in which she was posted, the impact of medical and communications technologies on the work of the district nurse, and professionalization of district nursing through regulation and education. In this last theme, the authors point to the changing emphasis in the way that district nursing developed, with the pendulum swinging between professionalism and managerialism, and to the constraints that attended these divergent models. Also examined is the theme of caring and professionalism; in this connection the authors point out that although district nurses tended to emphasize caring as an essential focus of their role, they were not "caught up in notions of caring and professionalism as conflicting concepts" (p. 185). In the final theme, Sweet and Dougall consider how images of the district nurse used in recruitment and public information campaigns shaped both public understandings and nurses' own self-concept, and they consider how these images contained encoded values and beliefs, such as the implied distinction between male and female members of the community care team and the distinction between the various gender-ascribed functions they each performed.

The authors draw a number of conclusions from their examination of the history of district nursing in Britain. From the viewpoint of the district nurse, Britain's great geographical variations could determine not only the content and scope of district nurses' work but also interprofessional working relationships and conditions of employment. As health care technology advanced, the role of the district nurse changed, and a key feature of district nursing was its ability to adapt to new situations and new technologies. A major thesis of the book is that the idea of care as a crucial aspect of the district nurse's work has shifted from one in which linguistic and practical expressions of caring were central to the work, to one in which caring has been dissipated and displaced among a larger team of community health professionals. Sweet and Dougall point to a much-altered role and function of the modern district nurse, who today is much less *of* his/her community and more a member of a multidisciplinary public health team, defined with reference to local administrative arrangements for organizing public health services.

GERARD M. FEALY, RGN, PHD
Associate Professor
UCD School of Nursing, Midwifery & Health Systems
Health Sciences Centre
University College Dublin
Belfield, Dublin 4
Ireland

Notes

1. Monica Baly, *A History of the Queen's Nursing Institute: 100 Years 1887–1987* (Kent: Croom Helm, 1987).

2. Mary Stocks, *A Hundred Years of District Nursing* (London: Allen & Unwin, 1960).

Three Generations, No Imbeciles: Eugenics, the Supreme Court, and *Buck v. Bell*

By Paul A. Lombardo
(Baltimore: Johns Hopkins University Press, 2008)
(384 pages; $29.95 cloth)

Paul Lombardo's book begins in the foothills of central Virginia in 1924. A small courthouse in Amherst became the center of a national discourse on eugenics and individuals' rights to control their reproductive abilities. Esteemed eugenicists Harry Laughlin and Alfred Estabrook, Virginia surgeon and administrator Albert Priddy, and state legislator Aubrey Strode mounted a joint defense of a law that allowed state officials to sterilize patients without their consent.

Three Generations, No Imbeciles chronicles the political and personal paths that led to the Amherst County Circuit Court and beyond. In opening chapters, Lombardo builds the social, scientific, and biological context of the American eugenics movement. He surveys the family studies of the late nineteenth century that lent academic credibility to concepts of hereditary transmission, sexual promiscuity, and the propriety of forced segregation and sterilization. Virginian representatives joined a cohort of lawmakers who created medical colonies for the epileptic, the mentally diseased, and the (usefully vague) "feebleminded." The possibility of coerced sterilization in Virginia emerged via a 1916 law allowing physicians the discretionary use of "moral, medical, and surgical treatment" (p. 60) to combat the spread of deficiencies.

The next section of the book considers the case of Carrie Buck. Once Strode ushered a sterilization law through the legislature in July 1924, he and Priddy manufactured a legal case to validate the law's constitutionality. Buck, a seventeen-year-old who had given birth four months earlier and had been committed to the Virginia Colony for Epileptics and Feebleminded shortly thereafter, made the ideal plaintiff for Strode and Priddy. Her mother was also incarcerated for "mental deficiency" and promiscuity; her foster parents openly reported her physical and mental deficiencies; and Estabrook detected signs of feeblemindedness in her infant daughter. Buck's attorney was even a good friend of both men and a firm believer that sterilization was "therapeutic." The teenager didn't stand a chance.

On appeal, Buck's case arrived at the Supreme Court in late 1926. Lombardo offers a detailed analysis of the Court and its 1927 decision that Buck posed a significant enough social threat to justify sterilization. Subsequent chapters survey editorial and legal reactions, the posttrial lives of the central figures, and the connection between the case and Nazi eugenics programs. The book ends by discussing the legal silence on *Buck v. Bell* after World War II, chronicling the end of Virginia's "sterilization era" (in 1985, via a state legal settlement), and connecting eugenics to recent developments in reproductive rights and genetics research.

Lombardo succeeds at moving between local, national, and international contexts. He traces professional linkages vividly, emphasizing both institutional leaders and those whom Lombardo describes as "foot soldiers in the battle to establish eugenic sterilization as public policy" (p. 90). The book reads well, with absorbing case studies and insightful biographical sketches of the lawyers, doctors, social scientists, and patients involved.

Although Lombardo gets much out of court documents, state records, and eugenics publications, the book is thin on argument. His goal is to excavate and contextualize the *Buck* case, not to provide an interpretive framework. His implied argument—that political, legal, and pseudo-scientific regimes can work against individuals in the name of the "greater good"—does not suffice. The suggestion that the case can only be understood in a long continuum, encompassing both the decades that came before and those that followed, is more illuminating, but Lombardo could have made it more explicit.

The book ultimately succeeds in three ways. First, Lombardo stresses the interplay between practitioners and popular audiences, especially people who had hazy conceptions of heredity. Too often in histories of eugenics, the ideas become disembodied actors. Lombardo demonstrates an actual give-and-take between proponents and those whom they attempted to persuade. Second, he offers remarkable details on the practice of eugenic surgery. Priddy sterilized inmates before lawmakers explicitly granted him such power. By explaining procedures as attempts to relieve pelvic pain—surgeries that incidentally necessitated sterilization once under way—Priddy drafted public policy himself. The spare, unflinching account of Buck's surgery is the most effective passage of the book. Finally, Lombardo demands that historians pay attention to the legacies of eugenics after 1945. Another writer might have ended the narrative in 1927, with an epilogue to treat briefly the material that Lombardo covers in one hundred pages. That would be a mistake. Lombardo convincingly shows that the eugenics of the 1920s, despite professional reversals and government apologies, still echoes in discussions of designer babies, grumbling about the costs of social programs and attempts to calculate the financial value of life.

EDWARD SLAVISHAK, PHD
Assistant Professor, History
Susquehanna University
Selinsgrove, PA 17870

Mary Breckinridge: The Frontier Nursing Service and Rural Health in Appalachia
By Melanie Beals Goan
(Chapel Hill, North Carolina:
University of North Carolina Press, 2008)
(348 pages; $45.00 cloth)

Melanie Beals Goan's *Mary Breckinridge: The Frontier Nursing Service and Rural Health in Appalachia* traces the life of Mary Breckinridge and her establishment of the Frontier Nursing Service in rural Kentucky. Goan does a fine job placing Breckinridge, her life, her ideas, and her achievements in their historical and cultural contexts. The author admirably shows how this historical case study of Mary Breckinridge and the Frontier Nursing Service enlarges our understanding of Appalachia, social reform, and scientific medicine in the twentieth century.

Coming from a long line of prestigious American leaders, Mary Breckinridge established the Frontier Nursing Service, an organization designed to meet the medical, emotional, and social needs of the residents of rural Kentucky. Originally intended to serve women and children, the Frontier Nursing Service soon offered medical care to the men of Leslie County too. Breckinridge emphasized the right of every human being to health care, realized that nurses had important roles in providing that care, and appreciated the wisdom of preventive medicine (252).

Goan's biography of Breckinridge and her institutional history of the Frontier Nursing Service pay close attention to the historical and cultural context from which Breckinridge and the organization came. Goan recognizes that Breckinridge's drive to provide medical care was shaped by both maternalist philosophy and the ideal of the New Woman. Goan takes great pains to elucidate Breckinridge's class and racial bias; she acknowledges that such bias emerged from Breckinridge's upbringing by parents who promoted the Lost Cause of the South. Goan maps out how Breckinridge navigated the difficulties that the Frontier Nursing Service experienced as a result of events like the Great Depression and World War II.

In addition to contextualizing Breckinridge's achievements as well as her shortcomings, Goan succeeds in placing the story of Breckinridge and the Frontier Nursing Service into the historiography of Appalachia, social reform, and scientific medicine. Goan says that her study is "another attempt to complicate . . . Appalachian reform"

(8). She asserts that Breckinridge "offers an important reminder that the female reformers who came to Appalachia, while often initially naïve, developed an increasingly sophisticated understanding of the region's problems as time went on" (8). Goan also maintains that her case study contributes to the history of American medicine by demonstrating the "ways in which scientific medicine established its supremacy over folk healing and" allows readers "to witness the struggles that developed as competing groups of medical practitioners sought legitimacy and to gain patients' trust" (9). Goan shows that "the struggle for professional legitimacy depended . . . on patients' recognition that seeking medical assistance not only benefited their health but also advanced their class aspirations" (9). The author says the history of the Frontier Nursing Service illustrates how nurse midwives battled with lay midwives as well as with female doctors (9).

Goan's history of scientific medicine in rural Kentucky is commendable; however, the minimal amount of time she spends discussing how rural residents negotiated between folk medicine and scientific medicine was a missed opportunity. Goan's primary source evidence largely depends on traditional sources including publications by Breckinridge and newspapers. Sources drawn directly from the lived experiences of rural Kentucky residents might have allowed Goan to develop more fully the response of residents to Breckinridge and the Frontier Nursing Service, the main focus of "Chapter Six: Winning Patients' Trust."

Goan's book will be embraced eagerly by medical and lay readers. Historians of Appalachia, social reform, and the rise of scientific medicine will welcome this volume. Nurse midwives and nurse practitioners will appreciate this history of a woman who contributed to the rise of their medical specialties in the United States. Finally, sections of the text can be incorporated into an array of classroom settings including courses on women and medicine, the history of the U.S. South, and the history of medicine.

Karol K. Weaver, PhD
Associate Professor, History
Susquehanna University
514 University Avenue
Selinsgrove, PA 17870

An Officer and a Lady: Canadian Military Nursing and the Second World War

By Cynthia Toman
(Vancouver, British Columbia: UBC Press, 2007)
(396 pages; $85.00 CAD cloth; $32.95 CAD paper)

The Second World War ended in 1945, and as we approach the sixty-fifth anniversary of that war, our veterans are now in their mid-eighties to mid-nineties. The call to mobilize Canadian Active Service Forces medical units came in September 1939, and the first

Nursing Sisters recruited tended to be an older cohort than the average soldier. Those who are left are aging and some are in poor health. Cynthia Toman, acutely aware of the dwindling numbers of Second World War nurses and the lack of historical record, seized the opportunity to capture and write their story. In her book, *An Officer and a Lady: Canadian Military Nursing and the Second World War*, Toman provides the reader with a compelling story of Canadian nurses at war. Based on her Ph.D. research and thesis, the author argues that Canadian Nursing Sisters were an "expandable" (p. 57) and "expendable" (p. 87) feminine workforce. She contends their presence on the frontlines was legitimized by medical technology, nursing knowledge, and skills. Toman claims that at the end of the war, nurses' gender and war experience facilitated a sense of community and a social memory as military nurses. A feminist and social historian with a keen interest in medical technologies, Toman uses these lenses to analyze how age, gender, class, race, education, ethnicity, Canadian identity, and marital status intersected to shape World War II (WWII) nurses' experience of war. In doing so, she makes a significant contribution to the historiography of nursing, military nursing, military history, and war as work.

Toman situates these "second generation" military nurses in time and place by describing nurses' contribution in the First World War as members of the Canadian Expeditionary Force (CEF); the interwar years including the Great Depression and nurses' socioeconomic struggles; the war years; and the postwar experience. The author builds a strong case to support her thesis. Using a systematic approach, she lays out a reasoned argument, supported with firsthand accounts, and easily convinces her readers of her assertions. However, in my opinion, "expandable and expendable" was not unique to females and nurses nor isolated to the Second World War, but characterizes the Canadian military experience and is a manifestation of Canadian ambivalence to involvement in international geopolitical affairs and warfare.

Following Germany's invasion of Poland, Canada declared war on Germany on September 10, 1939. Canadian nurses volunteered for military service in overwhelming numbers, easily filling the allotted nursing positions. Toman's research is meticulous. In 1939, Canada's population was only 11,267,000; there were approximately 54,491 trained nurses and at least 4,381 nurses (3.7 percent) served (p. 27). The author reviewed 1,145 military records, representing a sample size of 26 percent (p. 9). She read countless military and government documents and accessed multiple archival sources. In addition, the author interviewed twenty-one WWII nursing sisters, giving voice to a group of nurses who had, for too long, been silent. Toman conducted an exhaustive professional literature review. She is not reticent in criticizing the existing literature as hagiographic, perpetuating the stereotype of nurses as exceptional women and heroines.

Toman dispels many myths about Canadian Nursing Sisters. First and foremost, they were not members of a religious order and they were not all nurses. Some were dietitians, physiotherapists, laboratory assistants, and home sisters (house mothers). The first cohort of Second World War Nursing Sisters came to the military with considerable experience, especially in teaching, supervising, and administration. Gender was integral to the selection of nurses and where and how they served in the military. They subsequently became soldiers and "one of the boys" (p. 201). The commissioned rank and pay grade reinforced class and professional status. Toman establishes that the enlistment of nurses was not responsible for the Canadian nurse shortage; however, she does indicate that at the end of the war nursing sisters were "reluctant to resume earlier roles and the practice constraints of hospital nursing" (p. 202). The Second World War was "less of a technological watershed for nurses than assumed in existing literature" (p. 201). A leadership theme permeates the text. Nurses were flexible, assuming and relinquishing expanded roles depending on the availability of medical officers (p. 201). Their servant leadership[1] was further characterized by the teamwork, mentoring and coaching, problem solving, decision making, risk taking, community building, listening, initiative, empathy, healing, and serving.

In terms of Canadian historical accounts on military nurses, there is little with which to compare Toman's work. For many years, Colonel Gerald W. L. Nicholson's book *Canada's Nursing Sisters*[2] stood as the only official history of military nurses in Canada. It is an organizational history that covers Canadian military nurses from the North West Rebellion to Korea. Toman adds to this account by sharing the WWII Nursing Sister's firsthand perspectives and exploring their stories using discourse analysis. In terms of compelling reading, Toman's book stands up well against Elizabeth Norman's two books, *We Band of Angels: The Untold Story of American Nurses Trapped on Bataan by the Japanese*[3] and *Women at War: The Story of Fifty Military Nurses Who Served in Vietnam.*[4] Evelyn Monahan and Rosemary Neidel-Greenee's book *And If I Perish*[5] also gives voice to WWII nurses; however, it is much more of a narrative of events than Toman's book. In my opinion, *An Officer and a Lady: Canadian Military Nursing and the Second World War* is academically rigorous while at the same time immensely readable.

While reading Toman's book, several of the nurse's names seemed very familiar. I realized that over the years I had met a few of these women. Others I recognized from watching Neil Bregman's 1994 documentary film *Angels of Mercy*,[6] and others I had watched on the Veterans Affairs Canada Web site, *Nursing Sisters Recollect.*[7] What I liked about this book is that Toman respected the voice of the nurses and created a convincing and intellectually stimulating interpretation of military nurses' experience in war. This book will appeal to a wide range of readers with an interest in military history, gender and war, women's history, medical history, and the history of nursing.

Stephanie Buckingham, CD, RN, BSN, MA
Nurse Educator
Vancouver Island University
Health and Human Services
900 Fifth Street
Nanaimo, BC V8R 5S5
Canada

Notes

1. Robert Greenleaf, *The Servant as Leader* (Indianapolis, Ind.: The Robert Greenleaf Center, 1991).

2. Gerald W. L. Nicholson, *Canada's Nursing Sisters* (Toronto, ON: Samuel Stevens Hakkert & Company, 1975).

3. Elizabeth M. Norman, *We Band of Angels: The Untold Story of American Nurses Trapped on Bataan by the Japanese* (New York: Pocket Books, a division of Simon & Schuster Inc., 1999).

4. Elizabeth M. Norman, *Women at War: The Story of Fifty Military Nurses Who Served in Vietnam* (Philadelphia: University of Pennsylvania Press, 1990).

5. Evelyn Monahan and Rosemary Neidel-Greenee, *And If I Perish: Frontline U.S. Army Nurses in World War II* (New York: Alfred A. Knopf, 2003).

6. Neil Bregman, Katherine A. Jeans, and John Tarzwell, *Angels of Mercy* (videorecording) (Port Credit, ON: Sound Venture Productions, 1991).

7. Government of Canada, Veterans Affairs Canada Web site, *Nursing Sister's Recollect*. http://www.vac-acc.gc.ca/remembers/sub.cfm?source=history/other/Nursing/recollect

Armies of Peace: Canada and the UNRRA Years

By Susan Armstrong Reid and David Murray
(Toronto: University of Toronto Press, 2008)
(482 pp; $20.00 USD cloth)

Armies of Peace encompasses much more than nursing history. This well-researched and comprehensive book focuses primarily on the Canadian involvement in the United Nations Relief and Rehabilitation Administration (UNRRA). Planned as a short-term project (and in operation only from 1943 to 1947), the Great Powers saw UNRRA as the first necessary step in the revitalization of war-torn Europe. This massive relief effort was designed to allow needy countries to draw on a pool of supplies and services, including repatriation support, which had been collected from the better-off nations. The Allied countries thus hoped to avoid the mistakes of the First World War that had led to a worldwide Depression by helping devastated countries get back on their economic feet. As the third-largest "supplier" nation, Canada's determination to bolster its position as a middle power on the international stage met with mixed success. Shut out of membership in the full council overseeing the program, Lester Pearson instead headed the important Commission on Supplies, where he honed his diplomatic skills to reconcile the increasingly divergent opinions of member countries. Gaining a solid reputation as a reliable and innovative supplier, Canada steered a course of "enlightened self-interest" that pragmatically weighed international commitments for UNRRA against its own domestic needs and goals for the postwar period.

During the program, UNRRA delivered $4 billion to more than twenty countries, including China, Greece, parts of Germany, and Eastern European nations, and aided in the relocation of 7 million refugees. As the authors ably demonstrate, the fact that UNRRA operated with any success at all is something of a miracle. Procurement and distribution of supplies created logistical nightmares because UNRRA's terms of agreement forced administrators and field operators to negotiate civilian relief with both the Allied military and often unstable governments. Relief became more politicized in the context of deepening East-West suspicion and the beginnings of the cold war. And despite international repatriation agreements in place, many people resisted returning to their homelands and refused to leave the refugee camps.

It was against this backdrop then that the UNRRAIDS—the field administrators, welfare officers, technical workers, and nurses—attempted to carry out their duties on the ground. Canadian nurses comprised fewer than 100 members of the 1,400-person Health Division, but they were an elite group for this time period in terms of educational background and professional experiences. Some, like Lyle Creelman, who was appointed chief nurse for the British Zone of Occupied Germany, held key administrative positions in the division. Others worked in the camps delivering public health care and setting up basic public health programs. They instituted training programs for auxiliary nurses from among the refugee populations and refresher courses to help displaced graduate nurses without any documents regain their credentials.

Mining official UNRRA reports, the *Canadian Nurse* journal, personal papers, and transcripts of oral interviews, the authors reconstructed the experiences of this select group of women. Although they are undoubtedly hard to find, one wishes for more photographs of the nurses and the places they worked. Canadian nurses joined UNRRA for the same mixture of adventure, economic opportunity, and humanitarianism as the rest of the UNRRAIDS, and like the others, found the chaotic environment into which they were plunged the most challenging of their careers.

Patients, UNRRA colleagues, supervisors, students, and physicians all had an impact on what they were able to accomplish. Responsible for the health of hundreds of thousands of war-ravaged and often psychologically scarred people in the huge displaced-persons camps, at times they celebrated small public health victories and at others despaired of resistance to even the most basic of measures. Surely one of the more complex tasks had to be supervising German nurses who cared for Jewish survivors of the concentration camp at Belsen. Complicating their work were arduous living conditions, delayed or nonexistent supplies, administrative ineptitude, political instability, and profound cultural differences, which forced these nurses, whether planned or not, to continually improvise and adapt their Westernized expectations of what constituted proper nursing. Establishing good working relationships and professional authority with physicians on the medical team was difficult when many doctors were continually on the move or held little regard for nurses and their work. The nurses' low pay grade within UNRRA—they were paid less than welfare officers with no special training—also undermined their status.

The nurses undoubtedly made a difference while they were present, but as the program wound down many of the camps and the people in them remained. The long-term significance of nursing work is thus as hard to assess as the entire UNRRA project itself. Perhaps, as the authors tentatively suggest, the greatest legacy of the nursing program lies in the impetus it appeared to give to the future involvement of some of these former UNRRA nurses in peace activism, social welfare issues, and leadership positions in agencies such as the World Health Organization.

The book itself, however, is an important reminder to historians of nursing that nurses and their work are part of a much larger context. The UNRRA nursing program deserves scholarly attention, and the authors have brought to light a little known aspect of Canadian nursing history. At the same time as they suggest that these nurses were a key element of the UNRRA story, they demonstrate that their successes and their failures, both professional and personal, cannot be fully understood without taking into account the political, economic, and military issues shaping events in the immediate postwar period.

JAYNE ELLIOTT, PHD
Research Facilitator, Administrator
AMS Nursing History Research Unit
Room 3245A, School of Nursing
University of Ottawa
451 Smyth Road
Ottawa, ON K1H 8M5 Canada

The W. K. Kellogg Foundation and the Nursing Profession: Shared Values, Shared Legacy

By Joan E. Lynaugh, Helen K. Grace, Gloria R. Smith, Roseni R. Sena, Maria Mercedes Duran de Villalobos, and Mary Malehloka Hlalele
(Indianapolis, Ind.: Sigma Theta Tau International Honor Society, 2007)
(428 pages, paper; $29.95)

W. K. Kellogg is a name recognized by millions as the worldwide maker of popular breakfast cereals, but for many health care professionals Kellogg is also recognized as a premier philanthropic foundation that funds innovative health care projects. *The W. K. Kellogg Foundation and Nursing Profession* offers readers a scholarly exposition of the history of the W. K. Kellogg Foundation and insiders' views of some of the decision-making policies that funded innovative and diverse health care projects for more than seventy-five years.

Nurse historian Joan Lynaugh opens the book with a succinct overview of the history of the W. K. Kellogg Foundation. Kellogg created the foundation in 1930 from cereal profits. His interest in the health of children motivated him to use the foundation to help communities find ways to empower their local leaders to create new ways to improve the health, education, and welfare of children. A firm believer in the power of education to change human behavior, Kellogg maintained that education was the means by which one generation could best improve the next generations' opportunities for better lives. This premise, put to the test in the 1931 Michigan Community Health Project, revealed the effectiveness of interdisciplinary collaboration in creating new public health services at the county and town levels and in persuading local health officials to permanently assume these services into their departments' mission. Elements of interdisciplinary collaboration between professional and lay personnel would become a stipulation in the foundation's guidelines for future health projects.

In tracing the history of the foundation through its archival records, Lynaugh offers readers not only the diversity of projects undertaken by the foundation, but she adeptly grounds these projects in the history of the nursing profession and the changing nature of the country's social and economic times. The Depression years and the country's involvement in World War II are depicted through the nation's changing needs for nurses and new health initiatives to meet the expanding needs of the country.

In addition to documenting the diverse projects and the organizations and communities involved in creating new ways to provide health services, Lynaugh captures the personalities of the Kellogg Foundation's leaders, its presidents, and directors. Each president brought different intellectual strengths and experiences to the foundation, and the shifting focus of Kellogg health initiatives reflected these changes and those occurring in society. For example, in the 1940s, instead of funding public health nursing projects the foundation moved to influencing national nursing and health policy. Later, changes in the foundation's focus included health projects that met the needs of hospitals for nurses, community health centers, and the elderly both in their homes and nursing homes, and those who were underserved and disenfranchised in society.

Helen Grace and Gloria Smith, both foundation vice presidents, provide information and personal insight about the actions of the foundation and the funded Kellogg projects they were involved in. This information dovetails and fleshes out the historical contributions of Lynaugh. I found their comments, especially Grace's, candid and revealing. She shares that there were times her nursing colleagues made her feel like a traitor to the profession when many of their submitted nursing projects were not selected. Their projects hadn't met the Kellogg criteria for grants and thus could not be funded no matter how important the projects were to the profession.

The book also documents the foundation's long involvement with nurses in Latin America and in southern Africa. Roseni Sena and Maria de Villalobos provided leadership to Kellogg projects in Latin America and the Caribbean for more than twenty years, and they share their analysis of the impact of the foundation's support in this area. Mary Hlalele, from a former program in Africa, writes of the impact of funding for nurses in this region.

This book, easy to read and well organized, reveals the power of a visionary and well-run philanthropic organization to significantly influence the health care of citizens in America and other regions of the world. And in so doing, it has significantly shaped the nursing profession. The book will appeal to medical historians, those interested in national and international health policy and health care, especially those involved in community health care. It is a case book on ways to develop and sustain collaborative interdisciplinary projects that lead to improvement in the health of society. In addition, the book is reasonably priced at $29.00 and will make a valuable addition to one's personal library.

BARBARA BRODIE, PhD, RN, FAAN
Madge M. Jones Professor Emerita
University of Virginia School of Nursing
McLeod Hall
202 Jeanette Lancaster Way
Charlottesville, VA 22903

Unnatural History: Breast Cancer and American Society

By Robert A. Aronowitz
(New York: Cambridge University Press, 2007)
(378 pp.; $30.00 cloth)

This historical study of breast cancer covering the past 200 years combines medical and cultural variables in the analysis of a serious human disease. Robert Aronowitz points out in the introduction that the title "Unnatural History," informs the reader that this analysis will go against the typical naturalistic approach to other social historical analyses such as parenting (p. 7). He accomplished his task. If you have ever wondered why women fear breast cancer more than heart disease, even though more die from the latter, then this book will give you the basic issues. The unique aspect of this study is that the author does not simply tell the story of our nation's battle to prevent and treat breast cancer over time. He delves into the cultural and social history of our response as a society to the perception of breast cancer and the fear that it has evoked in spite of advances in diagnosis and treatment. Breast cancer has a singular history, but the approach of this author would serve other analyses well as we expand our historical view from the individual to culture and society.

Perhaps the most significant sections of the book involve his extensive discussion of ideas about assessment and treatment of the disease along with the summary of statistical risk pattern development in the twentieth century. He lays out a clear argument that breast cancer screening and public education about the disease has heightened awareness but that there are still many for whom there is little control over the devastating impact of aggressive forms of the disease. He presents data showing that statistical increases in breast cancer risk for American women may lie in overdiagnosis as the result of mass screening and demographics rather than major environmental or lifestyle risks. He also points out the flaws in current risk programs used for clinical decision making and how women may be able to make choices, but the options may still be unclear.

Aronowitz demonstrates his skill as a historian, clearly enhanced by his wisdom as a physician, as he traces the lived experience of breast cancer across specific time frames and takes the reader through the pain and reality of this disease in individual women and the physicians who treated them. Nurse historians can infer the clinical practice of care at the bedside from the descriptions of treatments in the past. He also sensitively describes the sources of fear that this disease caused in women, their loved ones, and their physicians. He emphasizes the commonalities among the patients regardless of their historical era and the consistent issue of maintaining hope with each therapeutic strategy. Innovation and medical technological advances did not change many of the core human needs. He clearly noted the need of patients and doctors to maintain a sense of control over this invader and to continue efforts to do something in its wake. The limited options and poor outcomes for some of these women were haunting.

Aronowitz strips away the veneer of public education efforts to get women to early screening and treatment and then cites limitations of our current system in certain types of breast cancer. It is important that nurses committed to disease prevention and accurately reporting the clinical practice histories of our profession read this work and use the findings in this study to better inform both our clinical activities and our historical analysis of illness as a lived experience in American society.

LINDA E. SABIN, RNC, PHD
Professor of Nursing
University of Louisiana at Monroe
700 University Avenue
Monroe, LA 71209

Cancer in the Twentieth Century
Edited by David Cantor
(Baltimore: The Johns Hopkins University Press, 2008)
(350 pages; $25.00 paper)

Cancer in the Twentieth Century is a compilation of selected papers presented at a 2004 same-named workshop at the National Institutes of Health in 2004. As editor, David Cantor presents these papers organized into three themes: "Between Education and Marketing," "Therapeutics," and "Prevention and Risk." Focusing primarily on Britain and the United States, these selections provide a trajectory of thought to cancer approaches and treatments from the early 1900s to the 1980s. Only a few specific cancers are addressed, serving as global representations for this disease.

Whereas early American approaches to cancer focused on detection, treatment, and public education, the British approach differed in its focus geared more to the practitioner and therapies. Indeed, the British led the use of radium for cancer treatment in the 1920s and 1930s. The section "Between Education and Marketing" highlights the differences between these philosophical approaches to public cancer education. American approaches included the use of media for public education, particularly the movies. The American Cancer Society spearheaded funding movies, trailers, and shorts with mixed results. Increasing cancer awareness through publicizing children's cancers, most notably the "Jimmy Fund," spurred fundraising efforts geared to research and cure. Public education efforts in the British approach were not as valued or seen as effective as within the United States.

The "Therapeutics" section addresses various therapies and the development of clinical trials as a method to determine alternatives to surgery for cancer treatment. Feminist surgeons in 1920s Britain were in the forefront of establishing radium usage for cervical cancer treatment and sought to establish radiotherapy as an alternative to surgery for some cancers.

Clinical trials as an emerging development post-World War II in the United States and Europe with multisite research investigated various drug protocols for the best outcomes. A compelling essay within this group is the Barron H. Lerner paper of the noted breast cancer advocate Rose Kushner's attack on adjuvant chemotherapy, a gripping presentation of the dichotomy of blurred roles and conflict of interest of a successful advocate in addition to being spokesperson for a pharmaceutical company.

"Prevention and Risk" presents risk predictions, hereditary cancers, and British preventive efforts on lung cancers. Henry Lynch's research into hereditary colorectal cancer highlights the evolution of medical genetics from the 1960s to the present, which ultimately led to the registry establishment for specific cancers.

Cancer in the Twentieth Century provides a somewhat narrow overview to the approaches and treatments of this disease but in no way detracts from its organized themes and presented papers. The diversity of presentations underscores the breadth and depth of the dilemma of cancer itself: prevention, approaches, treatment, and public education. Extensive footnotes accompany each paper, which allows the reader to further investigate what has been presented. Readers interested in the historical trajectory of a disease approach will find this book interesting and useful. Those interested in feminist history will appreciate the efforts of women physicians and advocates to make women's cancers shift from a disfiguring surgical approach to those that yield the same or better results with minimal disfigurement. Cantor has assembled a collection that has appeal to those interested in the development and evolution of cancer treatments, the effect of gender and advocacy upon modifying or changing treatment protocols, and how public awareness and involvement has spurred cancer awareness and care.

TERESA M. O'NEILL, RNC, PHD
Professor
Our Lady of Holy Cross College
4123 Woodland Drive
New Orleans, LA 70131

Mania: A Short History of Bipolar Disorder
By David Healy
(Baltimore, Md.: Johns Hopkins University Press, 2008)
(296 pages; $24.95 cloth)

This well-written and compelling book goes well beyond the historical analysis of a single illness, bipolar disorder, once called manic depression, to fundamentally question the relationship between the science of psychiatry and the business of psychopharmacology. The author, David Healy, is a professor of psychiatry whose previous works, *The Antidepressant Era (1998)* and *Let Them Eat Prozac* (2004), raised serious concerns about the increased risk of suicide with certain medications. *Mania* draws from both primary historical sources and interviews to build on these previous accounts by arguing that pharmaceuticals have become less about breakthrough commodities, like penicillin and insulin, and more about marketing and manipulation of public views on health and illness.

In the book's first chapters, Healy takes on claims that bipolar disorder can be traced to the ancient Greeks. He points out that Greek physicians relied on publicly visible signs to make diagnoses—"the swelling, heat, and redness of a tumor, the smell of urine, the mute rigidity of stupor, the frenzy of delirium" (p. 12). In contrast, modern-day psychiatrists base diagnoses on the words of patients or even third parties, such as parents or teachers. Even the famous story of the woman from Thasos, frequently cited as an early case of bipolar disorder, was apparently a condition of nausea, fever, and spasms. Mania during this period was more likely delirium, according to Healy. Melancholia was stupor or lethargy. Against a background of the lethal epidemics of antiquity, Healy concludes, bipolar disorder "was almost an irrelevance" (p. 8).

A similar approach to debunking the idea that bipolar disorder was a widespread condition in past societies takes the reader through subsequent chapters on the evolution of medical science. During the Renaissance, for instance, attention within the European scientific community shifted from observable behavior to internal mental states. This was typified in Willis's anatomical work that revealed the brain as a solid organ, a new vision that in turn laid the groundwork for the fields of neurology and psychology. Sydenham's study of hysteria likewise contributed to the emphasis on the mind rather than the body in explaining psychiatric conditions. In threading these developments together, Healy moves on to consider "the brain in the asylum," noting how the building of asylums in the nineteenth century gave physicians unprecedented access to persons with various forms of mental illness. The first clear descriptions of bipolar disorder by French psychiatrists soon followed. However, this disorder remained quite rare, according to Healy. Reviewing nearly 3,500 admissions to the asylum in North Wales between 1875 and 1924, he found only 123 individuals who were admitted for what we would now call bipolar disorder.

Manic depression continued to be seen as a curious and rare condition until the 1990s, when reports began circulating that 5 percent of the U.S. population had some type of bipolar disorder. As Healy moves into this more recent discussion, his tone also becomes more impassioned, particularly in focusing on "the latest mania"— young children diagnosed with bipolar disorder. Healy confronts what he describes as the muddle in his profession, one in which clinicians diagnose patients by proxy, relying on reports of symptoms as vague as nightmares, temper tantrums, and sadness to substantiate a diagnosis of bipolar disorder. The diagnostic criteria are so vague that "in the absence of judgment, this exercise differs little from reading a horoscope" (p. 202). This might not be significant except for the fact that meeting the criteria for a disease brings with it the expectation of treatment, including potent antidepressants and antipsychotics.

The combination of a muddled psychiatry and a hugely profitable pharmaceutical industry is what has fueled the sudden epidemic of psychiatric illnesses like bipolar disorder, charges Healy. Pharmaceutical companies have largely succeeded in sequestering data and marketing "selected parts of it back to us under the banner of science" (p. 251). This has been done with the key assistance of willing academics. What has resulted is a system that inhibits our abilities to find cures "while encouraging companies to seek short-term profits by co-opting bipolar disorder for the purposes of increasing the sales of major tranquilizers to infants" (p. 252).

Mania is a fascinating and provocative account that should appeal to a wide range of readers, including those whose primary interest is health-related history and general readers interested in understanding the competing interests that have shaped our understanding of mental health and mental illness. Those without a health care background may find parts of the discussion involving specific illnesses, drugs, and research methodologies to be somewhat daunting. However, this should not diminish the vital nature of this work. At its core is the increasing tension between science and commerce, as well as a key debate in the history of diseases—whether our focus as historians should be on the pure disease entity or whether we should focus on people who are "dis-eased." Has bipolar disorder existed in unchanged form since the Greeks, Healy posits, or is this view of history inadequate? I encourage you to read this exceptional book to answer this question for yourself.

TOM OLSON, PHD, PMHCNS-BC
Professor and Executive Associate Dean
College of Nursing
New York University
246 Greene Street, 8th Floor
New York, NY 10003–6677

NEW DISSERTATIONS

Compiled for the *Nursing History Review* by Jonathon Erlen, PhD, history of medicine librarian, Health Sciences Library System, and assistant professor, Graduate School of Public Health at the University of Pittsburgh, Pittsburgh, Pennsylvania. These dissertations can be obtained through Proquest Dissertations.

Sebastien Normandin, "Visions of Vitalism: Medicine, Philosophy and the Soul in Nineteenth Century France," 2006 PhD dissertation, McGill University (Canada) (Publication Number: AAT NR25222).

Keaghan Kane Turner, "In Perfect Sympathy: Representations of Nursing in New Woman Fiction," 2006 PhD dissertation, University of South Carolina (Publication Number: AAT 3262044).

Eike Reichardt, "Health, "Race" and Empire: Popular-scientific Spectacles and National Identity in Imperial Germany, 1871–1914," 2006 PhD dissertation, State University of New York at Stony Brook (Publication Number: AAT 3258933).

Cynthia Dianne Creagh, "Benevolent Leverage: Substitute Mothers and Autonomy at the New York Foundling Hospital, 1869–1939," 2006 PhD dissertation, State University of New York at Stony Brook (Publication Number: AAT 3258938).

Amy Beth Gangloff, "Medicalizing the Automobile: Public Health, Safety, and American Culture, 1920–1967," 2006 PhD dissertation, State University of New York at Stony Brook (Publication Number: AAT 3258930).

Bradford Wilson Sample, "Firmly and Conscientiously Attached to the Cause of Temperance": The Anti-Alcohol Movement in Indianapolis, 1825—1856," 2006 PhD dissertation, Purdue University (Publication Number: AAT 3260013).

Jeffrey M. Jentzen, "Death Investigation in America: Coroners, Medical Examiners, and the Pursuit of Medical Certainty," 2007 PhD dissertation, The University of Wisconsin–Madison (Publication Number: AAT 3261437).

Robert Kevin Thomas, "An Analysis of the Development of the Seventh-Day Adventist Health, Physical, Education, Recreation Association (1981–2005)," 2007 PhD dissertation, Boston University (Publication Number: AAT 3259895).

Trisha Diane Carter Posey, "Poverty Encounters: Unitarians, the Poor, and Poor Relief in Antebellum Boston and Philadelphia," 2007 PhD dissertation, University of Maryland, College Park (Publication Number: AAT 3260343).

Andrew Jonathan Noymer, "Studies in the Historical Demography and Epidemiology of Influenza and Tuberculosis Selective Mortality," 2006 PhD dissertation, University of California, Berkeley (Publication Number: AAT 3254008).

Cindy L. Linden, "'An Element of Blank': Reading Silences in Post-World War II American Narratives of Pain," 2007 PhD dissertation, Syracuse University (Publication Number: AAT 3266300).

Ian Hamilton Offord, "The Discourse of Hygiene in French Fascist Literature," 2007 PhD dissertation, University of Minnesota (Publication Number: AAT 3263127).

John Matthew Kinder, "Encountering Injury: Modern War and the Problem of the Wounded Soldier," 2007 PhD dissertation, University of Minnesota (Publication Number: AAT 3263109).

Sok Chul Hong, "The Health and Economic Burdens of Malaria: The American Case," 2007 PhD dissertation, The University of Chicago (Publication Number: AAT 3262247).

Sean Michael Smith, "From Charitable to Public Assistance: Late Eighteenth-Century Transformations of Assistance in Buenos Aires, Lima, and Madrid," 2007 PhD dissertation, The University of Chicago (Publication Number: AAT 3262302).

Joseph Charles Wicentowski, Policing Health in Modern Taiwan, 1895–1949," 2007 PhD dissertation, Harvard University (Publication Number: AAT 3265216).

Matthew L. Newsom Kerr, "Fevered Metropolis: Epidemic Disease and Isolation in Victorian London," 2007 PhD dissertation, University of Southern California (Publication Number: AAT 3262682).

Howell Williams, "Homosexuality and the American Catholic Church: Reconfiguring the Silence, 1971–1999," 2007 PhD dissertation, The Florida State University (Publication Number: AAT 3301609).

Xiangyin Yang, "Colonial Power and Medical Space: The Transformation of Chinese and Western Medical Services in the Tung Wah Group of Hospitals, 1894–1941," 2007 PhD dissertation, The Chinese University of Hong Kong (Hong Kong) (Publication Number: AAT 3302416).

Simone Ameskamp, "On Fire—Cremation in Germany, 1870s–1934," 2006 PhD dissertation, Georgetown University (Publication Number: AAT 3302096).

Deirdre M. Bryan, "A 'Peculiarly Fitting' Institute: The Origins of Marie Martin's Medical Missionaries of Mary," 2007 PhD dissertation, Boston College (Publication Number: AAT 3301785).

Thomas Iain Faith, "Under a Green Sea: The US Chemical Warfare Service 1917–1929," 2008 PhD dissertation, George Washington University (Publication Number: AAT 3297069).

Shelley Conroy Hirsekorn, "Interest Groups and Institutional Change: Health Policy and the House Reforms of the 104th Congress," 2008 PhD dissertation, Cornell University (Publication Number: AAT 3300217).

June Samuel, "Adapting to Norms at the United Nations: The Abortion-Rights and Anti-Abortion Networks," 2007 PhD dissertation, University of Maryland, College Park (Publication Number: AAT 3297256).

Carrie C. Sheehan, "Securitizing the HIV/AIDS Pandemic in U.S. Foreign Policy," Proquest Dissertations and Theses 2008. Section 0008, Part 0615 385 pages; [PhD dissertation]. United States–District of Columbia: The American University; 2008. Publication Number: AAT 3302229.

Cynthia C. Adams, "Dying with Dignity in America: The Transformational Leadership of Florence Wald," 2008 EdD dissertation, University of Hartford (Publication Number: AAT 3302016).

Sarah Raphael Lawrence, "On Their Own Terms: African Americans and Birth Control in the Rural South, 1900–1942," 2007 PhD dissertation, The Pennsylvania State University (Publication Number: AAT 3266149).

Marcos Luna, "The Biomedicalization of Public Health and the Marginalization of the Environment: A Policy History from the Environment to the Hospital and Back Again," 2007 PhD dissertation, University of Delaware (Publication Number: AAT 3267192).

Paul W. White, "Kennedy General Hospital: Its Impact on Memphis in War and Peace," 2007 PhD dissertation, The University of Memphis (Publication Number: AAT 3263718).

Noemi R. Tousignant, "Pain and the Pursuit of Objectivity: Pain-Measuring Technologies in the United States, c. 1890–1975," 2006 PhD dissertation, McGill University (Canada) (Publication Number: AAT NR27851).

Ashby F. Walker, "Creating Gateways to the Home Circle: Food, Gender and Domesticity in American Magazines," 2007 PhD dissertation, Emory University (Publication Number: AAT 3264111).

Nuning Tassanee Murphy, "The Experiences of Surviving World War II: Memories, Attitudes, and Motivation in Engaging a World War," 2007 PsyD dissertation, Massachusetts School of Professional Psychology (Publication Number: AAT 3265860).

Robin E. Jensen, "The Birth of Public Sexual Education in the United States: Women, Rhetoric, and the Progressive Era," 2007 PhD dissertation, University of Illinois at Urbana-Champaign (Publication Number: AAT 3269925).

Katherine Lynn Castles, "Little 'Tardies'": Mental Retardation, Race, and Class in American Society, 1945–1965," 2006 PhD dissertation, Duke University (Publication Number: AAT 3269504).

Anu King Dudley, "What Was in the Doctor's Bag: A Material Culture Study of the Performance of Medicine in Antebellum New England," 2007 PhD dissertation, The University of Maine (Publication Number: AAT 3267951).

Janet McShane Galley, "Infanticide in the American Imagination, 1860–1920," 2007 PhD dissertation, Temple University (Publication Number: AAT 3268147).

Kari Suzanne McLeod, "Health Matters: Public Understandings of Health in 1950s America," 2007 PhD dissertation, Yale University (Publication Number: AAT 3267318).

Heather MacGibbon, "The Abortion Narrative in American Film: 1900–2000," 2007 PhD dissertation, New York University (Publication Number: AAT 3269798).

Marguerite Letourneau, "Trends in Basic Diploma Nursing Programs within the Provincial Systems of Education in Canada, 1964 to 1974," 1975 PhD dissertation, University of Ottawa, Canada (Publication Number: AAT DC52541).

Donna B. Searles, "Medicalizing Motherhood: San Carlos Apache Women and Birth," 2007 PhD dissertation, Brown University (Publication Number: AAT 3272050).

Lee Kennedy Pennington, "Wartorn Japan: Disabled Veterans and Society, 1931–1952," 2005 PhD dissertation, Columbia University (Publication Number: AAT 3271882).

Sean J. Harris, "Found Insane in 'the Holy Land': Psychiatry and the African American Experience in Illinois, 1870–1910," 2007 PhD dissertation, University of Illinois at Chicago (Publication Number: AAT 3274129).

Karen E. Huber, "Sex and its Consequences: Abortion, Infanticide, and Women's Reproductive Decision-Making in France, 1901–1940," 2007 PhD dissertation, Ohio State University (Publication Number: AAT 3275257).

Ana Maria Prata Amaral Pereira, "Women's Movements, the State, and the Struggle for Abortion Rights: Comparing Spain and Portugal in Times of Democratic Expansion (1974–1988)," 2007 PhD dissertation, University of Minnesota (Publication Number: AAT 3273155).

"Bringing the Movement Home: Black Social Workers' Struggle for Power in the Profession, 1966–1976," 2007 PhD dissertation, University of Minnesota (Publication Number: AAT 3273112).

Mary Eckenrode Gibson, "From Charity to an Able Body: The Care and Treatment of Disabled Children in Virginia, 1910–1935," 2007 PhD dissertation, University of Pennsylvania (Publication Number: AAT 3271755).

Kimberly Ann Hamlin, "Beyond Adam's Rib: How Darwinian Evolutionary Theory Redefined Gender and Influenced American Feminist Thought, 1870–1920," 2007 PhD dissertation, The University of Texas at Austin (Publication Number: AAT 3277529).

Jalynn Olsen Padilla, "Army of 'Cripples': Northern Civil War Amputees, Disability, and Manhood in Victorian America," 2007 PhD dissertation, University of Delaware (Publication Number: AAT 3277826).

Dominique Padurano, "Making American Men: Charles Atlas and the Business of Bodies, 1892–1945," 2007 PhD dissertation, Rutgers The State University of New Jersey (Publication Number: AAT 3277314).

Kendra D. Smith-Howard, "Perfecting Nature's Food: A Cultural and Environmental History of Milk in the United States, 1900–1970," 2007 PhD dissertation, The University of Wisconsin–Madison (Publication Number: AAT 3278896).

Ethan G. Sribnick, "Rehabilitating Child Welfare: Children and Public Policy, 1945–1980," 2007 PhD dissertation, University of Virginia (Publication Number: AAT 3280024).

Eve Fine, "Pathways to Practice: Women Physicians in Chicago, 1850–1902," 2007 PhD dissertation, The University of Wisconsin–Madison (Publication Number: AAT 3278791).

Elizabeth Popp Berman, "Creating the Market University: Science, the State, and the Economy, 1965–1985," 2007 PhD dissertation, University of California, Berkeley (Publication Number: AAT 3275345).

Julianne Gray Ludlam, "The Double-Edged Sword of Posttraumatic Stress Disorder: A Historical Analysis of Trauma Diagnoses," 2007 PhD dissertation, Alliant International University (Publication Number: AAT 3276581).

Shelly McKenzie, "Mass Movements: A Cultural History of Physical Fitness and Exercise, 1953–1989," 2008 PhD dissertation, The George Washington University (Publication Number: AAT 3295059).

Elizabeth Ann Mackay, "'Mother Wits and Rhetorics': Representations of Maternal Instruction in Early Modern England," 2007 PhD dissertation, Ohio: Miami University (Publication Number: AAT 3282341).

Matthew Warner Osborn, "The Anatomy of Intemperance: Alcohol and the Diseased Imagination in Philadelphia, 1784–1860," 2007 PhD dissertation, University of California, Davis (Publication Number: AAT 3283017).

Timothy Archibald Yates, "Unmade in America: The Cultural Construction of the Alcohol Abuser in the Industrializing United States," 2007 PhD dissertation, University of California, Davis (Publication Number: AAT 3283059).

Stuart Green, "Patient-Centered Medical Education: The Breast Cancer Teaching Team Project," 2007 DMH dissertation, Drew University (Publication Number: AAT 3284519).

Jennifer Casavant Telford, "American Red Cross Nursing during World War I: Opportunities and Obstacles," 2007 PhD dissertation, University of Virginia (Publication Number: AAT 3282483).

Deanna L. Pucciarelli, "The Medicinal Use of Chocolate: Past, Present and Future (1776–2007)," 2007 PhD dissertation, University of California, Davis (Publication Number: AAT 3283027).

Sarah Carlene Glassford, "Marching As to War: The Canadian Red Cross Society, 1885–1939," 2007 PhD dissertation, York University, Canada (Publication Number: AAT NR32048).

Michael Zdenek David, "The White Plague in the Red Capital: The Control of Tuberculosis in Russia, 1900–1941," 2007 PhD dissertation, The University of Chicago (Publication Number: AAT 3287036).

Jennifer Lyn Cote, "'Nobody Ever Paid Me for Anything': Crafting a Professional Social Work Identity in Progressive-era Boston," 2007 PhD dissertation, Boston College (Publication Number: AAT 3283906).

Margot Lynn Iverson, "Blood Types: A History of Genetic Studies of Native Americans, 1920–1955," 2007 PhD dissertation, University of Minnesota (Publication Number: AAT 3285656).

Marcella M. Rutherford, "More Than Good, Kind Angels: The Daughters of Charity's Relationship to Valuation, Mission and Money, 1916 to 1994," 2007 PhD dissertation, Florida Atlantic University (Publication Number: AAT 3287383).

Rhiannon Stephens, "A History of Motherhood, Food Procurement and Politics in East-Central Uganda to the Nineteenth Century," 2007 PhD dissertation, Northwestern University (Publication Number: AAT 3284148).

Hillary Jean Bracken, "Maternity and Child Welfare Reform in North India, 1900–1947," 2007 PhD dissertation, University of Virginia (Publication Number: AAT 3289613).

Marti M. Lybeck, "Gender, Sexuality, and Belonging: Female Homosexuality in Germany, 1890–1933," 2007 PhD dissertation, University of Michigan (Publication Number: AAT 3287575).

Virginia Rose Espino, "Women Sterilized As They Give Birth: Population Control, Eugenics, and Social Protest in the Twentieth-Century United States," 2007 PhD dissertation, Arizona State University (Publication Number: AAT 3287938).

James A Schafer, Jr., "Finding a Niche: Doctors, Urban Change, and the Business of Private Medical Practice in Philadelphia, 1900–1940," 2008 PhD dissertation, The Johns Hopkins University (Publication Number: AAT 3288529).

Zoe Burkholder, "With Science as His Shield: Teaching Race and Culture in American Public Schools, 1900–1954," 2008 PhD dissertation, New York University (Publication Number: AAT 3295334).

Jennifer Emerling Bone, "When Publics Collide: The Rhetorical Strategies of Margaret Sanger's Early Arguments on Birth Control," 2007 PhD dissertation, University of Colorado at Boulder (Publication Number: AAT 3293913).

Shelly McKenzie, "Mass Movements: A Cultural History of Physical Fitness and Exercise, 1953–1989," 2008 PhD dissertation, The George Washington University (Publication Number: AAT 3295059).

Joseph John Murray, "'One Touch of Nature Makes the Whole World Kin': The Transnational Lives of Deaf Americans, 1870–1924," 2007 PhD dissertation, The University of Iowa (Publication Number: AAT 3290674).

Gerald J. Pierce, "Public and Private Voices: The Typhoid Fever Experience at Camp Thomas: 1898," 2007 PhD dissertation, Georgia State University (Publication Number: AAT 3293833).

David Andrew Silkenat, "Suicide, Divorce, and Debt in Civil War Era North Carolina," 2007 PhD dissertation, The University of North Carolina at Chapel Hill (Publication Number: AAT 3289084).

Karen L. Walloch, "'A Hot-Bed of the Anti-Vaccine Heresy': Opposition to Compulsory Vaccination in Boston and Cambridge, 1890–1905," 2007 PhD dissertation, The University of Wisconsin–Madison (Publication Number: AAT 3294105).

Allison Patricia Squires, "A Case Study of the Professionalization of Mexican Nursing: 1980 to 2005," 2007 PhD dissertation, Yale University (Publication Number: AAT 3293410).

Todd Green, "Secularization and the Public Sphere: The Social Significance of Swedish Deaconesses in Education, Health Care, and Poor Relief, 1851–1901," 2007 PhD dissertation, Vanderbilt University (Publication Number: AAT 3300686).

Adrian Lopez Denis, "Disease and Society in Colonial Cuba, 1790–1840," 2007 PhD dissertation, University of California, Los Angeles (Publication Number: AAT 3295782).

Toni A. Lang, "Changing Maternal Profile and the Rise of Short Gestation and Low Birth Weight Rates in the United States between 1981 and 2002," 2007 PhD dissertation, State University of New York at Albany (Publication Number: AAT 3298389).

Christopher Ellis Hayden, "Of Medicine and Statecraft: Smallpox and Early Colonial Vaccination in French West Africa (Senegal-Guinea)," 2008 PhD dissertation, Northwestern University (Publication Number: AAT 3303521)

New Dissertations

Gretchen Kristine Pierce, "Sobering the Revolution: Mexico's Anti-Alcohol Campaigns and the Process of State-Building, 1910–1940," 2008 PhD dissertation, The University of Arizona (Publication Number: AAT 3303755).

Simon Finger, "Epidemic Constitutions: Public Health and Political Culture in the Port of Philadelphia, 1735–1800," 2008 PhD dissertation, Princeton University (Publication Number: AAT 3305758).

David A. Loving, "The Development of American Public Health, 1850–1925," 2008 PhD dissertation, The University of Oklahoma (Publication Number: AAT 3303520).

Theodore Wisniewski, "Experimenting with Power: Liberal Psychologists and the Challenge of Social Reform: 1945–1975," 2008 PhD dissertation, City University of New York (Publication Number: AAT 3303801).

SPRINGER PUBLISHING COMPANY

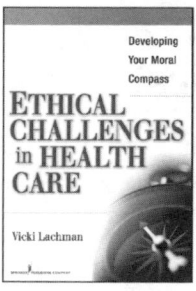

Ethical Challenges in Health Care
Developing Your Moral Compass

Vicki Lachman, PhD, MBE, APRN, Editor

"Stand up for what you believe in, even if it means standing alone."
—**Nelson Mandela**

This book provides the knowledge, insight, strategies, and encouragement necessary for developing moral courage in health care practice, even in the face of adversity.

Lachman outlines both personal and organizational strategies to help nurses, physicians, physical therapists, and health care leaders develop moral courage, and face difficult ethical challenges in health care practice and management head-on. Lachman presents numerous, real-life case examples to illustrate skills and opportunities for developing moral courage in the workplace. Also included are tips for executives on how to develop their ethical leadership skills.

Key Features:

- Presents guidelines for developing moral courage for organization leaders as well as for individual practitioners
- Discusses topics of critical concern to nurses and physicians, including patient autonomy, informed consent, and the importance of truth-telling
- Highlights pressing issues for health care leaders, including the uninsured in America, managing disruptive practitioners, and promoting patient safety
- Includes guidelines for "standing up and speaking out" against unethical practices
- Reiterates "Key Points to Remember" at the end of each chapter

June 2009 · 288 pp · Paperback · 978-0-8261-1089-3 · $50.00

11 West 42nd Street, New York, NY 10036-8002 • Fax: 212-941-7842
Order Toll-Free: 877-687-7476 • Order Online: www.springerpub.com

The Penn Center Guide to Bioethics

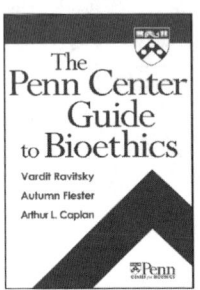

Vardit Ravitsky, PhD;
Autumn Fiester, PhD;
Arthur L. Caplan, PhD, Editors

The Center for Bioethics at the University of Pennsylvania is the internationally recognized leader in bioethical education and research. Its interdisciplinary faculty is drawn from the fields of medicine, law, nursing, education, philosophy, psychology, and religious studies. Arthur L. Caplan, the Center's founding director, is recognized as one of the most influential experts in bioethics. He has authored numerous books and articles, and served as the Chair of the Advisory Committee to the United Nations on human cloning.

The Penn Center's leading fellows, Autumn Fiester and Vardit Ravitsky, have combined their expertise with Dr. Caplan and over 80 other contributors to create *The Penn Center Guide to Bioethics*—the foremost authority on both traditional and cutting-edge bioethical issues. *The Penn Guide* navigates uncharted ethical terrains, undoubtedly shaping both academic and public discourses on the challenging controversies generated by new technologies, theories, and medical advances.

This volume represents the Penn Center's distinct, pioneering approach to bioethics, one that emphasizes empirical treatment of bioethical issues, and the integration of bioethical scholarship with practical application.

Learn what the Penn Center has to say about:
- Neuroethics and brain imaging: Is my mind mine?
- Choosing future people: reproductive technologies and identity
- Eugenics and survival of the fittest in the modern world
- Bioethics and national security
- Vaccination, abortion, nanotechnology, organ transplantation, end-of-life issues, and more

The Penn Guide will be the definitive text for policy makers, health practitioners, researchers, and students. This book will also inform the general public, patients, and family members as they seek answers to the bioethical issues of the day.

April 2009 · 700 pp · Hardback · 978-0-8261-1522-5

---

11 West 42nd Street, New York, NY 10036-8002 • Fax: 212-941-7842
Order Toll-Free: 877-687-7476 • Order Online: www.springerpub.com

SPRINGER PUBLISHING COMPANY

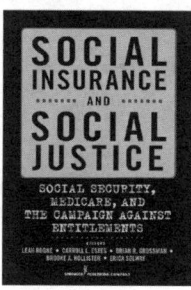

Social Insurance and Social Justice
Social Security, Medicare and the Campaign Against Entitlements

Leah Rogne, PhD; **Carroll Estes**, PhD; **Brian Grossman**, ScM; **Brooke Hollister**; **Erica Solway**, MSW, MPH, Editors

This politically charged, provocative text serves as an introduction to social insurance programs, examining all aspects of these hotly debated policies. The editors cover cutting-edge topics, including Social Security and privatization, universal health insurance, and how America's changing demographics will impact social security in the years to come.

Five key sections cover the critical topics:

- **Social Insurance: History, Politics, and Prospects** examines the foundational social insurance principles upon which Social Security, Medicare, and other programs are based

- **What's at Stake** identifies the risks posed to women, minorities, and the elderly if they could no longer depend on social insurance programs

- **The Ongoing Debates on Social Insurance** discusses public opinions of social insurance programs, and responds to arguments supporting privatization

- **Critical Perspectives on Social Insurance Reform** presents international experiences and policy trends, and analyzes reform movements from a social justice perspective

- **Teaching Social Insurance: Critical Pedagogy and Social Justice** presents pedagogical strategies to help students understand, influence, and engage in an informed debate about social policy

March 2009 · 488 pp · Hardback · 978-0-8261-1614-7

11 West 42nd Street, New York, NY 10036-8002 • Fax: 212-941-7842
Order Toll-Free: 877-687-7476 • Order Online: www.springerpub.com

SPRINGER PUBLISHING COMPANY

Nursing in the Storm
Voices from Hurricane Katrina

Denise Danna

"It's amazing how dedicated nurses are. If there is a need, here we come! We will be the first ones there and the last ones to leave"

—**John Jones** (Charity Hospital)

"I would like to hear about other nurses' stories. People...won't believe half of what they're reading because it's so incredible. It is something you could not imagine happening..."

—**Donna Sciortino** (Chalmette Medical Center)

This book documents first-hand accounts of nurses' and health professionals' experiences during Hurricane Katrina.

Structured thematically per hospital—before the storm, during the storm, and the aftermath—this book features testimony from nurses and health professionals who were there, and who remain in the city serving patient populations. The book—written in collaboration with a nurse historian, Dr. Barbara Mann Wall—includes a brief history of nursing in New Orleans with a focus on previous natural and man-made disasters endured by the city, its residents, and health care communities. It is also a vital resource for Registered Nurses (RNs), graduate students, and doctorally-prepared healthcare educators and managers/administrators.

Key Features:

- Offers suggestions on how to restore primary and critical care services in New Orleans
- Utilizes the Katrina catastrophe to discuss nurse disaster preparations nationally
- Features the stories about health care delivery that nurses need to know in a city in crisis
- Presents lessons learned and guidance for future disaster response

December 2009 · 264 pp (est.) · Paperback · 978-0-8261-1837-0

11 West 42nd Street, New York, NY 10036-8002 • Fax: 212-941-7842
Order Toll-Free: 877-687-7476 • Order Online: www.springerpub.com

SPRINGER PUBLISHING COMPANY

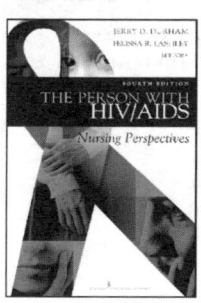

The Person With HIV/AIDS
Nursing Perspectives, Fourth Edition

Jerry D. Durham, PhD, RN, FAAN
Felissa R. Lashley, RN, PhD, ACRN, Editors

HIV/AIDS is no longer a certain death sentence. Patients fighting the chronic symptoms of HIV/AIDS are now living longer, fuller lives due to recent scientific and pharmaceutical breakthroughs. As a result, the new generation of caregivers must keep pace with cutting-edge, evidence-based practices to better serve patients who may live with HIV/AIDS for several decades.

This updated edition is a vital resource for nurses and other health care professionals providing care to HIV-positive persons in the 21st century. The contributors present essential information on the medical assessment and management of symptoms, the prevention of infection, ethical and legal dimensions of care, and much more. With a greater emphasis on the international dimensions of the HIV pandemic and the treatment of minority populations, this book serves as an essential guide for nurses and health care practitioners serving patients with HIV/AIDS.

Key topics include:

- HIV screening, testing, and counseling
- HIV/AIDS nursing case management within the global community
- HIV and gay, lesbian, bisexual, and transgender persons
- Children and HIV prevention and management
- HIV in corrections facilities and the care of incarcerated patients
- Sex workers and the transmission of HIV

September 2009 · 624 pp · Hardback · 978-0-8261-2137-0

---

11 West 42nd Street, New York, NY 10036-8002 • Fax: 212-941-7842
Order Toll-Free: 877-687-7476 • Order Online: www.springerpub.com

Subscription Order Form

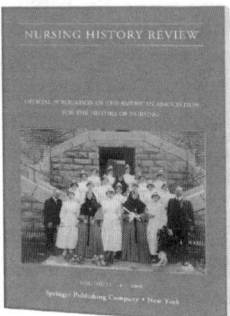

Official Journal of the American Association for the History of Nursing

Editor:
Patricia D'Antonio

❏ **Yes! Start my subscription to *Nursing History Review* with the current issue.**

	Individuals	Institutions
Print	❏ $85	❏ $150
Online	❏ $75	❏ $140
Print and Online	❏ $130	❏ $225

Outside the United States please add $40.

Nursing History Review, an annual peer-reviewed publication, is a showcase for the most significant current research on nursing and the health care history. Contributors include national and international scholars who represent many different disciplinary backgrounds.

Subscribe to the online edition and receive access to all back issues!

International subscriptions are also available. Please visit www.springerpub.com/nhr for more information.

4 Easy Ways to Order
- Web: www.springerpub.com
- Toll Free Phone: 1-877-687-7476
- Fax This Form: 212-941-7842
- Mail this form to address below

❏ Start my subscription to **Nursing History Review**

Checks or International Money Orders must be in U.S. dollars drawn on a U.S. bank made payable to Springer Publishing Company. All prices are subject to change, and are slightly higher outside the U.S.

Check or money order enclosed: $ _____ payable to Springer Publishing Company

Charge to: ❏ Visa ❏ MasterCard ❏ American Express ❏ Discover

Card No. _____ Exp. date _____

Signature _____

Name _____

Institution _____

Address _____

City _____ State _____ Zip _____

Telephone _____ E-mail _____

By providing us with your e-mail address, you agree to receive occasional book and journal announcements. You may unsubscribe at any time.

SPRINGER PUBLISHING COMPANY
11 West 42nd Street, 15th floor, New York, NY 10036